Law & Ethics

for Health Professions

EIGHTH EDITION

Karen Judson, BS

Carlene Harrison, EdD, CMA (AAMA)

Mc Graw Hill Education

LAW & ETHICS FOR HEALTH PROFESSIONS, EIGHTH EDITION

Published by McGraw-Hill Education, 2 Penn Plaza, New York, NY 10121.

This book is printed on acid-free paper.
1 2 3 4 5 6 7 8 9 LMN 21 20 19 18

ISBN 978-1-259-84471-3
MHID 1-259-84471-4

Portfolio Manager: *William Mulford*
Product Developer: *Yvonne Lloyd*
Executive Marketing Manager: *Roxan Kinsey*
Content Project Manager: *Ann Courtney*
Buyer: *Susan K. Culbertson*
Lead Designer: *David W. Hash*
Content Licensing Specialist: *Lori Hancock*
Cover Image: *Leonardo da Vinci's Vetruvian Man: ©vitstudio/Shutterstock.com; Themis at Sunset: ©Andrii Bielov/Shutterstock.com; stethoscope: ©ktsdesign/Shutterstock.com; columns: ©Nice_Media/ Shutterstock.com*
Compositor: *Lumina Datamatics, Inc.*

Library of Congress Cataloging-in-Publication Data

Names: Judson, Karen, 1941- author. | Harrison, Carlene, author.
Title: Law & ethics for health professions / Karen Judson, BS, Carlene Harrison, EdD, CMA (AAMA).
Other titles: Law and ethics for health professions
Description: Eighth edition. | New York, NY : McGraw-Hill Education, [2018] | Includes bibliographical references and index.
Identifiers: LCCN 2017021338| ISBN 9781259844713 (alk. paper) | ISBN 1259844714 (alk. paper)
Subjects: LCSH: Medical ethics. | Medical jurisprudence.
Classification: LCC R725.5 .J83 2018 | DDC 174.2–dc23
LC record available at https://lccn.loc.gov/2017021338

mheducation.com/highered

Brief Contents

Contents

About the Authors

Karen Judson, BS

Karen Judson has taught college and high school sciences and grades kindergarten, one, and three. Judson has also worked as a laboratory and X-ray technician and completed two years of nursing while earning a degree in biology. Judson has also published numerous science and relationship articles and books for adult and young adult readers.

Carlene Harrison, EdD, CMA (AAMA)

Carlene Harrison was an administrator in a variety of outpatient health care facilities for 20 years in Colorado, Texas, and Florida. She became a full-time faculty member at Hodges University in 2000 serving first as a professor and program chair in both medical assisting and health administration. In 2007, she was named Dean of the School of Allied Health. During her 15 years at Hodges, she was responsible for adding six academic programs to the School of Allied Health, retiring in 2015. Her doctorate is from Argosy University. Her dissertation research looked at improvement in critical thinking in adult learners.

Preface

Law and Ethics: For Health Professions explains how to navigate the numerous legal and ethical issues that health care professionals face every day. Topics are based upon real-world scenarios and dilemmas from a variety of health care practitioners. Through the presentation of Learning Outcomes, Key Terms, From the Perspective of . . ., Ethics Issues, Chapter Reviews, Case Studies, Internet Activities, Court Cases, and Videos, students learn about current legal and ethical problems and situations. In the eighth edition, material has been revised to reflect the current health care environment. As students progress through the text, they will get the opportunity to use critical thinking skills to learn how to resolve real-life situations and theoretical scenarios and to decide how legal and ethical issues are relevant to the health care profession in which they will practice.

Law & Ethics is also available with McGraw-Hill Education's revolutionary adaptive learning technology, McGraw-Hill LearnSmart®and now SmartBook®! You can study smarter, spending your valuable time on topics you don't know and less time on the topics you have already mastered. Succeed with LearnSmart. . . . Join the learning revolution and achieve the success you deserve today!

New to the Eighth Edition

A number of updates have been made in the eighth edition to enrich the user's experience with the product:

- Chapter 3, "Working in Health Care," has been updated to reflect the changing configuration of health care management. Additionally, the types of accreditation in health care are explained in more detail.
- Chapter 7, "Medical Records, Informed Consent, and Health Information Technology" provides more coverage of meaningful use, social media, and telemedicine.
- Chapter 8, "Privacy, Security, and Fraud," includes coverage of not only privacy of the health care record but also more detail on the security requirements for health care records. There is now information about security breaches, as well as information about the increasing cost of fraud in health care.
- Chapter 10, "Workplace Legalities," updates appropriate Centers for Disease Control and Occupational Safety and Health Administration regulations, as well as best practices in hiring employees.
- Chapter 12, "Death and Dying," provides information about careers in palliative care, as well as updated information about "Death with Dignity" legislation in the states.
- Chapter 13, "Health Care Trends and Forecasts," has been updated to evaluate the current status of health care stakeholders in the United States and to inform students of today's trends in health care that may affect our health care in the future.
- All statistics and court cases have been updated, as well as content relevant to laws passed since the seventh edition.
- The interior design and layout have been refreshed to make it easier for students to navigate through the content.
- *McGraw-Hill Connect® Law & Ethics* has been updated to reflect updates in the chapters and feedback from customers. Additional Case Studies are included in Connect, as well as Video Case Scenarios, to allow students to apply important skills learned from the text. Both the Case Studies and the Video Cases include related questions with immediate feedback for the students.

For a detailed transition guide between the seventh and eighth editions of *Law & Ethics*, visit the Instructor Resources in *Connect!*

To the Student

As you study to become a health care provider, you have undoubtedly realized that patients are more than the sum of their medical problems. In fact, they are people with loved ones, professions, worries, hobbies, and daily routines that are probably much like your own. However, because patients' lives and well-being are at stake as they seek and receive health care, in addition to seeing each patient as an individual, you must carefully consider the complex legal, moral, and ethical issues that will arise as you practice your profession. And you must learn to resolve such issues in an acceptable manner.

Law & Ethics provides an overview of the laws and ethics you should know to help you give competent, compassionate care to patients that is also within acceptable legal and ethical boundaries. The text can also serve as a guide to help you resolve the many legal and ethical questions you may reasonably expect to face as a student and, later, as a health care provider.

To derive maximum benefit from *Law & Ethics:*

- Review the Learning Outcomes and Key Terms at the beginning of each chapter for an overview of the material included in the chapter.
- Complete all Check Your Progress questions as they appear in the chapter, and correct any incorrect answers.
- Review the legal cases to see how they apply to topics in the text, and try to determine why the court ruled as it did.
- Study the Ethics Issues at the end of each chapter, and answer the discussion questions.
- Complete the Review questions at the end of the chapter, correct any incorrect answers, and review the material again.
- Review the Case Studies, and use your critical thinking skills to answer the questions.
- Complete the Internet Activities at the end of the chapter to become familiar with online resources and to see what additional information you can find about selected topics.
- Complete the *Connect* assignments from your instructor, including any LearnSmart or SmartBook modules assigned, as well as additional Case Studies and Video Case Scenarios.
- Study each chapter until you can answer correctly questions posed by the Learning Outcomes, Check Your Progress, and Review questions.

Law & Ethics Preparation in the Digital World: Supplementary Materials for the Instructor and Student

McGraw-Hill Education knows how much effort it takes for instructors to prepare for a new course. Through focus groups, symposia, reviews, and conversations with instructors like you, we have gathered information about what materials you need in order to facilitate successful courses. We are committed to providing you with high-quality, accurate instructor support. Knowing the importance of flexibility and digital learning, McGraw-Hill Education has created multiple assets to enhance the learning experience no matter what the class format: traditional, online, or hybrid. This product is designed to help instructors and students be successful, with digital solutions proven to drive student success.

Mc Graw Hill Education connect®

A ONE-STOP SPOT TO PRESENT, DELIVER, AND ASSESS DIGITAL ASSETS AVAILABLE FROM MCGRAW-HILL: MCGRAW-HILL *CONNECT* LAW & ETHICS

McGraw-Hill *Connect*® **Law & Ethics** provides online presentation, assignment, and assessment solutions. It connects your students with the tools and resources they'll need to achieve success. With *Connect,* you can deliver assignments, quizzes, and tests online. A robust set of questions and activities, including all of the Check Your Progress and End-of-Chapter Questions, additional Case Studies, Video Case Scenarios, and interactives are presented and aligned with the textbook's learning outcomes. As an instructor, you can edit existing questions and author entirely new problems. *Connect* enables you to track individual student performance—by question, by assignment, or in relation to the class overall—with detailed grade reports. You can integrate grade reports easily with learning management systems (LMSs), such as Blackboard, Desire2Learn, and eCollege, plus much more. ***Connect* Law & Ethics** also provides students with 24/7 online access to an ebook. This media-rich version of the textbook is available through the McGraw-Hill *Connect* platform and allows seamless integration of text, media, and assessments. To learn more, visit http://connect.mheducation.com.

Connect Insight™ is the first and only analytics tool of its kind, which highlights a series of visual data displays—each framed by an intuitive question—to provide at-a-glance information regarding how your class is doing. As an instructor or administrator, you receive an instant, at-a-glance view of student performance matched with student activity. It puts real-time analytics in your hands so you can take action early and keep struggling students from falling behind. It also allows you to be empowered with a more valuable, transparent, and productive connection between you and your students. Available on demand wherever and whenever it's needed, Connect Insight travels from office to classroom!

A SINGLE SIGN-ON WITH CONNECT AND YOUR BLACKBOARD COURSE: MCGRAW-HILL EDUCATION AND BLACKBOARD

Blackboard, the Web-based course management system, has partnered with McGraw-Hill Education to better allow students and faculty to use online materials and activities to complement face-to-face teaching. Blackboard features exciting social learning and teaching tools that foster active learning opportunities for students. You'll transform your closed-door classroom into communities where students remain connected to their educational experience 24 hours a day. This partnership allows you and your students access to McGraw-Hill's *Connect* and *Create* right from within your Blackboard course—all with a single sign-on. Not only do you get single sign-on with *Connect* and *Create,* but you also get deep integration of McGraw-Hill Education content and content engines right in Blackboard. Whether you're choosing a book for your course or building *Connect* assignments, all the tools you need are right where you want them—inside Blackboard. Gradebooks are now seamless. When a student completes an integrated *Connect* assignment, the grade for that assignment automatically (and instantly) feeds into your Blackboard grade center. McGraw-Hill Education and Blackboard can now offer you easy access to industry-leading technology and content, whether your campus hosts it or we do. Be sure to ask your local McGraw-Hill Education representative for details.

Still want a single sign-on solution using another learning management system? See how **McGraw-Hill Campus** (http://mhcampus.mhhe.com/) makes the grade by offering universal sign-on, automatic registration, gradebook synchronization, and open access to a multitude of learning resources—all in one place. MH Campus supports Active Directory, Angel, Blackboard, Canvas, Desire2Learn, eCollege, IMS, LDAP, Moodle, Moodlerooms, Sakai, Shibboleth, WebCT, BrainHoney, Campus Cruiser, and Jenzibar eRacer. Additionally, MH Campus can be easily connected with other authentication authorities and LMSs.

CREATE A TEXTBOOK ORGANIZED THE WAY YOU TEACH: MCGRAW-HILL CREATE

With **McGraw-Hill** *Create,* you can easily rearrange chapters, combine material from other content sources, and quickly upload content you have written, such as your course syllabus or teaching notes. Find the content you need in *Create* by searching through thousands of leading McGraw-Hill Education textbooks. Arrange your book to fit your teaching style. *Create* even allows you to personalize your book's appearance by selecting the cover and adding your name, school, and course information. Order a *Create* book and you'll receive a complimentary print review copy in three to five business days or a complimentary electronic review copy (eComp) via e-mail in minutes. Go to www.mcgrawhillcreate.com today and register to experience how McGraw-Hill *Create* empowers you to teach *your* students *your* way.

RECORD AND DISTRIBUTE YOUR LECTURES FOR MULTIPLE VIEWING: MY LECTURES—TEGRITY

McGraw-Hill Tegrity records and distributes your class lecture with just a click of a button. Students can view it anytime and anywhere via computer, iPod, or mobile device. It indexes as it records your PowerPoint presentations and anything shown on your computer, so students can use keywords to find exactly what they want to study. Tegrity is available as an integrated feature of **McGraw-Hill *Connect* Law & Ethics** and as a standalone product.

McGraw-Hill Connect® is a highly reliable, easy-to-use homework and learning management solution that utilizes learning science and award-winning adaptive tools to improve student results.

HOMEWORK AND ADAPTIVE LEARNING

- Connect's assignments help students contextualize what they've learned through application, so they can better understand the material and think critically.
- Connect will create a personalized study path customized to individual student needs through SmartBook®.
- SmartBook helps students study more efficiently by delivering an interactive reading experience through adaptive highlighting and review.

Over **7 billion questions** have been answered, making McGraw-Hill Education products more intelligent, reliable, and precise.

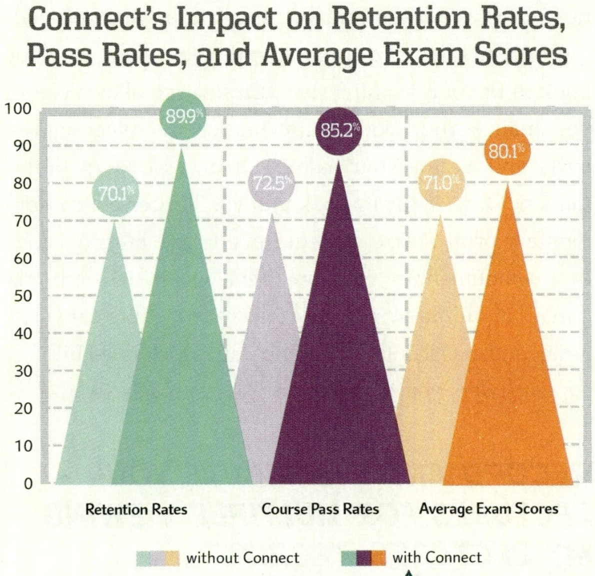

Using **Connect** improves retention rates by **19.8%**, passing rates by **12.7%**, and exam scores by **9.1%**.

QUALITY CONTENT AND LEARNING RESOURCES

- Connect content is authored by the world's best subject matter experts, and is available to your class through a simple and intuitive interface.
- The Connect eBook makes it easy for students to access their reading material on smartphones and tablets. They can study on the go and don't need Internet access to use the eBook as a reference, with full functionality.
- Multimedia content such as videos, simulations, and games drive student engagement and critical thinking skills.

73 percent of instructors who use **Connect** require it; instructor satisfaction **increases** by 28 percent when **Connect** is required.

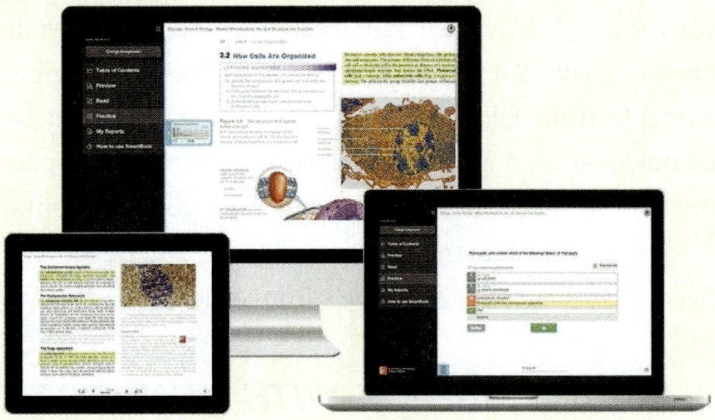

©McGraw-Hill Education

ROBUST ANALYTICS AND REPORTING

- Connect Insight® generates easy-to-read reports on individual students, the class as a whole, and on specific assignments.
- The Connect Insight dashboard delivers data on performance, study behavior, and effort. Instructors can quickly identify students who struggle and focus on material that the class has yet to master.
- Connect automatically grades assignments and quizzes, providing easy-to-read reports on individual and class performance.

More students earn **As** and **Bs** when they use McGraw-Hill Education **Connect.**

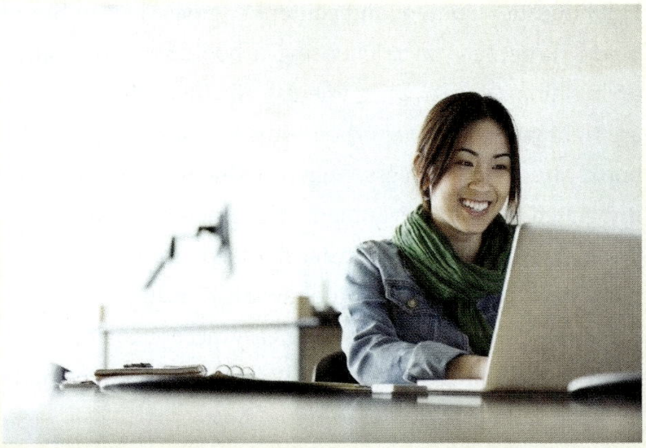

©Hero Images/Getty Images

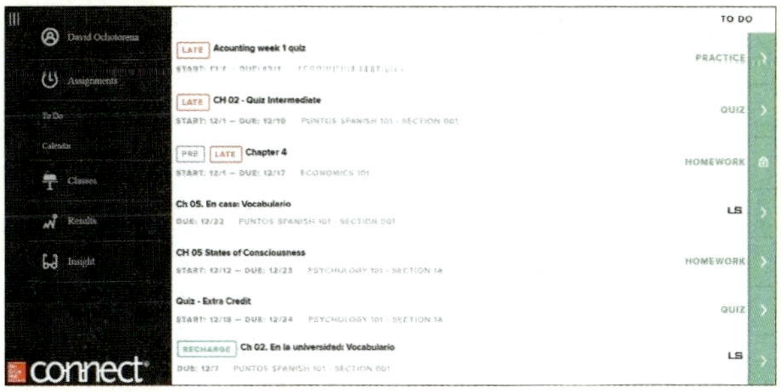

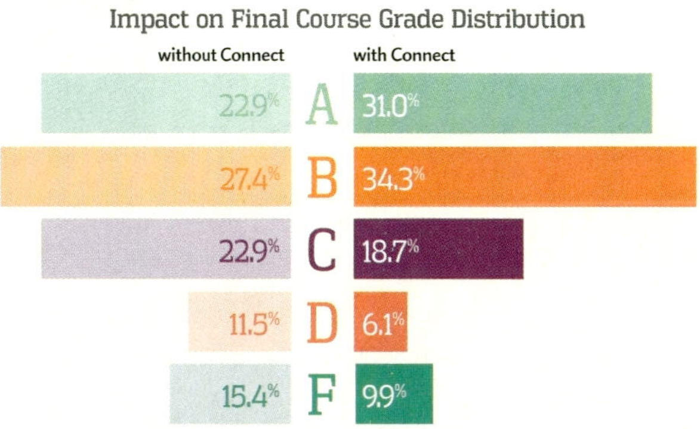

TRUSTED SERVICE AND SUPPORT

- Connect integrates with your LMS to provide single sign-on and automatic syncing of grades. Integration with Blackboard®, D2L®, and Canvas also provides automatic syncing of the course calendar and assignment-level linking.
- Connect offers comprehensive service, support, and training throughout every phase of your implementation.
- If you're looking for some guidance on how to use Connect, or want to learn tips and tricks from super users, you can find tutorials as you work. Our Digital Faculty Consultants and Student Ambassadors offer insight into how to achieve the results you want with Connect.

www.mheducation.com/connect

Instructor Resources

You can rely on the following materials to help you and your students work through the material in this book. All of the resources in the following table are available in the Instructor Resources under the Library tab in *Connect.*

Need help? Contact McGraw-Hill Education's Customer Experience Group (CXG). Visit the CXG Web site at www.mhhe.com/support. Browse our FAQs (frequently asked questions) and product documentation and/or contact a CXG representative. CXG is available Sunday through Friday.

Want to learn more about this product? Attend one of our online webinars. To learn more about the webinars, please contact your McGraw-Hill sales representative. To find your McGraw-Hill representative, go to www.mhhe.com and click "Find My Sales Rep."

Supplement	Features
Instructor's Manual	Each chapter includes: • Learning Outcomes • Overview of PowerPoint Presentations • Teaching Points • Answer Keys for Check Your Progress and End-of-Chapter Questions
PowerPoint Presentations	• Key Concepts • References to Learning Outcomes
Electronic Test Bank	• EZ Test Online (computerized) • Word version • These questions are also available through Connect • Questions are tagged with learning outcomes, level of difficulty, level of Bloom's taxonomy, feedback, topic, and the accrediting standards of ABHES and CAAHEP, where appropriate
Tools to Plan Course	• Transition Guide, by chapter, from *Law & Ethics,* 7e to 8e • Correlations by learning outcomes to ABHES, CAAHEP, and more • Sample syllabi • Asset Map—a recap of the key instructor resources, as well as information on the content available through *Connect*

BEST-IN-CLASS DIGITAL SUPPORT

Based on feedback from our users, McGraw-Hill Education has developed Digital Success Programs that will provide you and your students with the help you need, when you need it.

- *Training for Instructors:* Get ready to drive classroom results with our Digital Success Team—which is ready to provide in-person, remote, or on-demand training as needed.
- *Peer Support and Training:* No one understands your needs like your peers. Get easy access to knowledgeable digital users by joining our Connect Community, or speak directly with one of our Digital Faculty Consultants, who are instructors using McGraw-Hill Education digital products.
- *Online Training Tools:* Get immediate anytime, anywhere access to modular tutorials on key features through our Connect Success Academy.

Get started today. Learn more about McGraw-Hill Education's Digital Success Programs by contacting your local sales representative or visiting http://connect.customer.mheducation.com/start.

Guided Tour

Chapter Openers

The **chapter opener** sets the stage for what will be learned in the chapter. **Key terms** are first introduced in the chapter opener so the student can see them all in one place; they are defined in the margins throughout the chapter for easy review, as well as in the glossary. **Learning Outcomes** are written to reflect the revised version of Bloom's taxonomy and to establish the key points the student should focus on in the chapter. In addition, major chapter heads are structured to reflect the Learning Outcomes, and the Learning Outcomes for easy reference. **From the Perspective of . . .** boxes illustrate real-life experiences related to the text. Each quotes health care providers as they encounter problems or situations relevant to the material about to be presented in the chapter.

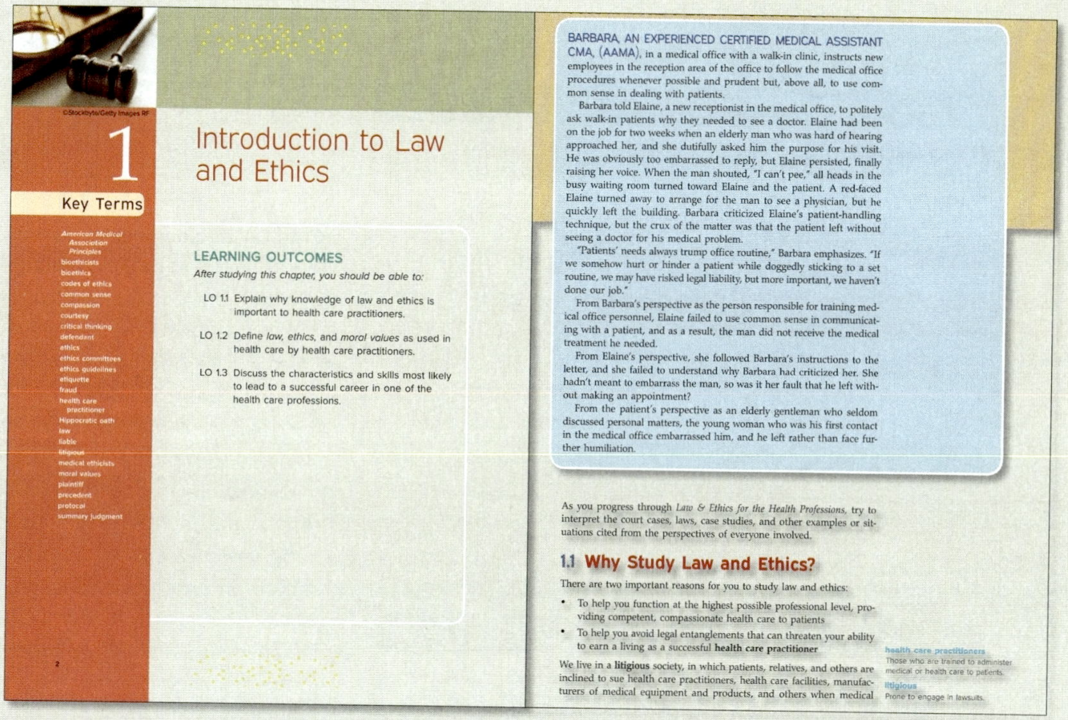

©Stockbyte/Getty Images RF

1

Key Terms

American Medical Association Principles
bioethicists
bioethics
codes of ethics
common sense
compassion
courtesy
critical thinking
defendant
ethics
ethics committees
ethics guidelines
etiquette
fraud
health care practitioner
Hippocratic oath
law
liable
litigious
medical ethicists
moral values
plaintiff
precedent
protocol
summary judgment

2

Introduction to Law and Ethics

LEARNING OUTCOMES

After studying this chapter, you should be able to:

LO 1.1 Explain why knowledge of law and ethics is important to health care practitioners.

LO 1.2 Define *law, ethics,* and *moral values* as used in health care by health care practitioners.

LO 1.3 Discuss the characteristics and skills most likely to lead to a successful career in one of the health care professions.

BARBARA, AN EXPERIENCED CERTIFIED MEDICAL ASSISTANT CMA, (AAMA), in a medical office with a walk-in clinic, instructs new employees in the reception area of the office to follow the medical office procedures whenever possible and prudent but, above all, to use common sense in dealing with patients.

Barbara told Elaine, a new receptionist in the medical office, to politely ask walk-in patients why they needed to see a doctor. Elaine had been on the job for two weeks when an elderly man who was hard of hearing approached her, and she dutifully asked him the purpose for his visit. He was obviously too embarrassed to reply, but Elaine persisted, finally raising her voice. When the man shouted, "I can't pee," all heads in the busy waiting room turned toward Elaine and the patient. A red-faced Elaine turned away to arrange for the man to see a physician, but he quickly left the building. Barbara criticized Elaine's patient-handling technique, but the crux of the matter was that the patient left without seeing a doctor for his medical problem.

"Patients' needs always trump office routine," Barbara emphasizes. "If we somehow hurt or hinder a patient while doggedly sticking to a set routine, we may have risked legal liability, but more important, we haven't done our job."

From Barbara's perspective as the person responsible for training medical office personnel, Elaine failed to use common sense in communicating with a patient, and as a result, the man did not receive the medical treatment he needed.

From Elaine's perspective, she followed Barbara's instructions to the letter, and she failed to understand why Barbara had criticized her. She hadn't meant to embarrass the man, so was it her fault that he left without making an appointment?

From the patient's perspective as an elderly gentleman who seldom discussed personal matters, the young woman who was his first contact in the medical office embarrassed him, and he left rather than face further humiliation.

As you progress through *Law & Ethics for the Health Professions*, try to interpret the court cases, laws, case studies, and other examples or situations cited from the perspectives of everyone involved.

1.1 Why Study Law and Ethics?

There are two important reasons for you to study law and ethics:

- To help you function at the highest possible professional level, providing competent, compassionate health care to patients
- To help you avoid legal entanglements that can threaten your ability to earn a living as a successful **health care practitioner**

We live in a **litigious** society, in which patients, relatives, and others are inclined to sue health care practitioners, health care facilities, manufacturers of medical equipment and products, and others when medical

health care practitioners Those who are trained to administer medical or health care to patients.

litigious Prone to engage in lawsuits.

COURT CASE Patients Sue Hospitals

In 2016, lawsuits against hospitals that were moving through various courts included:

- A Texas woman, 32, suffered a seizure at 5 AM inside her home. Her husband took her to the hospital ER, where she was diagnosed with a migraine and a sinus infection and sent home with a prescription. Once home, she suffered a second seizure. An ambulance transported her to the ER, and while en route, she had a third seizure that left her brain-dead.
- Two hospitals in Washington, DC, were sued for excessive charges when three patients received bills for several hundred dollars for copying their medical records.
- Patients of a Seattle hospital were discussing a class action lawsuit against the hospital when they learned that a former employee of the hospital, a surgical technician, may have exposed them to hepatitis or HIV when he used surgical syringes for administering drugs to himself, then returned the used syringes to surgical supply.

(All of the above cases were still in litigation as the eighth edition of *Law & Ethics for Health Professions* was prepared for publication, but perhaps the underlying reasons for filing the lawsuits are already apparent to you.)

Court Cases

Several **court cases** are presented in every chapter. Each summarizes a lawsuit that illustrates points made in the text and is meant to encourage students to consider the subject's relevance to their health care specialty. The legal citations at the end of each case indicate where to find the complete text for that case. "Landmark" cases are those that established an ongoing precedent.

Check Your Progress Questions

These questions appear at various points in the chapters to allow students to test their comprehension of the material they just read. These questions can also be answered in *Connect*.

Check Your Progress

1. Name two important reasons for studying law and ethics.
2. Which state laws apply specifically to the practice of medicine?
3. What purpose do laws serve?
4. How is the enforcement of laws made possible?
5. What factors influence the formation of one's personal set of ethics and values?
6. Define the term *moral values.*
7. Explain how one's moral values affect one's sense of ethics.

End-of-Chapter Resources

The **Chapter Summary** is in a tabular, step-by-step format organized by Learning Outcome to help with review of the material. **Ethics Issues** are issues and related discussion questions based on interviews conducted with ethics counselors within the professional organizations for health care providers, as well as with bioethics experts. Each **Chapter Review** includes Applying Knowledge questions that reinforce the concepts the students have just learned. These questions can be answered in *Connect.* **Case Studies** are scenarios with exercises that allow students to practice their critical thinking skills to decide how to resolve the real-life situations and theoretical scenarios presented. **Internet Activities** include exercises designed to increase students' knowledge of the chapter topics and help them gain more Internet research expertise. The **Resources** section presents a listing of additional references for the chapter.

Chapter Summary

Learning Outcome	Summary
LO 1.1 Explain why knowledge of law and ethics is important to health care practitioners.	Why study law and ethics? • Health care practitioners who function at the highest possible levels have a working knowledge of law and ethics. • Knowing the law relevant to your profession can help you avoid legal entanglements that threaten your ability to earn a living. Court cases illustrate how health care practitioners, health care facilities, and drug and medical device manufacturers can be held accountable in a court of law. • A knowledge of law and ethics will also help familiarize you with the following areas: • The rights, responsibilities, and concerns of health care consumers • The legal and ethical issues facing society, patients, and health care practitioners as the world changes
LO 1.2 Define *law, ethics,* and *moral values* as used in health care by health care practitioners.	

Chapter 2 Review

Applying Knowledge

LO 2.1

1. What is another term for your personal concept of right and wrong?
   a. Utilitarianism
   b. Beneficence
   c. Moral values

Ethics Issues Introduction to End-of-Chapter Ethics Discussions

Learning Outcomes for the Ethics Issues Feature at the End of Each Chapter

After studying the material in each chapter's Ethics Issues feature, you should be able to:

1. Discuss current ethical issues of concern to health care practitioners.
2. Compare ethical guidelines to the law as discussed in each chapter of the text.
3. Practice critical thinking skills as you consider medical, legal, and ethical issues for each situation presented.
4. Relate the ethical issues presented in the text to the health care profession you intend to practice.

Health care practitioners are bound by state and federal laws, but they are also bound by certain ethical standards—both personal standards and those set forth by professional codes of ethics and ethical guidelines and by bioethicists. Many professional organizations for health care practitioners employ an ethics consultant who is available to speak with organization members who need help with an ethical dilemma. "We serve as a third party who can stand outside a situation and facilitate communication," says Dr. Carmen Paradis, an ethics consultant with the Cleveland Clinic's Department of Bioethics. At the Cleveland Clinic, ethics consultations are available to health care pra…

Case Studies

Use your critical thinking skills to answer the questions that follow each case study.

LO 2.3

Susan, a nursing student, is arguing with her friend Linda, also a nursing student, over the benefits of getting a flu shot.

"I'm not getting a flu shot this year," Linda declares. "I paid $14 for one last year, and I still got sick. I had a horrible sinus infection that kept me out of school for days."

…ople in the clinic—especially …ould be immunized against

Internet Activities

LO 2.3

Complete the activities and answer the questions that follow.

24. Locate the Web site for the organization representing the profession you plan to practice. Check the organization's code of ethics. Does the code conform to the seven principles of health care ethics? Explain your answer.
25. Visit the Web site for th… ethicsresources.asp. Unc…

Resources

LO 2.1 and 2.3

Value Development Theories and the Seven Principles of Health Care Ethics

Edge, R., and J. Groves. *Ethics of Health Care: A Guide for Clinical Practice.* 3rd ed. New York: Thomson Delmar Learning, 2006.

Mappes, T., and D. Degrazia. *Biomedical Ethics.* 6th ed. Boston: McGraw-Hill, 2006.

LO 2.2

Acknowledgments

Author Acknowledgments

Karen Judson

Thank you to the editorial team and production staff at McGraw-Hill and all the reviewers and sources who contributed their time and expertise to making the eighth edition of Law & Ethics for Health Professions *the best ever. Thank you, too, Carlene, for your hard work on this eighth edition.*

Carlene Harrison

A big thank you to Karen Judson for getting me started on this marvelous adventure called textbook writing over 10 years ago.

To our reviewers, your contributions really make a difference. The editorial and production staff at McGraw-Hill did a great job. And last, to my husband, Bill, your support and love keeps me going.

Reviewer Acknowledgments

Suggestions have been received from faculty and students throughout the country. This is vital feedback that is relied on for product development. Each person who has offered comments and suggestions has our thanks. The efforts of many people are needed to develop and improve a product. Among these people are the reviewers and consultants who point out areas of concern, cite areas of strength, and make recommendations for change. In this regard, the following instructors provided feedback that was enormously helpful in preparing the book and related products.

8e Reviewers

Multiple instructors reviewed the product while it was in development, providing valuable feedback that directly impacted the product. They include the following individuals:

Tammy Albright, CMA (AAMA)
Wake Technical Community College

Michaelann Allen, MAEd
North Seattle College

Wilfredo Barreto, MD
Florida Technical College

Valerie Brock, MBA, EdS, RHIA, CDIP, CPC, CCP, CPAR
Tennessee State University

Pamela A. Burton, EdM, CMA(AAMA), LRT, CPT (ASPT)
Ivy Tech Community College

Melissa Cotten, RHIA, CCS, CAHIMS
Southwest Mississippi Community College

Sarah Darrell, BSN, RN, CNOR
Ivy Tech Community College

Darlene R. Dulin, MSN, RN
Ivy Tech Community College

Jim Dunson
Xavier University of Louisiana

Cindy Fietzer, MBS, BSN, RN
Fox Valley Technical College

Terri Fleming, MS, BSN
Ivy Tech Community College

Karen Garcia, RMA, RHIA, RPT, CPT
Front Range Community College

Linda Gobis, JD, MN, RN
University of Wisconsin–Oshkosh

Kristina Guo, PhD
University of Hawaii–West Oahu

Valentina Holder, MAEd, RHIA
Pitt Community College

Lina Jawad
Wayne County Community College

Mary Juenemann, MS, RHIA, CCS
Rochester Community & Technical College

Sherry Marvin, NCMA, CPSI, CST, CET
Alaska Career College

Shannon Mitchell, CMA (AAMA)
Surry Community College

Elizabeth Pratt, MSN, RNC-OB, CNE
State University of New York at Delhi

Pamela B. Primrose, PhD, MLS (ASCP)
Ivy Tech Community College

Linda Pristelski, RHIT
Northeast Wisconsin Technical College

Nicole Procise, BS, CMA (AAMA), PBT (ASCP)
Ivy Tech Community College

Lenette Thompson, CST, AS
Piedmont Technical College

Marianne Van Deursen
Warren County Community College

Devoncia Vaught, MSHI, RHIA
Indian River Community College

Wanda Ziemba, EJD, MFA, BA, RHIT, CCS, CHCO/CHCC, CPC
City College of San Francisco

7e Reviewers

Multiple instructors reviewed the product while it was in development, providing valuable feedback that directly impacted the product. They include the following individuals:

Yvonne Alles, DHA
Davenport

Theresa Allyn, MEd, BS
Edmonds Community College

Doris Beran, MPH
Coconino Community College

Chantalle Blakesley-Boddie, BS, CMA (AAMA)
Lake Washington Institute of Technology

Marianne Bovee, CCMA, CET, CHI
Duluth Business University

Joey L. Brown, MA/MS
Great Lakes Institute of Technology

Myra Brown, MBA, RHIA
East Carolina University

Patricia Brown Raphiel, MEd, MT/PBT (ASCP)
Southern University of Shreveport

Deborah Bryant, MS/EdPSY, CMA (AAMA)
Chattahoochee Technical College

Cyndi Caviness, AAS, AHI, CMA (AAMA), CRT
Montgomery Community College

Christine Christensen, AAS, CCA, BAS
Williston State College

Marsha Eriks, BS, CST
Ivy Tech Community College

Kim Ford, MA, AAS
Catawba Valley Community College

Rebecca French, RN, BS, CRNI, MSN, ARNP-C, GNP-BC
Allen Community College (Iola, KS)

Brenda Garrett, MHA, CAM, CMOM, RMC
Danville Community College

Diane Gryglak, AA, BS, CMA (AAMA)
College of DuPage

Angela Hennessy, BS, MS
Corning Community College

Sandy Hunter, BS, MEd, PhD
Eastern Kentucky University

Robert Kieffer
Trocaire College

Karmon Kingsley, BS, CMA (AAMA)
Cleveland State Community College

Rhonda S. Lazette, BS, CMA (AAMA), CPC (AAPC)
Stautzenberger College

Kathy Locke, BA, CMA (AAMA), MS
Northwestern College

Sharon Luczu Thompkins
Gateway Community College

Erica Matteson, RHIA, BPS
Alfred State College

Mindy McDonald, BS, CMA (AAMA)
University of Northwest Ohio

Kelly Meyer, MEd, BS, CPhT, PhTR
Cisco College

Robert Micallef, MA
Madonna University

Pat Moody, MSN, RN
Athens Technical College (GA)

Brigitte Niedzwiecki, MSN, BSN, RN
Chippewa Valley Technical College

Cynthia S. Nivens
Forsyth Technical Community College

Ruth O'Brien, AAS, BA, CPFT, MHA, RRT, CPT, CPC-A
Miami-Jacobs Career College (OH)

Julie Pepper, CMA (AAMA)
Chippewa Valley Technical College

Berta Powers, AA, CCMA, CMA (AAMA)
De Anza College

Debra Pressley, MBA, BA
Blue Ridge Community College

Sue Pylant, CCS-P
Sanford-Brown College–San Antonio

Adrienne Reaves, EdD, RMA
Westwood College–DuPage

Starra Robinson-Herring, AAS, AHI, BA, BSHA, MS
Stanly Community College

Donna Rowan, MA, RMA
Community College of Baltimore County

Mary Ann Schaefer, MBA, MJ, RNC, BAABS
William Rainey Harper College

Jeanne Smoczyk, MS, RHIT
Chippewa Valley Technical College

Marlene Suvada, MHPE, RRT
National-Louis University

Charlene Thiessen
GateWay Community College

L. Joleen VanBibber, CDPMA, CFRDA
Davis Applied Technology College

Stacey Wanovich, MLT
Anoka Technical College

Gail Warchol
Mohawk Valley Community College

Claudia Williams, MS
Campbell University

Veronica Zurcher, BSAS, CMA (AAMA)
National College (Youngstown, OH)

Technical Editing/Accuracy Panel

A panel of instructors completed a technical edit and review of the content in the book page proofs to verify its accuracy.

Lynnae Lockett, RMA, CMRS, RN
Bryant and Stratton College

Marta Lopez, MD, LM, CPM, RMA, BMO
Miami Dade College

Angela M. B. Oliva, BS, CMRS
Heald College and Boston Reed College

Luz P. Rios-Garcia, CMA (AAMA)
Branford Hall Career Institute

Wendy Schmerse, CMRS
Charter College

Digital Tool Development

Special thanks to the instructors who helped with the development of *Connect,* LearnSmart, and SmartBook. They include:

Chantalle Blakesley-Boddie, BS, CMA (AAMA)
Lake Washington Institute of Technology

William Travis Butler, MHA, RMA
ECPI University

Gloryvee Diaz, MA
Branford Hall Career Institute

Terri Gilbert, BSBA
ECPI University

Debra Glover, BSN, RN
Goodwin College

Susan Harrison-Grant, EdD, MS, RN,
William Rainey Harper College

Judy Hurtt, MEd
East Central Community College

Kelli Lewis, MSHI, RHIA
Valencia College

Lynnae Lockett, RMA, RN, CMRS
Bryant and Stratton College

Carrie Mack, AS, CMA (AAMA)
Branford Hall Career Institute

Angela M. B. Oliva, BS, CMRS
Heald College and Boston Reed College

Luz P. Rios-Garcia, CMA (AAMA)
Branford Hall Career Institute

Wendy Schmerse, CMRS
Charter College

Mia C. Small, MBA, AHI, RMA, CMRS
Bryant & Stratton College

Linda Sorensen, MPA, RHIA, CHPS
Davenport University

Alice L. Spencer, MS, BS MT, CQA (ASQ)
National College

Stacey Wanovich, MLT
Anoka Technical College

Art Witkowski, MEd
Chemeketa Community College

PART ONE

The Foundations of Law and Ethics

©Stockbyte/Getty Images RF

1

Introduction to Law and Ethics

Key Terms

American Medical Association Principles
bioethicists
bioethics
codes of ethics
common sense
compassion
courtesy
critical thinking
defendant
ethics
ethics committees
ethics guidelines
etiquette
fraud
health care practitioner
Hippocratic oath
law
liable
litigious
medical ethicists
moral values
plaintiff
precedent
protocol
summary judgment

LEARNING OUTCOMES

After studying this chapter, you should be able to:

LO 1.1 Explain why knowledge of law and ethics is important to health care practitioners.

LO 1.2 Define *law, ethics,* and *moral values* as used in health care by health care practitioners.

LO 1.3 Discuss the characteristics and skills most likely to lead to a successful career in one of the health care professions.

FROM THE PERSPECTIVE OF. . .

BARBARA, AN EXPERIENCED CERTIFIED MEDICAL ASSISTANT CMA, (AAMA), in a medical office with a walk-in clinic, instructs new employees in the reception area of the office to follow the medical office procedures whenever possible and prudent but, above all, to use common sense in dealing with patients.

Barbara told Elaine, a new receptionist in the medical office, to politely ask walk-in patients why they needed to see a doctor. Elaine had been on the job for two weeks when an elderly man who was hard of hearing approached her, and she dutifully asked him the purpose for his visit. He was obviously too embarrassed to reply, but Elaine persisted, finally raising her voice. When the man shouted, "I can't pee," all heads in the busy waiting room turned toward Elaine and the patient. A red-faced Elaine turned away to arrange for the man to see a physician, but he quickly left the building. Barbara criticized Elaine's patient-handling technique, but the crux of the matter was that the patient left without seeing a doctor for his medical problem.

"Patients' needs always trump office routine," Barbara emphasizes. "If we somehow hurt or hinder a patient while doggedly sticking to a set routine, we may have risked legal liability, but more important, we haven't done our job."

From Barbara's perspective as the person responsible for training medical office personnel, Elaine failed to use common sense in communicating with a patient, and as a result, the man did not receive the medical treatment he needed.

From Elaine's perspective, she followed Barbara's instructions to the letter, and she failed to understand why Barbara had criticized her. She hadn't meant to embarrass the man, so was it her fault that he left without making an appointment?

From the patient's perspective as an elderly gentleman who seldom discussed personal matters, the young woman who was his first contact in the medical office embarrassed him, and he left rather than face further humiliation.

As you progress through *Law & Ethics for the Health Professions,* try to interpret the court cases, laws, case studies, and other examples or situations cited from the perspectives of everyone involved.

1.1 Why Study Law and Ethics?

There are two important reasons for you to study law and ethics:

- To help you function at the highest possible professional level, providing competent, compassionate health care to patients
- To help you avoid legal entanglements that can threaten your ability to earn a living as a successful **health care practitioner**

We live in a **litigious** society, in which patients, relatives, and others are inclined to sue health care practitioners, health care facilities, manufacturers of medical equipment and products, and others when medical

health care practitioners
Those who are trained to administer medical or health care to patients.

litigious
Prone to engage in lawsuits.

outcomes are not acceptable. This means that every person responsible for health care delivery is at risk of being involved in a health care–related lawsuit. It is important, therefore, for you to know the basics of law and ethics as they apply to health care, so you can recognize and avoid those situations that might not serve your patients well or that might put you at risk of legal liability.

In addition to keeping you at your professional best and helping you avoid litigation, knowledge of law and ethics can also help you gain perspective in the following three areas:

1. *The rights, responsibilities, and concerns of health care consumers.* Health care practitioners not only need to be concerned about how law and ethics impact their respective professions but they must also understand how legal and ethical issues affect the patients they treat. With the increased complexity of medicine has come the desire of consumers to know more about their options and rights and more about the responsibilities of health care providers. Today's health care consumers are likely to consider themselves partners with health care practitioners in the healing process and to question fees and treatment modes. They may ask such questions as, Do I need to see a specialist? If so, which specialist can best treat my condition? Will I be given complete information about my condition? How much will medical treatment cost? Will a physician treat me if I have no health insurance?

   In addition, as medical technology has advanced, patients have come to expect favorable outcomes from medical treatment, and when expectations are not met, lawsuits may result.

2. *The legal and ethical issues facing society, patients, and health care practitioners as the world changes.* Nearly every day the media report news events concerning individuals who face legal and ethical dilemmas over biological/medical issues. For example, a grief-stricken husband must give consent for an abortion in order to save the life of his critically ill and unconscious wife. Parents must argue in court their decision to terminate life-support measures for a daughter whose injured brain no longer functions. Patients with HIV/AIDS fight to retain their right to confidentiality.

   While the situations that make news headlines often involve larger social issues, legal and ethical questions are resolved daily, on a smaller scale, each time a patient visits his or her physician, dentist, physical therapist, or other health care practitioner. Questions that must often be resolved include these: Who can legally give consent if the patient cannot? Can patients be assured of confidentiality, especially since telecommunication has become a way of life? Can a physician or other health care practitioner refuse to treat a patient? Who may legally examine a patient's medical records?

   Rapid advances in medical technology have also influenced laws and ethics for health care practitioners. For example, recent court cases have debated these issues: Does the husband or the wife have ownership rights to a divorced couple's frozen embryos? Will a surrogate mother have legal visitation rights to the child she carried to term? Should modern technology be used to keep those patients alive who are diagnosed as brain-dead and have no hope of recovery? How should parenthood disputes be resolved for children resulting from reproductive technology?

3. *The impact of rising costs on the laws and ethics of health care delivery.* Rising costs, both of health care insurance and of medical treatment in general, lead to questions concerning access to health care services and allocation of medical treatment. For instance, should the uninsured or underinsured receive government help to pay for health insurance? And should everyone, regardless of age or lifestyle, have the same access to scarce medical commodities such as organs for transplantation or very expensive drugs?

COURT CASES ILLUSTRATE RISK OF LITIGATION

As you will see in the court cases used throughout this text, sometimes when a lawsuit is brought, the trial court or a higher court must first decide if the **plaintiff** has a legal reason to sue, or if the **defendant** is **liable.** When a court has ruled that there is a standing (reason) to sue and that a defendant can be held liable, the case may proceed to resolution. Often, once liability and a standing to sue have been established, the two sides agree on an out-of-court settlement. Depending on state law, an out-of-court settlement may not be published. For this reason, the final disposition of a case is not always available from published sources. The published cases that have decided liability, however, are still case law, and such cases have been used in this text to illustrate specific points.

plaintiff
The person bringing charges in a lawsuit.

defendant
The person or party against whom criminal or civil charges are brought in a lawsuit.

liable
Legally responsible or obligated.

In addition, sometimes it takes time after the initial trial for a case to be settled. For example, perhaps a patient dies after surgery in 2012, and the family files a wrongful death suit soon after. The case may go through several appeals and finally be settled in 2016.

It is also important to remember that while the final result of a case is important to the parties involved, from a legal standpoint, the most important aspect of a court case is not the result but whether the case represents good law and will be persuasive as other cases are decided.

COURT CASE Patients Sue Hospitals

In 2016, lawsuits against hospitals that were moving through various courts included:

- A Texas woman, 32, suffered a seizure at 5 AM inside her home. Her husband took her to the hospital ER, where she was diagnosed with a migraine and a sinus infection and sent home with a prescription. Once home, she suffered a second seizure. An ambulance transported her to the ER, and while en route, she had a third seizure that left her brain-dead.
- Two hospitals in Washington, DC, were sued for excessive charges when three patients received bills for several hundred dollars for copying their medical records.
- Patients of a Seattle hospital were discussing a class action lawsuit against the hospital when they learned that a former employee of the hospital, a surgical technician, may have exposed them to hepatitis or HIV when he used surgical syringes for administering drugs to himself, then returned the used syringes to surgical supply.

(All of the above cases were still in litigation as the eighth edition of *Law & Ethics for Health Professions* was prepared for publication, but perhaps the underlying reasons for filing the lawsuits are already apparent to you.)

COURT CASE 911 Operators Sued

In 2006, just before 6 PM, a five-year-old boy called 911. He told the 911 operator that his "mom has passed out." When the operator asked to speak to the boy's mother, he said, "She's not gonna talk." The operator scolded the boy and logged the call as a child's prank. Three hours later, the boy called 911 again. A different operator answered, and she also scolded the boy for playing a prank, but she did send a police officer to the boy's home. The officer discovered the boy's mother lying unresponsive on the floor and summoned emergency medical services. The EMS workers arrived 20 minutes later and determined that the woman was dead and had probably died within the past two hours.

The boy's older sister sued the two 911 operators on behalf of the dead woman's estate and on behalf of her son. The lawsuit alleged gross negligence causing a death and intentional infliction of emotional distress.

The 911 operators argued that they were entitled to government immunity, that they owed no duty to provide assistance to the woman who died, and that their failure to summon medical aid was not gross negligence.

A trial court and an appeals court found for the plaintiff, and the case was appealed to the Michigan Supreme Court, where in January 2012, the court denied further appeals.

Source: *Estate of Turner v. Nichols*, 807 N.W.2d 164, 490 Mich. 988 (2012).

Although recent cases published have been sought for illustration in this text, sometimes a dated case (1995, 1985, 1970, etc.) is used because it established important **precedent.**

precedent
Decisions made by judges in the various courts that become rule of law and apply to future cases, even though they were not enacted by a legislature; also known as case law.

summary judgment
A decision made by a court in a lawsuit in response to a motion that pleads there is no basis for a trial.

Court cases appear throughout each chapter of the text to illustrate how the legal system has resolved complaints brought by or against health care service providers and product manufacturers. Some of these cases involve summary judgment. **Summary judgment** is the legal term for a decision made by a court in a lawsuit in response to a motion that pleads there is no basis for a trial because there is no genuine issue of material fact. In other words, a motion for summary judgment states that one party is entitled to win as a matter of law. Summary judgment is available only in a civil action. (Chapter 4 distinguishes between criminal and civil actions.)

The following court cases illustrate that a wide variety of legal questions can arise for those engaged directly in providing health care services, whether in a hospital, in a medical office, or in an emergency situation. Health care equipment and product dealers and manufacturers can be held indirectly responsible for defective medical devices and products through charges of the following types:

- Breach of warranty
- Statements made by the manufacturer about the device or product that are found to be untrue
- Strict liability, for cases in which defective products threaten the personal safety of consumers
- **Fraud** or intentional deceit (Fraud is discussed in further detail in Chapter 4.)

fraud
Dishonest or deceitful practices in depriving, or attempting to deprive, another of his or her rights.

LANDMARK COURT CASE

Supreme Court Shields Medical Devices from Lawsuits

An angioplasty was performed on a patient, Charles Riegel, in New York. During the procedure, the catheter used to dilate the patient's coronary artery failed, causing serious complications. The patient sued the catheter's manufacturer, Medtronic, Inc., under New York state law, charging negligence in design, manufacture, and labeling of the device, which had received Food and Drug Administration (FDA) approval in 1994. Medtronic argued that Riegel could not bring state law negligence claims because the company was preempted from liability under Section 360k(a) of the Medical Device Amendments (MDA) of the U.S. Food, Drug, and Cosmetic Act. State requirements are preempted under the MDA only to the extent that they are "different from, or in addition to" the requirements imposed by federal law. Thus, 360k(a) does not prevent a state from providing a damages remedy for claims premised on a violation of FDA regulations; the state duties in such a case "parallel," rather than add to, federal requirements (*Lohr,* 518 U.S., at 495, 116 S.Ct. 2240).

The *Riegel* case reached the U.S. Supreme Court, where the question to be decided was this: Does Section 360k(a) of the Medical Device Amendments to the Food, Drug, and Cosmetic Act preempt state law claims seeking damages for injuries caused by medical devices that received premarket approval from the Food and Drug Administration?

In February 2008, the U.S. Supreme Court held in this case that makers of medical devices are immune from liability for personal injuries as long as the FDA approved the device before it was marketed and it meets the FDA's specifications.

Source: Appeals Court Case: *Riegel v. Medtronic, Inc.,* 451 F.3d 104 (2006); Supreme Court Case: *Riegel v. Medtronic, Inc.,* 552 U.S. 312, 128 S.Ct. 999, 2008.

The extent of liability for manufacturers of medical devices and products may be changing, however, since a 2008 U.S. Supreme Court decision held that makers of medical devices such as implantable defibrillators or breast implants are immune from liability for personal injuries as long as the Food and Drug Administration (FDA) approved the device before it was marketed and it meets the FDA's specifications. (See the previous *Medtronic Inc.* case.)

Drugs and medical devices are regulated under separate federal laws, and an important issue in deciding drug injury cases is whether or not the drug manufacturer made false or misleading statements to win FDA approval. For example, the case *Warner-Lambert Co. v. Kent,* filed in 2006, involved a group of Michigan residents who claimed injury after taking Warner-Lambert's Rezulin diabetes drug. The case was brought under a Michigan tort reform law that said a drug company could be liable for product injury if it had misrepresented the product to win FDA approval. In this case, the question before the court was, Does a federal law prohibiting fraudulent communications to government agencies preempt a state law permitting plaintiffs to sue for faulty products that would not have reached the market absent the fraud?

A federal appeals court eventually heard the case and ruled that the Michigan "fraud on the FDA" law was preempted by a federal law that allowed the FDA itself to punish misrepresentations. This decision was appealed to the U.S. Supreme Court, and in a March 2008 decision, the Supreme Court affirmed the appeals court, thus leaving the previous state of the law unchanged and unclarified.

In this case, the people who sued the drug manufacturer were not allowed to collect damages. But when courts find that drugs are misrepresented so that developers can win FDA approval, drug manufacturers

Table 1-1 Damage Awards Can Be Substantial

- Drug: Yasmin (2012): Bayer paid $110 million to settle more than 500 lawsuits. Consumers who took the prescription drug for birth control experienced blood clots.
- Drug: Prempro (2011): Pfizer agreed to pay $330 million to settle more than 2,200 lawsuits. The company was accused of hiding the menopause drug's cancer risks.
- Drug: Avandia (2010): GlaxoSmithKline agreed to pay $460 million to settle 10,000 lawsuits. Claimants said the company hid heart attack risks associated with the diabetes drug.
- Drug: Vioxx (2008): Merck paid $4.85 billion to settle a reported 50,000 claims. People who took the painkiller suffered heart attacks and strokes.

Source: www.drugwatch.com/drug-lawsuits.php.

could be held legally responsible and forced to pay damages. Table 1-1 lists several settlements.

Federal preemption—a doctrine that can bar injured consumers from suing in state court when the products that hurt them had met federal standards—has become an important concern in product liability law. One such case, *Wyeth v. Levine,* decided by the U.S. Supreme Court in 2009, will become precedent for future cases involving drug manufacturers and consumers.

COURT CASE

Patient Sues over Drug-Labeling Issue

In 2000, Diana Levine, a Vermont woman in her fifties, sought medical help for migraine headaches. As part of the treatment, the antinausea drug Phenergan, made by Wyeth, was injected in her arm. An artery was accidentally damaged during the injection, gangrene set in, and Levine's right arm was amputated. The amputation was devastating for Levine, a professional musician who had released 16 albums, and she filed a personal injury action against Wyeth in Vermont state court.

Levine asserted that Wyeth should have included a warning label describing the possible arterial injuries that could occur from negligent injection of the drug. Wyeth argued that because the warning label had been deemed acceptable by the FDA, a federal agency, any Vermont state regulations making the label insufficient were preempted by the federal approval. The Superior Court of Vermont found in favor of Levine and denied Wyeth's motion for a new trial. Levine was awarded $7 million in damages for the amputation of her arm. The Supreme Court of Vermont affirmed this ruling on appeal, holding that the FDA requirements merely provide a floor, not a ceiling, for state regulation. Therefore, states are free to create more stringent labeling requirements than federal law provides.

The U.S. Supreme Court eventually heard the case and issued a decision in March 2009. Wyeth had argued that because the warning label had been accepted by the FDA, any Vermont state regulations making the label insufficient were preempted by the federal approval. The U.S. Supreme Court affirmed the Vermont Supreme Court, holding that federal law did not preempt Levine's state law claim that Wyeth's labeling of Phenergan failed to warn of the dangers of intravenous administration.

Source: *Wyeth v. Levine,* 555 U.S. 555, 173 L.Ed.2d 51 (2009).

1.2 Comparing Aspects of Law and Ethics

To understand the complexities of law and ethics, it is helpful to define and compare a few basic terms. Table 1-2 summarizes the terms described in the following sections.

Table 1-2 Comparing Aspects of Law and Ethics

	Law	Ethics	Moral Values
Definition	Set of governing rules	Principles, standards, guide to conduct	Beliefs formed through the influence of family, culture, and society
Main purpose	To protect the public	To elevate the standard of competence	To serve as a guide for personal ethical conduct
Standards	Minimal—promotes smooth functioning of society	Builds values and ideals	Serves as a basis for forming a personal code of ethics
Penalties of violation	Civil or criminal liability. Upon conviction: fine, imprisonment, revocation of license, or other penalty as determined by courts	Suspension or eviction from medical society membership, as decided by peers	Difficulty in getting along with others
	Bioethics	**Etiquette**	**Protocol**
Definition	Discipline relating to ethics concerning biological research, especially as applied to medicine	Courtesy and manners	Rules of etiquette applicable to one's place of employment
Main purpose	To allow scientific progress in a manner that benefits society in all possible ways	To enable one to get along with others	To enable one to get along with others engaged in the same profession
Standards	Leads to the highest standards possible in applying research to medical care	Leads to pleasant interaction	Promotes smooth functioning of workplace routines
Penalties of violation	Can include all those listed under "Law," "Ethics," and "Etiquette"; as current standards are applied and as new laws and ethical standards evolve to govern medical research and development, penalties may change	Ostracism from chosen groups	Disapproval from one's professional colleagues; possible loss of business

LAW

A **law** is defined as a rule of conduct or action prescribed or formally recognized as binding or enforced by a controlling authority. Governments enact laws to keep society running smoothly and to control behavior that could threaten public safety. Laws are considered the minimum standard necessary to keep society functioning.

law
Rule of conduct or action prescribed or formally recognized as binding or enforced by a controlling authority.

Enforcement of laws is made possible by penalties for disobedience, which are decided by a court of law or are mandatory as written into the law. Penalties vary with the severity of the crime. Lawbreakers may be fined, imprisoned, or both. Sometimes lawbreakers are sentenced to probation. Other penalties appropriate to the crime may be handed down by the sentencing authority, as when offenders must perform a specified number of hours of volunteer community service or are ordered to repair public facilities they have damaged.

Many laws affect health care practitioners, including criminal and civil statutes as well as state medical practice acts. Medical practice acts apply specifically to the practice of medicine in a certain state. Licensed health care professionals convicted of violating criminal, civil, or medical practice laws may lose their licenses to practice. (Medical practice acts are discussed further in Chapter 3. Laws and the court system are discussed in more detail in Chapter 4.)

ETHICS

ethics
Standards of behavior, developed as a result of one's concept of right and wrong.

moral values
One's personal concept of right and wrong, formed through the influence of the family, culture, and society.

An illegal act by a health care practitioner is always unethical, but an unethical act is not necessarily illegal. **Ethics** are concerned with standards of behavior and the concept of right and wrong, over and above that which is legal in a given situation. **Moral values**—formed through the influence of the family, culture, and society—serve as the basis for ethical conduct.

The United States is a culturally diverse country, with many residents who have grown up within vastly different ethnic environments. For example, a Chinese student in the United States brings to his or her studies a unique set of religious and social experiences and moral concepts that will differ from that of a German, Japanese, Korean, French, Italian, or Canadian classmate. Therefore, moral values and ethical standards can differ for health care practitioners, as well as patients, in the same setting.

In the American cultural environment, however, acting morally toward another usually requires that you put yourself in that individual's place. For example, when you are a patient in a physician's office, how do you like to be treated? As a health care provider, can you give care to a person whose conduct or professed beliefs differ radically from your own? In an emergency, can you provide for the patient's welfare without reservation?

Check Your Progress

1. Name two important reasons for studying law and ethics.
2. Which state laws apply specifically to the practice of medicine?
3. What purpose do laws serve?
4. How is the enforcement of laws made possible?
5. What factors influence the formation of one's personal set of ethics and values?
6. Define the term *moral values*.
7. Explain how one's moral values affect one's sense of ethics.

CODES OF ETHICS AND ETHICS GUIDELINES

code of ethics
A list of principles intended to govern behavior—here, the behavior of those entrusted with providing care to the sick.

ethics guidelines
Publications that detail a wide variety of ethical situations that professionals (in this case, health care practitioners) might face in their work and offer principles for dealing with the situations in an ethical manner.

While most individuals can rely on a well-developed personal value system, organizations for the health occupations also have formalized **codes of ethics** to govern behavior of members and to increase the level of competence and standards of care within the group. Included among these are the American Nurses Association Code for Nurses, American Medical Association Code of Medical Ethics, American Health Information Management Association Code of Ethics, American Society of Radiologic Technologists Code of Ethics, and the Code of Ethics of the American Association of Medical Assistants. Codes of ethics generally consist of a list of general principles and are often available to laypersons as well as members of health care practitioner organizations.

Many professional organizations for health care practitioners also publish more detailed **ethics guidelines,** usually in book form, for members.

Generally, ethics guideline publications detail a wide variety of ethical situations that health care practitioners might face in their work and offer principles for dealing with the situations in an ethical manner. They are routinely available to members of health care organizations and are typically available to others for a fee.

One of the earliest medical codes of ethics, the code of Hammurabi, was written by the Babylonians around 2250 B.C.E. This document discussed the conduct expected of physicians at that time, including fees that could be charged.

Sometime around 400 B.C.E., a pledge for physicians known as the **Hippocratic oath** was published. The oath was probably not actually written by Hippocrates, the Greek physician known as the Father of Medicine. Authorship has been attributed to one or more of his students and to the Pythagoreans, but scholars indicate it was probably derived from Hippocrates's writings (see Figure 1-1).

Hippocratic oath
A pledge for physicians, influenced by the practices of the Greek physician Hippocrates.

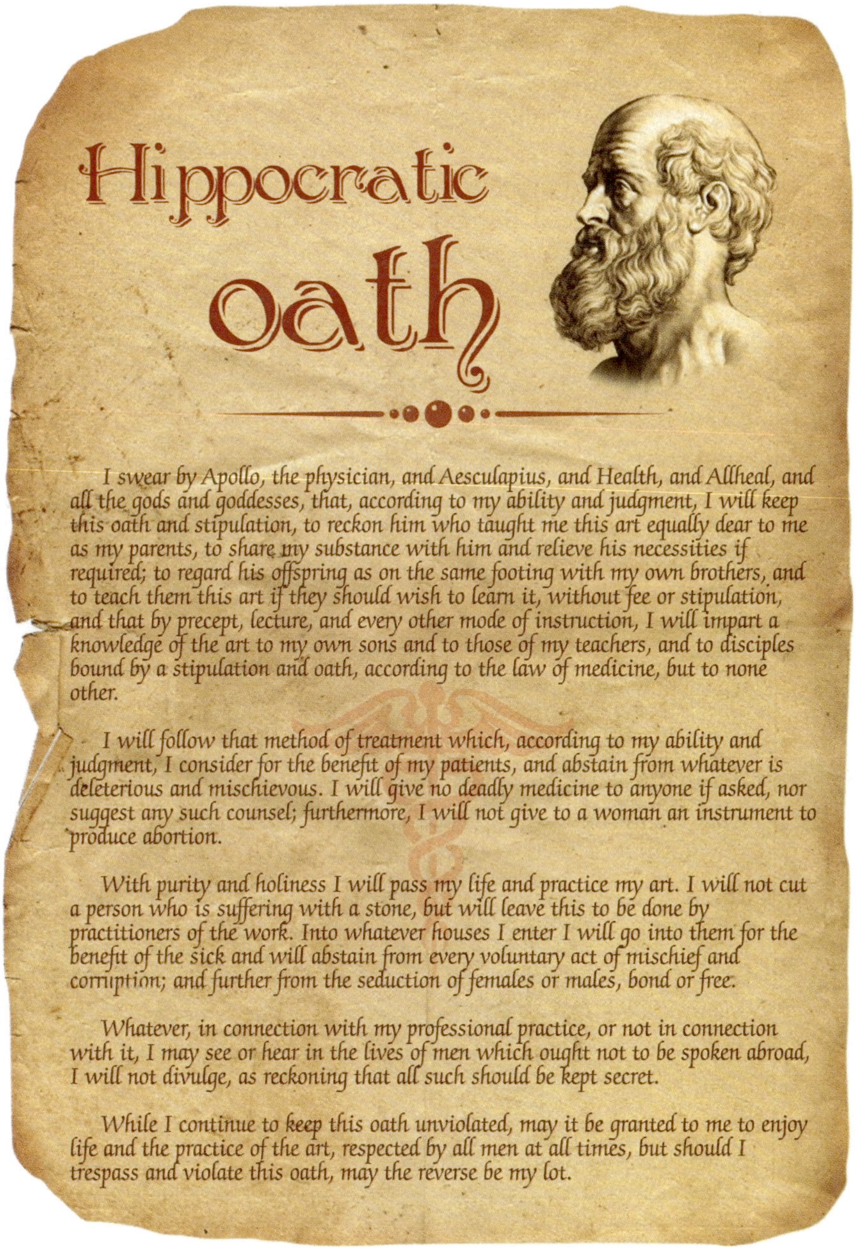

FIGURE 1-1
Hippocratic Oath

Source: Rijksmuseum, Amsterdam.

Percival's Medical Ethics, written by the English physician and philosopher Thomas Percival in 1803, superseded earlier codes to become the definitive guide for a physician's professional conduct. Earlier codes did not address concerns about experimental medicine, but according to Percival's code, physicians could try experimental treatments when all else failed, if such treatments served the public good.

When the American Medical Association met for the first time in Philadelphia in 1847, the group devised a code of ethics for members based on Percival's code. The resulting ***American Medical Association Principles,*** currently called the *American Medical Association Principles of Medical Ethics,* has been revised and updated periodically to keep pace with changing times. The *American Medical Association Principles of Medical Ethics* briefly summarizes the position of the American Medical Association (AMA) on ethical treatment of patients, while the more extensive *Code of Medical Ethics: Current Opinions with Annotations* provides more detailed coverage. The AMA Ethics statement can be read online at www.ama-assn.org/sites/default/files/media-browser/public/ethics/principles-of-medical-ethics-20160627.pdf.

American Medical Association Principles
A code of ethics for members of the American Medical Association, written in 1847. (American Medical Association Web site: www.ama-assn.org/ama/pub/physicianresources/medical-ethics/code-medical-ethics/principles-medical-ethics.page.)

While the AMA code pertains solely to physicians, the National Association for Healthcare Quality has compiled a Code of Ethics and Standards of Practice that applies specifically to Healthcare Quality Professionals, and could perhaps apply more generally to all health care practitioners. The list can be read in its entirety at http://nahq.org/about/code-of-ethics. The list below reflects some of the statements that could be included in any health care practitioners code of ethics:

- Practice [your] profession with honesty, integrity, and accountability.
- Maintain [an acceptable/legal] level of competency for your profession.
- Seek the trust and confidence of all customers.
- Respect all laws and avoid involvement in any false, fraudulent, or deceptive activity.
- Promote the right of privacy for all individuals and protect the maintenance of confidential information to the fullest extent permitted [and mandated] by law.
- Facilitate informed decision-making.
- Give credit for the work of others to whom it is due.
- Aid the professional development and advancement of colleagues.
- Maintain membership in professional organizations as a means of promoting quality and professional growth.
- [Maintain a] primary commitment to the health, well-being, and safety of patients.
- Take appropriate actions regarding any instances of incompetent, unethical, illegal, or impaired practice.
- Encourage the reporting of events that may result in actual or potential harm to patients or others.

including photocopying, recording, or by any means of information storage and retrieval system, without written permission from the copyright holder.

When members of professional associations such as the AMA and the AAMA are accused of unethical conduct, they are subject to peer council review and may be censured by the organization. Although a professional group cannot revoke a member's license to practice, unethical members may be expelled from the group, suspended for a period of time, or ostracized by other members. Unethical behavior by a medical practitioner can result in loss of income and eventually the loss of a practice if, as a result of that behavior, patients choose another practitioner. Figure 1-2 is an example of a code of ethics from the American Association of Medical Assistants.

FIGURE 1-2 Code of Ethics and Creed of the American Association of Medical Assistants (AAMA)

The Medical Assisting Code of Ethics of the AAMA sets forth principles of ethical and moral conduct as they relate to the medical profession and the particular practice of medical assisting.

Members of AAMA dedicated to the conscientious pursuit of their profession, and thus desiring to merit the high regard of the entire medical profession and the respect of the general public which they serve, do pledge themselves to strive always to:

A. Render service with full respect for the dignity of humanity.

B. Respect confidential information obtained through employment unless legally authorized or required by responsible performance of duty to divulge such information.

C. Uphold the honor and high principles of the profession and accept its disciplines.

D. Seek to continually improve the knowledge and skills of medical assistants for the benefit of patients and professional colleagues.

E. Participate in additional service activities aimed toward improving the health and well-being of the community.

The Medical Assisting Creed of the AAMA sets forth medical assisting statements of belief:

I. I believe in the principles and purposes of the profession of medical assisting.

II. I endeavor to be more effective.

III. I aspire to render greater service.

IV. I protect the confidence entrusted to me.

V. I am dedicated to the care and well-being of all people.

VI. I am loyal to my employer.

VII. I am true to the ethics of my profession.

VIII. I am strengthened by compassion, courage and faith.

Source: www.aama-ntl.org/about/overview#.

BIOETHICS

bioethics
A discipline dealing with the ethical implications of biological research methods and results, especially in medicine.

Bioethics is a discipline dealing with the ethical implications of biological research methods and results, especially in medicine. As biological research has led to unprecedented progress in medicine, medical practitioners have had to grapple with issues such as these:

- What ethics should guide biomedical research? Do individuals own all rights to their body cells, or should scientists own cells they have altered? Is human experimentation essential, or even permissible, to advance biomedical research?
- What ethics should guide organ transplants? Although organs suitable for transplant are in short supply, is the search for organs dehumanizing? Should certain categories of people have lower priority than others for organ transplants?
- What ethics should guide fetal tissue research? Some say such research, especially stem cell research, is moral because it offers hope to disease victims, while others argue that it is immoral.
- Do reproductive technologies offer hope to the childless, or are they unethical? Are the multiple births that sometimes result from taking fertility drugs an acceptable aspect of reproductive technology, or are those multiple births too risky for women and their fetuses and even immoral in an allegedly overpopulated world?
- Should animals ever be used in research?
- How ethical is genetic research? Should the government regulate it? Will genetic testing benefit those at risk for genetic disease, or will it lead to discrimination? Should cloning of human organs for transplantation be permitted? Should cloning of human beings ever be permitted?

Society is attempting to address these questions, but because the issues are complicated, many questions may never be completely resolved.

THE ROLE OF ETHICS COMMITTEES

Health care practitioners may be able to resolve the majority of the ethical issues they face in the workplace from their own intuitive sense of moral values and ethics. Some ethical dilemmas, however, are not so much a question of right or wrong, but more a question of "Which of these alternatives will do the most good and the least harm?" In these more ambiguous situations, health care practitioners may want to ask the advice of a medical ethicist or members of an institutional ethics committee.

medical ethicist or bioethicist
Specialists who consult with physicians, researchers, and others to help them make difficult ethical decisions regarding patient care.

ethics committee
Committee made up of individuals who are involved in a patient's care, including health care practitioners, family members, clergy, and others, with the purpose of reviewing ethical issues in difficult cases.

Medical ethicists or **bioethicists** are specialists who consult with physicians, researchers, and others to help them make difficult decisions, such as whether to resuscitate brain-damaged premature infants or what ethics should govern privacy in genetic testing. Hospital or medical center ethics committees usually consist of physicians, nurses, social workers, clergy, a patient's family, members of the community, and other individuals involved with the patient's medical care. A medical ethicist may also sit on the ethics committee if such a specialist is available. When difficult decisions must be made, any one of the individuals involved in a patient's medical care can ask for a consultation with the ethics committee. Larger hospitals have standing ethics committees, while smaller facilities may form ethics committees as needed.

When a case is referred to the ethics committee, the members meet and review the case. The committee does not make binding decisions but helps the physician, nurse, patient, patient's family, and others clarify the issue and understand the medical facts of the case and the alternatives available to resolve the situation. Ethics committees may also help with conflict resolution among parties involved with a case. They do not, however, function as institutional review boards or morals police looking for health care workers who have committed unethical acts.

See Chapter 2 for a more detailed discussion of the processes involved in making ethical decisions.

ETIQUETTE

While professional codes of ethics focus on the protection of the patient and his or her right to appropriate, competent, and humane treatment, **etiquette** refers to standards of behavior that are considered good manners. Every culture has its own ideas of common courtesy. Behavior considered good manners in one culture may be bad manners in another. For example, in some Middle Eastern countries, it is extremely discourteous for one male acquaintance to ask another, "How is your wife?" In Western culture, such a question is well received. Similarly, within nearly every profession, there are recognized practices considered to be good manners for members.

etiquette
Standards of behavior considered to be good manners among members of a profession as they function as individuals in society.

Most health care facilities have their own policies concerning professional etiquette that staff members are expected to follow. Policy manuals written especially for the facility can serve as permanent records and as guidelines for employees in these matters.

By the same token, health care practitioners are expected to know **protocol,** standard rules of etiquette applicable specifically to their place of employment. For example, when another physician telephones, does the receptionist put the call through without delay? What is the protocol in the diagnostic testing office when the technicians get behind because of a late patient or a repair to an X-ray machine?

protocol
A code prescribing correct behavior in a specific situation, such as a situation arising in a medical office.

Within the health care environment, all health care practitioners are, of course, expected to treat patients with the same respect and courtesy afforded others in the course of day-to-day living. Politeness and appropriate dress are mandatory.

1.3 Qualities of Successful Health Care Practitioners

Successful health care practitioners have a knowledge of techniques and principles that includes an understanding of legal and ethical issues. They must also acquire a working knowledge of and tolerance for human nature and individual characteristics, since daily contact with a wide variety of individuals with a host of problems and concerns is a significant part of the work. Courtesy, compassion, and common sense are often cited as the "three Cs" most vital to the professional success of health care practitioners.

COURTESY

courtesy
The practice of good manners.

The simplest definition of **courtesy** is the practice of good manners. Most of us know how to practice good manners, but sometimes circumstances make us forget. Maybe we're having a rotten day—we overslept and dressed in a hurry but were still late to work; the car didn't start so we had to walk, making us even more late; we were rebuked at work for coming in late . . . and on and on. Perhaps we're burned out, stressed out, or simply too busy to think. Regardless of a health care practitioner's personal situation, however, patients have the right to expect courtesy and respect, including self-introduction. ("Hi, I'm Maggie, and I'll be taking care of you" is one nursing assistant's way of introducing herself to new patients in the nursing home where she works.)

Think back to experiences you have had with health care practitioners. Did the receptionist in a medical office greet you pleasantly, or did he or she make you feel as though you were an unwelcome intruder? (Remember Elaine in the chapter's opening scenario?) Did the laboratory technician or phlebotomist who drew your blood for testing put you at ease or make you more anxious than you already were? If you were hospitalized, did health care practitioners carefully explain procedures and treatments before performing them, or were you left wondering what was happening to you? Chances are that you know from your own experiences how important common courtesy can be to a patient.

COMPASSION

compassion
The identification with and understanding of another's situation, feelings, and motives.

Compassion is empathy—the identification with and understanding of another's situation, feelings, and motives. In other words, compassion is temporarily putting oneself in another's shoes. It should not be confused with sympathy, which is feeling sorry for another person's plight—typically a less deeply felt emotion than compassion. While "I know how you feel" is not usually the best phrase to utter to a patient (it too often earns the retort, "No, you don't"), compassion means that you are sincerely attempting to know how the patient feels.

COMMON SENSE

common sense
Sound practical judgment.

Common sense is simply sound practical judgment. It is somewhat difficult to define because it can have different meanings for different people, but it generally means that you can see which solution or action makes good sense in a given situation. For example, if you were a nursing assistant and a gasping, panicked patient told you he was having trouble breathing, common sense would tell you to immediately seek help. You wouldn't simply enter the patient's complaint in his medical chart and wait for a physician or a nurse to see the notation. Likewise, if a patient spilled something on the floor, common sense would tell you to wipe it up (even if you were not a member of the housekeeping staff) before someone stepped in it and possibly slipped and fell. While it's not always immediately obvious that someone has common sense, it usually doesn't take long to recognize its absence in an individual.

Additional capabilities that are helpful to those who choose to work in the health care field include those that are listed in the following sections "People Skills" and "Technical Skills."

PEOPLE SKILLS

People skills are those traits and capabilities that allow you to get along well with others and to relate well to patients or clients in a health care setting. They include such attributes as the following:

- A relaxed attitude when meeting new people
- An understanding of and empathy for others
- Good communication skills, including writing, speaking, and listening
- Patience in dealing with others and the ability to work as a member of a health care team
- Tact, or sensitivity when dealing with others or with difficult issues
- The ability to impart information clearly and accurately
- The ability to keep information confidential
- The ability to leave private concerns at home
- Trustworthiness and a sense of responsibility

TECHNICAL SKILLS

Technical skills include those abilities you have acquired in your course of study, including but not limited to the following:

- Computer literacy
- Proficiency in English, science, and mathematics.
- A willingness to learn new skills and techniques.
- An aptitude for working with the hands.
- Ability to document well.
- Ability to think critically.

CRITICAL THINKING SKILLS

When faced with a problem, most of us worry a lot before we finally begin working through the problem effectively, which means using fewer emotions and more rational thinking skills. As a health care practitioner, you will be expected to approach a problem at work in a manner that lets you act as ethically, legally, and helpfully as possible. Sometimes solutions to problems must also be found as quickly as possible, but solutions must always be within the scope of your training, licensure, and capabilities. This problem-solving process is called **critical thinking.** Here is a five-step aid for approaching a problem using critical thinking:

critical thinking
The ability to think analytically, using fewer emotions and more rationality.

1. **Identify and clarify the problem.** It's impossible to solve a problem unless you know the exact nature of the problem. For example, imagine that patients in a medical office have frequently complained that the wait to see physicians is too long, and several have protested

loudly and angrily that their time "is valuable too." Rhea is the waiting room receptionist and the person who faces angry patients first, so she would like to solve this problem as quickly as possible. Rhea has recognized that a problem exists, of course, but her apologies to patients have been temporary fixes, and the situation continues.

2. **Gather information.** In the previous situation, Rhea begins to gather information. She first checks to see exactly why patients have been kept waiting and considers the following questions: Are all the physicians simply oversleeping and beginning the day behind schedule? (Not likely, but an easy solution if this were the case would be to buy the physicians new alarm clocks.) Are the physicians often delayed in surgery or because of hospital rounds? Is the clinic understaffed? How long, on average, has each patient who has complained been waiting beyond his or her appointment time?
3. **Evaluate the evidence.** Rhea evaluates the answers she has gathered to the earlier questions and determines that too many patients are, indeed, waiting too long beyond appointment times to see their physicians. The next step in the critical thinking process is to consider all possible ways to solve the problem.
4. **Consider alternatives and implications.** Rhea has determined that the evidence supports the fact that a problem exists and begins to formulate alternatives by asking herself these questions: Could the waiting room be better supplied with current reading material or perhaps television sets and a children's corner, so that patients both with and without children are less likely to complain about waiting? Is the waiting room cheery and comfortable, so waiting does not seem interminable? What solution would best serve the goals of physicians, other medical office personnel, and patients? Rhea must consider costs of, objections to, and all others' opinions of each alternative she considers.
5. **Choose and implement the best alternative.** Rhea selects an alternative and implements it. As a medical office receptionist, she cannot act alone, but she has brought the problem to the attention of those who can help, and her suggestions have been heard. As a result of Rhea's research, acceptable solutions to patients' complaints that they are forced to wait too long to see physicians might include the following:
   - Patients are asked to remind receptionists when they have been waiting more than 15 minutes so receptionists can check to see what is causing the delay.
   - Additional personnel are hired to see patients.
   - The waiting room is stocked with current news publications, television sets, and/or a child play center for patient comfort while waiting.

   Critical thinking is not easy, but, like any skill, it improves with practice.

Check Your Progress

8. Describe how each of the following characteristics relates to law and ethics in the health care professions:
   The ability to be a good communicator and listener
   The ability to keep information confidential
   The ability to impart information clearly and accurately
   The ability to think critically
9. List and discuss each of the steps helpful to developing critical thinking skills
10. Explain how you, as a health care practitioner, would use the critical thinking steps listed previously to reach a solution to the following problem: A patient from a different culture believes he has been cursed with a "liver demon" and will die unless the organ is surgically removed

DETERMINING IF A DECISION IS ETHICAL

While considering the legality of a certain act, health care practitioners must also consider ethical implications. According to many ethics experts, the following questions can help you determine if an act you have decided on via critical thinking skills is ethical:

- If you perform this act, have you followed relevant laws and kept within your employing organization's policy?
- Will this act promote a win–win situation for as many of the involved individuals as possible?
- How would you feel if this act were to be publicized in the newspapers or other media?
- Would you want your family members to know?
- If you perform this act, can you look at yourself in a mirror?

The health care practitioner who demonstrates these qualities and skills, coupled with a working knowledge of law and ethics, is most likely to find success and job satisfaction in his or her chosen profession.

Chapter Summary

Learning Outcome	Summary

LO 1.1 Explain why knowledge of law and ethics is important to health care practitioners.	Why study law and ethics?
	• Health care practitioners who function at the highest possible levels have a working knowledge of law and ethics.
	• Knowing the law relevant to your profession can help you avoid legal entanglements that threaten your ability to earn a living. Court cases illustrate how health care practitioners, health care facilities, and drug and medical device manufacturers can be held accountable in a court of law.
	• A knowledge of law and ethics will also help familiarize you with the following areas:
	  • The rights, responsibilities, and concerns of health care consumers
	  • The legal and ethical issues facing society, patients, and health care practitioners as the world changes
	  • The impact of rising costs on the laws and ethics of health care delivery

LO 1.2 Define *law, ethics,* and *moral values* as used in health care by health care practitioners.	What are the basic aspects of law and ethics, and how do they compare? • Laws are considered the minimum standard necessary to keep society functioning. Many laws govern the health care professions, including criminal and civil statutes and medical practice acts. • Ethics are principles and standards that govern behavior. Most health care professions have a code of ethics members are expected to follow. • Bioethics is the discipline dealing with the ethical implications of biological research methods and results, especially in medicine. • Moral values define one's personal concept of right and wrong. • Etiquette refers to manners and courtesy. • Protocol is a code prescribing correct behavior in a specific situation, such as in a medical office.
LO 1.3 Discuss the characteristics and skills most likely to lead to a successful career in one of the health care professions.	What characteristics and skills will most likely help a health care practitioner achieve success? • People skills, such as listening to others and communicating well, are an asset to health care practitioners. • Technical skills, including a basic knowledge of computers, and a foundation in science and math are necessary to achieve an education in the health care sciences. • Critical thinking skills are required for you to correctly assess a situation and provide the proper response. Solving problems through critical thinking involves: 1. Identifying and clarifying the problem 2. Gathering information 3. Evaluating the evidence 4. Considering alternatives and implications 5. Choosing and implementing the best alternative What questions can help you determine if a decision is ethical? 1. If you perform this act, have you followed relevant laws and kept within your employing organization's policy? 2. Will this act promote a win-win situation for as many of the involved individuals as possible? 3. How would you feel if this act were to be publicized in the newspapers or other media? 4. Would you want your family members to know? 5. If you perform this act, can you look at yourself in a mirror?

Chapter 1 Review

Applying Knowledge

LO 1.1

1. List three areas where health care practitioners can gain insight through studying law and ethics.
2. Define *summary judgment.*

LO 1.2

3. Define *bioethics.*
4. Define *law.*
5. Define *ethics.*
6. How is unethical behavior punished?
7. Define *etiquette.*
8. How are violations of etiquette handled?
9. What is the purpose of a professional code of ethics?
10. Name five bioethical issues of concern in today's society.
11. What duties might a medical ethicist perform?
12. Decisions made by judges in the various courts and used as a guide for future decisions are called what?
13. Written codes of ethics for health care practitioners
    a. Evolved primarily to serve as moral guidelines for those who provided care to the sick
    b. Are legally binding
    c. Did not exist in ancient times
    d. None of these
14. What Greek physician is known as the Father of Medicine?
    a. Hippocrates
    b. Percival
    c. Hammurabi
    d. Socrates
15. Name the pledge for physicians that remains influential today.
    a. Code of Hammurabi
    b. Babylonian Ethics Code
    c. Hippocratic oath
    d. None of these
16. What ethics code superseded earlier codes to become the definitive guide for a physician's professional conduct?
    a. Code of Hammurabi
    b. Percival's Medical Ethics
    c. Hippocratic oath
    d. Babylonian Ethics Code

17. Unethical behavior is always

 a. Illegal

 b. Punishable by legal means

 c. Unacceptable

 d. None of these

18. Unlawful acts are always

 a. Unacceptable

 b. Unethical

 c. Punishable by legal means

 d. All of these

19. Violation of a professional organization's formalized code of ethics

 a. Always leads to prosecution in a court of law

 b. Is ignored if one's membership dues in the organization are paid

 c. Can lead to expulsion from the organization

 d. None of these

20. Law is

 a. The minimum standard necessary to keep society functioning smoothly

 b. Ignored if transgressions are ethical, rather than legal

 c. Seldom enforced by controlling authorities

 d. None of these

21. Conviction of a crime

 a. Cannot result in loss of license unless ethical violations also exist

 b. Is always punishable by imprisonment

 c. Always results in expulsion from a professional organization

 d. Can result in loss of license

22. Sellers and manufacturers can be held legally responsible for defective medical devices and products through what charges?

 a. Fraud

 b. Breach of warranty

 c. Misrepresentation of the product through untrue statements made by the manufacturer or seller

 d. All of these

23. The basis for ethical conduct includes

 a. One's morals

 b. One's culture

 c. One's family

 d. All of these

24. What is bioethics concerned with?
    a. Health care law
    b. Etiquette in medical facilities
    c. The ethical implications of biological research methods and results
    d. None of these

LO 1.3

25. Critical thinking skills include
    a. Assessing the ethics of a situation
    b. First clearly defining a problem
    c. Determining the legal implications of a situation
    d. None of these

Ethics Issues Introduction to End-of-Chapter Ethics Discussions

Learning Outcomes for the Ethics Issues Feature at the End of Each Chapter

After studying the material in each chapter's Ethics Issues feature, you should be able to:

1. Discuss current ethical issues of concern to health care practitioners.
2. Compare ethical guidelines to the law as discussed in each chapter of the text.
3. Practice critical thinking skills as you consider medical, legal, and ethical issues for each situation presented.
4. Relate the ethical issues presented in the text to the health care profession you intend to practice.

Health care practitioners are bound by state and federal laws, but they are also bound by certain ethical standards—both personal standards and those set forth by professional codes of ethics and ethical guidelines and by bioethicists. Many professional organizations for health care practitioners employ an ethics consultant who is available to speak with organization members who need help with an ethical dilemma. "We serve as a third party who can stand outside a situation and facilitate communication," says Dr. Carmen Paradis, an ethics consultant with the Cleveland Clinic's Department of Bioethics. At the Cleveland Clinic, ethics consultations are available to health care practitioners, patients, family members, and others involved with patient decisions.

Medical facility ethics committees can also serve as consultants. In larger health care facilities, such committees usually deal with institutional matters, but in smaller communities where ethics consultants may not be available, members of an ethics committee may also function as ethics consultants.

Keep in mind as you read the Ethics Issues feature for each chapter that ethical guidelines are not law but deal solely with ethical conduct for health care practitioners. Most guidelines published for professional health care practitioner organizations emphasize this difference. For example, as stated in *Guidelines for Ethical Conduct for the Physician Assistant Profession:*

> Generally, the law delineates the minimum standard of acceptable behavior in our society. Acceptable ethical behavior is usually less clearly defined than law and often places greater demands on an individual. . . .
>
> Ethical guidelines for health care practitioners are not meant to be used in courts of law as legal standards to which practitioners will be held. Ethical guidelines are, rather, meant to guide health care practitioners and to encourage them to think about their individual actions in certain situations.

The ethical guidelines for various health care professions have several points in common, but first and foremost is that health care practitioners are obligated to provide the best care possible for every patient and to protect the safety and welfare of every patient.

State and federal law may differ somewhat from an ethical principle. For example, a state's law may not require physicians to routinely inquire about physical, sexual, and psychological abuse as part of a patient's medical history, but the physician may feel an ethical duty to his or her patients to do so.

Furthermore, the fact that a health care practitioner who has been charged with illegal conduct is acquitted or exonerated does not necessarily mean that the health care practitioner acted ethically.

The term *ethical* as used here refers to matters involving the following:

1. Moral principles or practices
2. Matters of social policy involving issues of morality in the practice of medicine

The term *unethical* refers to professional conduct that fails to conform to these moral standards or policies.

The ethical issues raised are from the real-life experiences of a variety of health care practitioners and are recounted throughout the text to raise awareness of the ethical dilemmas many practitioners face daily and to stimulate discussion.

Ethics Issues Introduction to Law and Ethics

Use your critical thinking skills to answer the questions that follow each ethics issue.

Ethics ISSUE 1:

A physician assistant (PA) in a medical practice with several physicians contacts his professional association, the American Academy of Physician Assistants (AAPA), to report that one of his employing physicians often recommends chiropractic treatment for patients with persistent back pain issues that have resisted medical solutions. The PA knows it is legal to refer a patient for chiropractic treatments, but he adamantly opposes the practice, considering it "bogus medicine." The physician declines to discuss the matter.

Discussion Questions

26. In your opinion, how might the situation be resolved?

27. Is it ethical for the PA to continue working for the physician when their opinions differ so widely on this issue?

Ethics ISSUE 2:

A registered nurse calls her professional organization's ethics consultant to ask for resources she can present to her employing medical clinic to support her intention to quit working with a physician she feels is providing sloppy and possibly dangerous care.

Discussion Questions

28. What is the most important principle for the nurse to consider here?

29. In your opinion, are there legal issues inherent in this situation, as well as ethical issues? Explain your answer.

Ethics ISSUE 3:

A physician assistant has been helping treat a patient awaiting a heart transplant. The patient is depressed and says he no longer wants to live. The PA is doubtful that the patient will cooperate in the demanding regimen required for post-transplantation patients.

Discussion Question

30. Is it ethical for the PA to say nothing to the patient's attending physician, or should he chart the patient's remarks and discuss the matter with the patient's physician?

Ethics ISSUE 4:

Family members of a certified medical assistant (CMA) (AAMA) employed by a medical clinic in a small community often ask the CMA for medical advice. Two of her family members have asked her to bring antibiotic samples home for them.

Discussion Question

31. In your opinion, would it be ethical for the CMA to give medical advice to her own family members? To bring drug samples home for them? Explain your answers.

Ethics ISSUE 5:

A radiology technician practicing in a small community is interested in dating a person he has seen as a patient.

Discussion Question

32. In your opinion, would it be ethical for the radiology technician to date one of his patients? Would it be ethical for him to date a coworker? Explain your answers.

Case Studies

LO 1.2

Use your critical thinking skills to answer the questions that follow each case study. Indicate whether each situation is a question of law, ethics, protocol, or etiquette.

You are employed as an assistant in an ophthalmologist's office. Your neighbor asks you to find out for him how much another patient was charged for an eye examination at the eye clinic that employs you. Your neighbor also asks you how much the patient was charged for his prescription eyeglasses (the eye clinic also sells lenses and frames).

33. Can you answer either of your neighbor's questions? Explain your answer.

A physician employs you as a medical assistant. Another physician comes into the medical office where you work and asks to speak with your physician/employer.

34. Should you seat the physician in the waiting room, or show her to your employer's private office? Why?

You are employed as a licensed practical nurse (LPN) in a small town. (In California and Texas, the term for this profession is *licensed vocational nurse,* abbreviated as LVN.) A woman visits the clinic where you work, complaining of a rash on her body. She says she recently came in contact with a child who had the same symptoms, and she asks, "What did this child see the doctor for, and what was the diagnosis?" She explains that she needs to know so that she can be immunized, if necessary. You explain that you cannot give out this information, but another LPN overhears, pulls the child's chart, and gives the woman the information she requested.

35. Did both LPNs in this scenario act ethically and responsibly? Explain your answer.

LO 1.3

A physician admitted an elderly patient to the hospital, where she was treated for an irregular heartbeat and chest pain. The patient was competent to make her own decisions about a course of treatment, but her opinionated and outspoken daughter repeatedly second-guessed the physician's recommendations with medical information she had obtained from the Internet.

36. In your opinion, what responsibilities, if any, does a physician or other health care practitioner have toward difficult family members or other third parties who interfere with a patient's medical care?
37. What might the physician in this situation have said to her patient's daughter to help resolve the situation?

Internet Activities

LO 1.1 and LO 1.2

Complete the activities and answer the questions that follow.

38. Use a search engine to conduct a search for Web sites on the Internet concerned with bioethics. Name two of those sites you think are reliable sources of information. Explain your choices. How does each site define the term *bioethics?*
39. Locate the Web site for the organization that represents the health care profession you intend to practice. Does the site provide guidance on ethics? If so, how? Does the site link to other sites concerning ethics? If so, list three ethics links, and then explore these links.
40. Visit this Web site sponsored by the National Institutes of Health: https://oir.nih.gov/sourcebook/ethical-conduct/responsible-conduct-research-training/annual-review-ethics-case-studies. Pick a case study from the list and review it. Do you agree or disagree with the conclusions reached about the issue? Explain your answer.

Resources

LO 1.1

Drug and medical device lawsuits: www.drugwatch.com/drug-lawsuits.php.

Lindgren, Jennifer. "Family of Fort Worth Mom Sues Hospital for Medical Malpractice." *ASC Communications,* July 6, 2015.

LO 1.2

Difference between medical ethics and medical etiquette: www.answers.com/Q/How_do_medical_ethics_differ_from_medical_etiquette.

LO 1.3

Sanchez, M. A. "Using Critical-Thinking Principles as a Guide to College-Level Instruction." *Teaching of Psychology* 22, no 1. (1995), pp. 72–74.

Telephone interview with Dr. Carmen Paradis, Department of Bioethics, Cleveland Clinic.

Ten qualities of a great health care professional: http://allhealthcare.monster.com/benefits/articles/3854-top-10-qualities-of-a-great-health-care-professional?page=6%22.

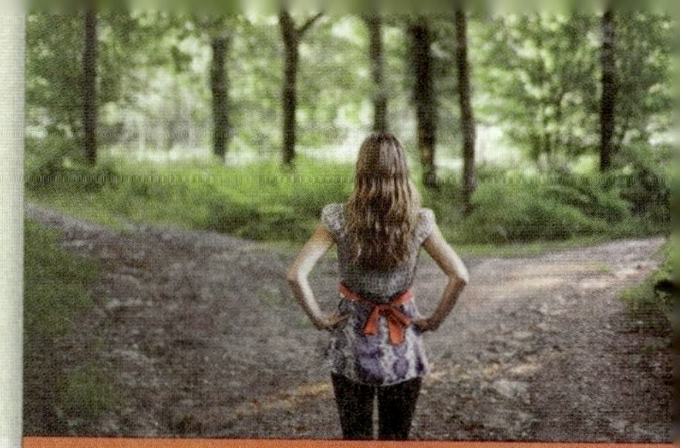

©Tim Robberts/The Image Bank/Getty Images

Making Ethical Decisions

2

Key Terms

autonomy
beneficence
categorical imperative
confidentiality
deontological or duty-oriented theory
fidelity
justice
needs-based motivation
nonmaleficence
principle of utility
teleological or consequence-oriented theory
utilitarianism
veracity
virtue ethics

LEARNING OUTCOMES

After studying this chapter, you should be able to:

LO 2.1 Describe and compare need and value development theories.

LO 2.2 Identify the major principles of contemporary consequence-oriented, duty-oriented, and virtue ethics reasoning.

LO 2.3 Define the basic principles of health care ethics.

FROM THE PERSPECTIVE OF. . .

TOM AND BILL ARE RADIOLOGY TECHNICIANS at a 300-bed hospital in a large metropolitan area. Tom has been employed by the hospital for 10 years, and Bill is a recent graduate from radiology technician school and has been on the job for four months. Their supervisor, Anna, has been with the hospital for 20 years, moving up the ranks from radiology technician to manager of the department. Because they are short staffed, Anna has been helping the staff complete the required X-rays throughout the day.

One afternoon, Bill notices that Anna is late coming back from lunch. He doesn't give it a second thought because Anna is the boss and often has lunch meetings. However, while working with her that afternoon, Bill realizes that he smells alcohol on Anna's breath. He decides not to say anything. Several days later, Bill once again smells alcohol when around Anna.

Bill decides to talk with Tom about the problem. Tom confirms that he has noticed the problem also. Tom advises Bill not to say anything and offers three pieces of advice. First, Anna's behavior is not Bill's problem. Second, Anna is a supervisor, and it is difficult to understand the pressure she is under. For his final piece of advice, Tom reminds Bill that the last person hired is often the first person fired.

From Bill's perspective, he has seen a clear violation of hospital policy on the part of his supervisor.

From Tom's perspective, he has already decided he doesn't want to get involved in what could be a messy situation. The department is already short staffed, and if Anna were fired, that would mean he would have to work even harder until a new manager was found.

From Anna's perspective, she may not realize that she has a problem with alcohol. Even if she does realize that she has a problem, she may believe that the problem is not serious or she would never be fired because she has been with the hospital for so long.

Ethical decision making requires you to tap into your values, morals, and sense of fair play, so that you can be comfortable with the decisions you implement and so that your decisions do not harm others. Study the following theories for further understanding of your own decision-making process.

2.1 Value Development Theories

In Chapter 1, the differences between law, ethics, and etiquette were briefly discussed. *Ethics* was defined as standards of behavior developed as a result of one's concept of right and wrong. One's personal concept of right and wrong, called *moral values,* is formed through the influence of the family, culture, and society. Because each individual experiences different family, cultural, and societal influences, like Tom and Bill in the opening scenario, individuals may see the same situation yet determine different methods to handle the problem.

Psychologists, philosophers, and social scientists all study human behavior. Many subscribe to the idea that human behavior is a reflection of our attention to our needs or to our values. A classic work by Abraham Maslow, *Motivation and Personality,* first published in 1954, identified a hierarchy of needs that motivates our actions (see Figure 2-1). According to Maslow's theory, there are five stages of need that influence our behavior. We must satisfy each need in order, and the resulting progression is called a *hierarchy.* Maslow defined needs 1 to 3 as *deficiency,* or D-needs. Needs 4 and 5 are growth needs, also known as *being,* or B-needs.

1. The need for *basic life*—food and shelter
2. The need for a *safe and secure environment*
3. The need to *belong and to be loved*
4. The need for *esteem,* where status, responsibility, and recognition are important
5. The need for *self-actualization,* for personal growth and fulfillment

Originally, Maslow believed that the needs followed a strict order, but in his later years, he allowed for the possibility that some people may not require meeting all the D-needs before moving on to the B-needs.

FIGURE 2-1 Maslow's Hierarchy of Needs Pyramid

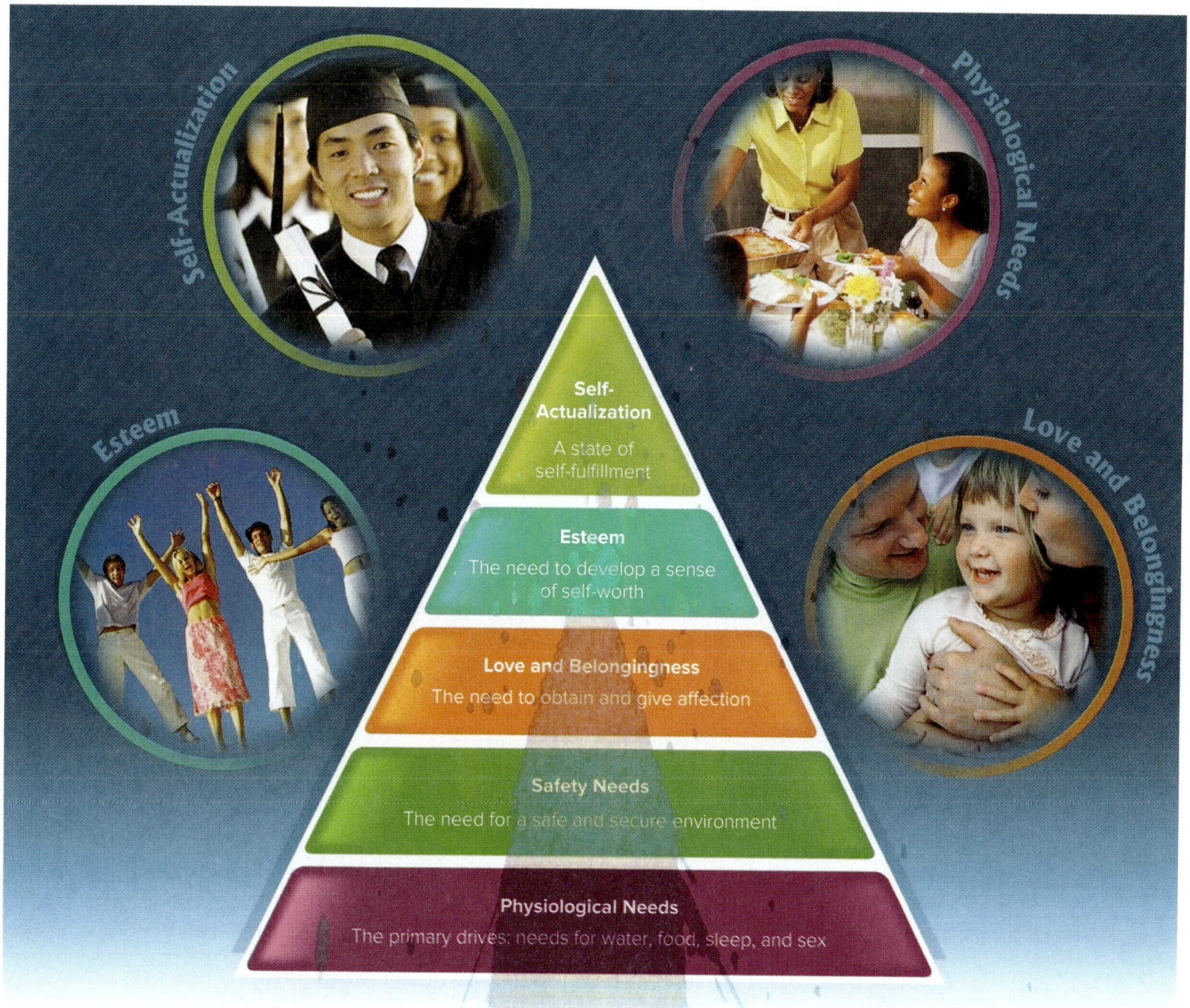

(*bottom left*): © BananaStock/age fotostock RF (*bottom right*): © Plush Studios/BrandX/Getty Images RF (*top right*): © Stockbyte/Getty Images RF (*top left*): © Mark Scott/Getty Images RF.

Maslow's theory may help us understand what motivates people, but it does not always help us determine how we developed the values that guide us in ethical decision making.

needs-based motivation
The theory that human behavior is based on specific human needs that must often be met in a specific order. Abraham Maslow is the best-known psychologist for this theory.

Many psychologists believe that individuals move from **needs-based motivation** to a personal value system that develops from childhood. When we are born, we have no values. The value system we develop as we grow and mature is dependent on the cultural framework in which we live. If one grows up in an Asian culture, for example, honoring ancestors and tradition may emerge as prominent values; growing up in a Western culture, such as in the United States, may encourage one to place more value on materialism.

A variety of theories exist about how we develop values. Most focus on our stages of development from childhood to adulthood. One of the most famous researchers in this area is Jean Piaget (see Figure 2-2). By observing children at play, Piaget described four levels of moral development.

FIGURE 2-2 Jean Piaget's Stages of Development from Childhood to Adulthood

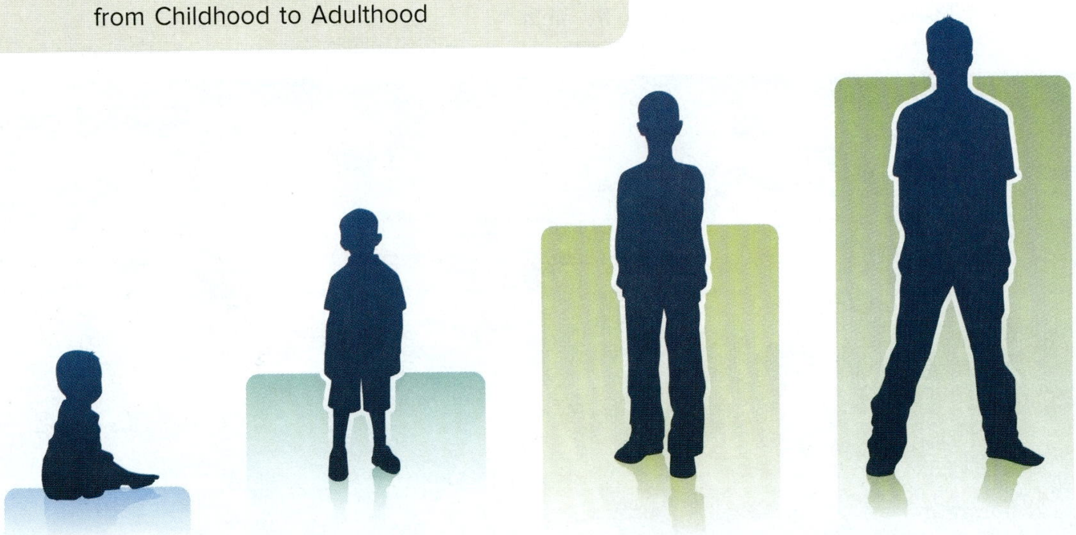

1. The first stage occurs from birth to age 2 and is called the *sensorimotor* stage, during which the child is totally self-centered. Children at this stage of development explore the world with their five senses, and cannot yet see from another's point of view.
2. As infants grow, they develop an awareness of things and people even if not in their direct sight, leading to the second stage, called the *preoperational* or egocentric stage, which extends from ages 2 to 7. During this time period, the child views the world from his or her own perspective. For example, when playing a game, the child is not particularly concerned with rules of play; the focus is on fun, not rules.
3. The third stage of Piaget's theory is called the *concrete operational* stage, extending from ages 7 to 12. In this stage, children tend to see things as either right or wrong, and to see adults as powerful and controlling.
4. Finally, during the *formal operational* stage, children develop abstract thought and begin to understand that there may be different degrees of wrongdoing. For example, children in earlier stages of development, when asked why telling a lie is wrong, may simply reply "because it's bad" whereas children in the formal operational stage can explain "because a lie isn't true." During this stage and through adulthood, intentions, such as lying (I intend to deceive you) and stealing (I intend to take that object) are central to decisions made.

Lawrence Kohlberg modified and expanded Piaget's work, laying the groundwork for modern studies on moral development. Consistent with Piaget, he proposed that children form ways of thinking through their experiences that include understandings of moral concepts such as justice, rights, equality, and human welfare. Kohlberg differed from Piaget in that he followed the development of moral judgment beyond the ages studied by Piaget, and he determined that the process of attaining moral maturity took longer and was more gradual than Piaget had proposed.

Kohlberg suggested that moral reasoning can best be understood as sequenced in six stages, grouped into three major levels:

1. Kohlberg's first major level is called *pre-conventional morality.* In the early stages of this level, children from ages 2 to 7 are egocentric, as in Piaget's first stage, and they accept the authority of others. In the second stage of pre-conventional morality, children begin to recognize that there may be more than just one view as to what is right or wrong. They begin to look at their own self-interest and begin to see advantages in the exchanging of favors.
2. The second level in Kohlberg's theory is called *conventional morality.* This level, with two stages, is when children ages 7 to 12 begin to conform to societal expectations as established by parents and social groups. The first stage in this level is sometimes referred to as "good boy/good girl" in which children focus on following the expected social conventions and demonstrating good intentions. In the second stage, children become more aware of doing one's duty. The focus is on the rules and respect for authority.
3. *Post-conventional morality* (ages 12 and above) is the last level of Kohlberg's moral development theory. There are two stages to this level:

   a. The first stage of post-conventional morality focuses on the social contract and individual rights. A social contract is accepted when people freely enter into work for the benefit of all and for a pleasant society. During this stage, individuals explore how to balance individual rights and a fair society for all.

   b. The second stage of post-conventional morality is called universal principles. In this stage, the individual makes a personal commitment to such universal principles as social justice, equal rights, and respect for the dignity of all people and realizes that conventional norms and conventions are necessary to uphold society. If there is a conflict between these values and the social contract, the individual follows his or her basic principles. Kohlberg believed that few individuals reached this stage as it requires a firm commitment to social justice and possible civil disobedience. For example, Martin Luther King, Jr. is sometimes cited as an example of stage 6. He believed that nonviolent civil disobedience was appropriate when the law was unjust. He was also willing to accept the penalties for his actions.

Kohlberg's theory has recently been criticized, since much of his data was gathered from observing young males. As a result, he revised his scoring methods to account for gender bias.

Check Your Progress

A pharmacist/researcher has invented a drug that is very effective against a certain type of cancer. He determines that he will sell the drug for $3,000 a treatment. The drug is effective only if it is taken once every week. Harry's young wife is dying from this specific type of cancer. Harry sells everything he can and borrows money from anyone who will lend it to him but cannot come up with enough money to pay for the drug. He approaches the pharmacist asking if the pharmacist will agree to payments or a lower fee. The pharmacist refuses, stating that he had worked very hard for many years to develop the drug and was entitled to profit from it. Harry decides to break into the pharmacy and steal the drug. (This dilemma was outlined in Kohlberg's writings and used as an example of how different levels of moral reasoning could be identified.)

1. Using Kohlberg's levels of pre-conventional, conventional, and post-conventional moral reasoning, complete the following table by filling in the moral reasoning.

Level	In Favor of Stealing the Drug	Against Stealing the Drug
Pre-conventional—reward and punishment		
Conventional—please others and maintain a good society		
Post-conventional—moral principles broader than any society		

2.2 Value Choices Theories

Maslow, Piaget, and Kohlberg devised theories to help explain how we develop our values, but their theories do not tell us why moral individuals often come to different conclusions based on reasoning. Tom and Bill, the radiology technicians presented in the chapter's opening scenario, illustrate how two moral individuals can reach different solutions for a problem they both face.

As health care practitioners, we know how to perform the tasks required in doing our jobs. That is, we know the right way to take a patient's history, give an injection, take an X-ray, draw blood, or bill the insurance company for the services provided. We know what is right or wrong in performing each medical procedure. That part of the job is straightforward.

Our values, however—our concepts of right or wrong, good or evil as related to our behavior—can be subjective. Universal ethics—problems such as abortion, stem cell research, and euthanasia—are discussed in later chapters, but it is the everyday problems like Bill and Tom faced that are frustrating. They frustrate us because individuals often come to different conclusions, and thus actions, based on their personal beliefs. When faced with a difficult problem, some of us will draw conclusions based on formal religious beliefs or philosophies, while others will place more emphasis on weighing the outcomes of actions, and still others will rely heavily on past experience.

Because no professional code of ethics can address every situation found in health care, we may often find ourselves facing a problem that has no perfect and specific right or wrong solution. Moral people may agree to differ; therefore, it is important to determine a common framework for examining our value decisions.

At least three frameworks or theories exist in the literature that determine how value choices are made: teleological or consequence-oriented theory, deontological or duty-oriented theory, and virtue ethics.

TELEOLOGICAL OR CONSEQUENCE-ORIENTED THEORY

Teleological or consequence-oriented theory judges the rightness of a decision based on the outcome or predicted outcome of the decision. **Utilitarianism** is the most well known of these theories. In *act-utilitarianism,* a person makes value decisions based on results that will produce the greatest balance of good over evil, everyone considered. In *rule-utilitarianism,* a person makes value decisions based on a rule that if generally followed would produce the greatest balance of good over evil, everyone considered (Mappes and Degrazia, 2006). In Tom and Bill's problem at the beginning of the chapter, Tom is perhaps using act-utilitarianism to decide that nothing should be done as there has been no harm done and by reporting Anna, harm may occur. Bill, on the other hand, may be using rule-utilitarianism because he knows there is a rule against drinking alcohol during work hours and intoxicated employees are potential safety hazards.

teleological or consequence-oriented theory
Decision-making theory that judges the rightness or wrongness based on the outcomes or predicted outcomes.

utilitarianism
A consequence-oriented theory that states that decisions should be made by determining what results will produce the best outcome for the most people.

Whether one uses act- or rule-utilitarianism, the process is the same. Once the person has described the problem and determined possible solutions, the solution will be based on which solution is best for all concerned. Often when describing utilitarianism, writers indicate that the solution that provides happiness or a net increase in pleasure over pain for those involved should be selected.

Supporters of the utilitarian theory have created a **principle of utility**. The principle of utility requires that the rule used to make the decision be a rule that brings about positive results when generalized to a wide variety of situations. There are, however, no absolute truths in utilitarianism.

principle of utility
Used in utilitarianism; requires that the rule used in making a decision must bring about positive results when generalized to a wide variety of situations.

DEONTOLOGICAL OR DUTY-ORIENTED THEORY

Deontological or duty-oriented theory focuses on the essential rightness or wrongness of an act, not the consequences of the act. Immanuel Kant (1724–1804) is considered the father of duty-oriented theory. He defined the **categorical imperative** as the guiding principle for all decision making. This principle means that there are no exceptions (categorical) from the rule (imperative). The right action is one based on a determined principle, regardless of outcome. The rule may come from religious or other beliefs, but it is a rule not to be ignored under any circumstances. A priest who maintains the absolute confidentiality of confession even if he knows harm has come to or will come to another human being is an example of using duty-oriented decision making.

deontological or duty-oriented theory
Decision-making theory that states that the rightness or wrongness of the act depends on its intrinsic nature and not the outcome of the act.

categorical imperative
A rule that is considered universal law binding on everyone and requiring action.

Kant argued that people may never be used as a means to an end. The Golden Rule ("do unto others as you would have them do unto you") is often cited in support of duty-oriented theory. Duty-oriented theories provide a foundation for rules of morality and for the idea of individual rights. However, critics of Kant find some of his ideas difficult to use in real life. For example, Kant argues that it is not permissible to lie or break a promise in an effort to save a third party from harm. These absolutes may create problems. For example, if a person promises to write a letter of recommendation for someone but has to stretch the truth in order to write a favorable recommendation, does not writing the letter make the person immoral? A terminally ill patient asks a nurse questions about physician-assisted death and asks that the nurse not say anything to the family about his questions. When the family asks if the patient has asked about euthanasia, should the nurse tell the truth, even if the patient has asked that his questions be kept confidential?

VIRTUE ETHICS

virtue ethics
Refers to the theory that people who have moral virtues will make the right decisions.

Rather than focusing on decision making or reasoning to arrive at a right action, **virtue ethics** focuses on the traits, characteristics, and virtues that a moral person should have. Virtue ethicists believe that someone who has appropriate moral virtues such as practical wisdom (common sense), a sense of justice, and courage will make the right decision. Ethicists who support this idea began with Aristotle (384 B.C.E.), but Alasdair MacIntyre (1929–present) is the most well-known ethicist to write about virtue ethics. MacIntyre argued that our practice of medicine has traditions and standards of practice that apply to every health care practitioner–whether one is a technician, medical assistant, physician, nurse, coder, or other professional. He stated that if we examine our actions in our roles as health care practitioners, we will see that we often follow the dictates of an idealized role. We ask ourselves, What would a perfect medical assistant (or physician or nurse) do in this situation? In virtue ethics, the loyalty to the role we play helps us make our decision. We look to what has been done in the past, assuming that it represents the right answer.

Like the other theories, virtue ethics has its critics. First, the past may not provide the right answer. As an example, the role of nurses or

Check Your Progress

The following questions involve making a decision. Answer each question with a *yes* or a *no*. Identify whether you arrived at your answer by consequence-oriented theory, duty-oriented theory, or virtue ethics.

2. Would it be acceptable to "stretch the truth" on insurance papers so that patients could get the care needed that they could not afford under their current insurance policy?
3. Is it acceptable to date a patient? Is it acceptable for a medical assistant or other staff member to date a physician?
4. A patient asks about a physician in the community. You think that particular physician is rude and doesn't care about his patients. Should you tell the patient who is asking about the physician what you think?
5. Would a surgical assistant with strong pro-life views be wrong in refusing to take part in a therapeutic abortion for a patient?
6. The radiology technician you work with has just done a chest X-ray on the wrong person. The patient was not hurt. Do you have to report the error to your manager?
7. A pharmacist believes that a prescription for a patient will do little to improve the patient's medical condition and may actually be contraindicated for the patient's problem. Does the pharmacist have a responsibility to talk with the physician?

medical assistants even 10 years ago is different than their roles today. Previously, virtues for nurses included always following the physician's orders and never questioning authority. Today, such virtues for nurses have been replaced with patient advocacy and education roles. Additionally, there are new situations coming up every day in health care that have never been at issue before, such as the possibility of cloning human organs for transplant and 3-D printing of human organs such as skin, so there is no established tradition. Last, practitioners may find themselves with conflicting roles. For example, in the case at the beginning of the chapter, Bill wants to be a team player, but he also may need to report Anna for violation of hospital policy.

Making ethical decisions is not easy, regardless of what model you choose to use. But whatever ethical framework is used, there are several steps that are common to them all. Figure 2-3 lists six steps to consider.

FIGURE 2-3 Ethical Problem-Solving Steps

I	Describe the problem. Identify the principles involved. Who will be affected by the decision? Who is ultimately in charge of making the decision?
II	Collect the facts. Be sure to differentiate between fact and opinion. Are there any legal problems? Has the problem been solved before? What documentation exists?
III	List the options—as many as possible.
IV	Evaluate the potential options from step 3. Who benefits by the decision? Who does not benefit? What principles are maintained? What principles may need to be sacrificed? Are you going to use utilitarianism, duty-oriented theory, or virtue ethics?
V	Make your decision and act.
VI	After a certain amount of time, assess the results.

2.3 Principles of Health Care Ethics

Several codes of ethics were quoted in Chapter 1. Each code, such as the AAMA Code or the AMA Code, addresses a specific profession, but there are common elements in all health care professional ethics codes. Health care ethicists agree that there are four ethical principles that are accepted as universal principles for all health care providers. Those four are autonomy, beneficence, nonmaleficence, and justice. However, confidentiality, role fidelity, and veracity are also found in many codes of ethics. All seven are defined below.

1. AUTONOMY OR SELF-DETERMINATION

The word **autonomy** comes from the Greek words *auto* (self) and *nomos* (governance). It is generally understood as the capacity to be one's own person, to make decisions based on one's own reasons and motives, not

autonomy
The capacity to be one's own person and make one's own decisions without being manipulated by external forces.

LANDMARK COURT CASE

Physician Charged in Assisted Suicide Case

In the late 1980s to early 1990s, Jack Kevorkian, a physician in Michigan, began helping terminally ill patients commit suicide. Janet Adkins, newly diagnosed with Alzheimer's disease, was Kevorkian's first public assisted suicide in 1989. Kevorkian was charged with murder, but the Oakland County District Court dropped charges on December 13, 1990, after a two-day preliminary hearing. The court ruled that Kevorkian did not break any law by helping Adkins commit suicide because there was, at that time, no Michigan law outlawing suicide or the medical assistance of it.

Prominent issues in the case were:

- Whether Adkins was in fact giving informed consent
- The fact that Kevorkian did not have an established professional relationship with Adkins
- The fact that Adkins was not terminally ill (facing death within six months)
- The issue of whether or not a person actually possesses the right to die
- The limits of autonomy

Source: *People v. Dr. Kevorkian*, No. 90-20157 52nd Dist. Ct. Mich. (1991); 534 N.W.2d. 172 (1995). Jack Kevorkian, nicknamed "Dr. Death," eventually claimed to have assisted with 130 suicides. In 1999, he was convicted of second-degree manslaughter, for which he served 8 years of a 10-to-25-year sentence. Kevorkian was released from prison in 2007, and allegedly remained unrepentant until his death on June 3, 2011.

manipulated or dictated to by external forces. Autonomous decisions are characterized by:

- Competency—a person must be competent to make his or her own decision.
- The ability to act on the decision.
- Respect for the autonomy of others.

Chapter 7 discusses informed consent, which derives from the principle of autonomy, as applied to health care. Paternalism, substituting the medical provider's opinion of what is "best" for the patient for the patient's own determination of his or her best interests, often threatens the concept of autonomy in health care. Because patients may disagree with medical providers about what is best and may not know or understand viable alternatives, informed consent is vital to preserving a health care consumer's autonomy.

Right-to-die cases, as discussed in Chapter 12, deal with a person's autonomy in making critical decisions.

The court case outlined in "Physician Charged in Assisted Suicide" is a landmark case that dealt with a patient's autonomy, as well as the issues of informed consent and the right to die.

2. BENEFICENCE

beneficence
Acts performed by a health care practitioner to help people stay healthy or recover from illness.

Although most dictionaries define **beneficence** as acts of charity and mercy, beneficence means more for the health care provider. Regardless of specialty, health care practitioners perform acts to help people stay healthy or recover from an illness. In fact, their first duty is to promote health for the patient above all other considerations. Modern medicine, however, has given rise to questions about the futility of care when discussing beneficence. For example, is it more beneficial for a patient in his nineties who is hospitalized after suffering a series of debilitating strokes to be maintained on a ventilator and drugs during his last days or to be allowed to die in comfort?

3. NONMALEFICENCE

Nonmaleficence, as paraphrased from the Hippocratic oath, means the duty to "do no harm." Technology has made this a difficult principle to follow, since many modern-day drugs and treatments have the potential to heal but also have serious side effects. A common example given when discussing nonmaleficence is the administration of morphine to reduce pain. Morphine is a powerful pain-killer, but it also suppresses respiration. When administering morphine, the provider's intent, of course, is to reduce pain, not to stop the patient's breathing. Accordingly, under the principle of double effect, secondary effects, such as reduced respiration or any other harmful outcome, must never be the intended result of medical treatment. The benefit to the patient must always outweigh the harm.

nonmaleficence
The duty to do no harm.

4. JUSTICE

Justice, defined as what is due an individual, seems simple when applied to the U.S. health care system, but it is often complicated. Many would argue, for example, that everyone is entitled to health care, regardless of the ability to pay for the care. Others argue that the distribution of scarce resources and the expense of providing them do not allow us to provide all care for all patients. Still others argue that people must take responsibility for their actions before assuming they can have justice. For example, should a lifelong smoker who refuses to quit and develops emphysema and continues to smoke be entitled to all available health care, regardless of cost? Should a motorcycle owner who refuses to wear a helmet while riding his or her motorcycle or an automobile driver who refuses to wear a seat belt be entitled to all available health care in the event of an accident, regardless of cost?

justice
Providing to an individual what is his or her due.

5. CONFIDENTIALITY

The Health Insurance Portability and Accountability Act (HIPAA), discussed in detail in Chapter 8, mandates privacy and **confidentiality** of medical records, but health care practitioners who take care to maintain confidentiality at all times are equally as effective as laws. Health care practitioners mindful of protecting privacy and confidentiality, for example, do not conduct conversations about patients in the hospital hallway, in the medical office break room, or with an acquaintance. They also take care to protect computerized medical information, as detailed in Chapter 7, and when patients ask that information be kept from concerned relatives, such requests are honored.

confidentiality
Keeping medical information strictly private.

Health care practitioners are in the most likely position to violate confidentiality rules, but others who have access to protected health care information, as defined under HIPAA, may also violate confidentiality, as in the case of unauthorized disclosure outlined in "Court Case" below.

Compensatory justice, a concept that applies to medical malpractice lawsuits, refers to an individual's right to seek monetary compensation in the form of damages for a wrong done. Compensatory justice is discussed in more detail in Chapters 5 and 6. The act of seeking compensatory justice—of suing for damages for medical malpractice—has become an important part of health care today.

COURT CASE

Unauthorized Disclosure of Medical Information Results in a $1.8 Million Award

As customers at the pharmacy, we expect our protected health information to be secure. However, the acts of a pharmacist in Indiana resulted in a $1.8 million award to a woman whose records were reviewed and given away by a pharmacist.

The plaintiff was engaged in an off-and-on relationship with a man. She became pregnant and delivered a son. The man also discovered that he had contracted genital herpes.

While the man was involved with the plaintiff, he also became involved with a pharmacist. She was employed by a large drugstore chain. The man told the pharmacist that she had been exposed to genital herpes. Upon her return to work, the pharmacist looked up the plaintiff's prescription profile to see if she could find any information about the plaintiff's sexually transmitted disease. The pharmacist checked a second time the next day. She printed out the prescription records of the plaintiff and gave them to the man.

The man contacted the plaintiff and told her that he had a copy of her prescription records and accused her of failing to renew her birth control pills. The plaintiff contacted the corporate headquarters of the drugstore chain. The drugstore chain had the pharmacist go through additional training about patient privacy. The plaintiff then filed suit against both the drugstore chain and the pharmacist alleging negligence/professional malpractice, invasion of privacy/public disclosure of private facts, and invasion of privacy/intrusion against the pharmacist and alleging the drugstore chain was responsible under *respondeat superior* as the pharmacists' employer. Additional claims against the drugstore chain included negligent training, negligent supervision, negligent retention, and negligence/professional malpractice. The claims were all based on state law. There was no mention of HIPAA, a federal law regarding privacy. *Respondeat superior* is Latin for "let the master answer," and you will learn more about this principle in Chapter 5.

A jury returned a verdict for the plaintiff for $1.8 million. The jury determined that the man was 20 percent responsible for the damages and the drugstore chain and the pharmacist were jointly responsible for the remaining 80 percent of damages. The drugstore chain appealed the verdict, but the Indiana Court of Appeals affirmed the verdict. The case was taken to the Indiana Supreme Court. The court declined to hear the case.

Source: *Walgreen Co. v. Abigail E. Hinchy,* Indiana Court of Appeals, Cause No. 49A02-1311-CT-950 2015.

6. ROLE FIDELITY

All health care practitioners have a specific scope of practice for which they are licensed, certified, or registered and from which the law says they may not deviate, as discussed in Chapters 3 and 5.

In addition to the laws that affect scope of practice, it is a basic ethical principle that a practitioner must be true to (have **fidelity** to) his or her role. For example, a medical assistant should not diagnose a patient's condition, and a nursing assistant should not administer an intravenous drug to a patient, since such acts are not within the scope of practice for either profession.

fidelity
Being faithful to the scope of practice for your profession.

7. VERACITY

Veracity, or truth telling, has always had an ambiguous place in the health care practitioner's world. Because medical providers want to do what is best for the patient, they may not always tell the whole truth.

veracity
Truth telling.

For example, consider the use of placebos—biologically inert substances that will do no harm but are sometimes given to patients under the guise of therapeutic treatment. Many studies have proven that if patients believe they are taking a drug that will help them, even if they are taking a placebo, their conditions may improve. In other cases, medical providers take a paternalistic view about truth telling, determining that what the patients don't know won't hurt them.

Health care ethics are drawn from the same pool of basic ethical principles that might be listed for any profession, but the nature of health care provides a unique focus. Primarily because a person's health is paramount to his or her living a successful and satisfying life, health care practitioners are routinely challenged to make sound decisions—concerning not only the appropriate medical care for each patient's condition but also the patient's future health and well-being and sometimes the health and well-being of the patient's family. In our changing world, the use of technology, scarce resources, and the ever-increasing cost of health care all require that health care practitioners constantly strive to provide the best possible care for patients.

Check Your Progress

For each of the following actions, name a principle of health care ethics that was followed or violated, adding whether the principle was followed or violated.

8. A nurse tells a patient faced with the dilemma of deciding for or against debilitating surgery what he thinks is "best" for her.
9. A patient's medical malpractice lawsuit against a physician is dismissed in court because her health maintenance organization employer lost the patient's medical records.
10. A physician who knows one of his patients always wants to hear the truth tells him treatment for his cancer has not cured him of the disease and he has less than a year to live.
11. An 85-year-old woman suffering from congestive heart failure is semiconscious and has been placed on a ventilator. Upon admission to the hospital, she filed a living will with the hospital detailing her end-of-life requests and signed a do-not-resuscitate (DNR) order. She is not expected to live beyond a matter of days, but her two daughters arrive from out of state and insist on overriding her DNR request. "Do everything to keep her alive," both daughters insist. The attending physician does not agree with the daughters but cannot dissuade them and is obligated to comply.
12. A nurse's physician/employer asks her to dress the burn on a patient's hand after debriding the wound. The nurse knows correct procedure for dressing the burn, but she finds gloves uncomfortable and fails to wear them. The patient's burn later becomes infected.
13. A medical assistant believes her mother has a thyroid condition, so she steals samples of the appropriate medication from the clinic where she works and takes them home for her mother.
14. A medical coder who works for a group of physicians knows, through her access to patients' medical records, that Melanie, a single friend, is pregnant. When another friend asks her why Melanie is seeing a doctor, she refuses to admit even that Melanie is a patient of one of her physician/employers.

Chapter Summary

Learning Outcome	Summary
LO 2.1 Describe and compare need and value development theories.	What classic needs development theory is discussed in this chapter? • Abraham Maslow, in *Motivation and Personality* first published in 1954, identified a hierarchy of needs that motivates our actions: • Deficiency or D-needs: 1. Need for basic life—food and shelter 2. Need for a safe and secure environment 3. Need to belong and to be loved • Being or B-needs: 4. Need for esteem, where status, responsibility, and recognition are important 5. Need for self-actualization, for personal growth and fulfillment What two value development theories are discussed in this chapter? • Jean Piaget's moral development stages: • Sensorimotor stage, during which the child is totally self-centered—birth to age 2. • Preoperational or egocentric stage, during which children view the world from their own perspective—ages 2 to 7. • Concrete operational stage, when children see things as right or wrong and adults as all powerful—ages 7 to 12. • Formal operational state, during which children practice more abstract thinking and learn there may be different degrees of wrongdoing—age 12, often extending into adulthood. • Lawrence Kohlberg's moral development stages: • Pre-conventional morality—children ages 2 to 7 accept others' authority; at end of stage, recognize their own interests. • Conventional morality—children ages 7 to 12 conform to others' expectations to win approval; at end of stage, focus on rules and respect for authority. • Post-conventional morality (ages 12 and above). a. Social contract and individual rights are balanced. b. Universal principles—personal commitment to larger issues of society.
LO 2.2 Identify the major principles of contemporary consequence-oriented, duty-oriented, and virtue ethics reasoning.	What is consequence-oriented ethics reasoning? • Best known is utilitarianism—judge the rightness of a decision based on the outcome or predicted outcome. • Act-utilitarianism—person makes value decisions based on results that will produce the greatest balance of good over evil. • Rule-utilitarianism—person makes value decisions based on a rule that should produce greatest balance of good over evil. What is the principle of utility? • Requires that the rule used to make a decision bring about positive results when generalized to a wide variety of situations. What is duty-oriented ethics reasoning? • Focuses on the essential rightness or wrongness of an act, not the consequences of the act. • The right action is one based on a determined principle, regardless of outcome. What is virtue ethics reasoning? • People who have appropriate moral virtues will make the right decisions. What ethical problem-solving steps are discussed in this chapter? • Describe the problem and identify the principles involved. • Collect the facts, differentiating between fact and opinion. • List as many options as possible. • Evaluate the potential options. • Make your decision and act. • After a certain amount of time, assess the results.

LO 2.3 Define the basic principles of health care ethics.	What are the basic principles of health care ethics? • Autonomy or self-determination • Beneficence • Nonmaleficence • Justice • Confidentiality • Role fidelity • Veracity

Chapter 2 Review

Applying Knowledge

LO 2.1

1. What is another term for your personal concept of right and wrong?
   a. Utilitarianism
   b. Beneficence
   c. Moral values
   d. Role fidelity
2. Why did Tom and Bill, in this chapter's opening scenario, come to different decisions?
   a. Because of their age differences
   b. Because of differences in their societal, cultural, and family influences
   c. Because of their different relationships with their supervisor
   d. None of these
3. How is Abraham Maslow's theory of needs-based motivation best defined?
   a. It is a five-step progression that sees pleasure as the primary motivation for all human behavior.
   b. It is a progression called beneficence.
   c. It is a theory that says human behavior is based on specific human needs that must often be met in a specific order.
   d. It is a system of moral values.
4. Which of the following is *not* true of Jean Piaget's theory of value development?
   a. Children in the sensorimotor stage of development see things as right or wrong.
   b. During the sensorimotor stage of development, children explore the world with their five senses.
   c. Children in the concrete operational stage of development see things as right or wrong.
   d. Children begin to see different degrees of wrongdoing during the formal operational stage.
5. How does Lawrence Kohlberg's theory of moral reasoning differ from Piaget's theory?
   a. Kohlberg theorized that moral development occurs more gradually and takes longer than Piaget proposed.
   b. Kohlberg studied adults instead of children.
   c. Kohlberg studied both boys and girls, whereas Piaget did not.
   d. Kohlberg does not break down moral development into stages, whereas Piaget did.

6. Which of the following is *not* true of Piaget's stages of value development?
   a. During the sensorimotor stage of development, children use their five senses to explore the world.
   b. The preoperational stage of development is characterized by abstract reasoning.
   c. During the concrete operational stage of development, children see certain behaviors as right or wrong.
   d. All of these are true statements concerning Piaget's stages of value development.
7. Which of the following is true of Lawrence Kohlberg's theory of the development of moral reasoning?
   a. During the pre-conventional morality stage, children reject the authority of others.
   b. A social contract is formed during the post-conventional morality stage.
   c. Children become rebellious during the conventional morality stage.
   d. None of these are true statements concerning Lawrence Kohlberg's theory.

LO 2.2

8. Teleological or consequence-oriented theories judge the rightness of a decision based on
   a. The feelings of the person making the decision
   b. The opinions of others who see the results of the decision
   c. How many people agree that the decision was right
   d. The outcome or predicted outcome of the decision
9. Which of the following best defines utilitarianism?
   a. It is the same as pre-conventional morality.
   b. It is a consequence-oriented theory that states that decisions should be made by determining what results will produce the best outcome for the most people.
   c. It is a duty-oriented theory that says everyone has a duty to behave correctly.
   d. It is a consequence-oriented theory that states that each individual should make decisions based on which outcome is best for him or her.
10. Which of the following best defines duty-oriented moral reasoning?
    a. Each individual's duty is to himself or herself first.
    b. Everyone should reject the authority of others and rely solely on self.
    c. It is a decision-making theory that states that the rightness or wrongness of the act depends on its intrinsic nature and not the outcome of the act.
    d. It is a form of post-conventional morality.
11. Immanuel Kant's categorical imperative states that
    a. Every rule has exceptions.
    b. Only the outcome is important in decision making.
    c. Feelings are not important in decision making.
    d. The right action is one based on a determined principle, regardless of outcome.
12. Virtue ethics focuses on
    a. The traits, characteristics, and virtues that a moral person should have
    b. The method one uses to make a moral decision
    c. Only the outcome of one's decisions
    d. The rule one uses in making a moral decision

13. Alasdair MacIntryc argues that

    a. All health care practitioners practice duty-oriented ethics reasoning.

    b. Virtue ethics is the only theory that makes sense.

    c. Individuals who have certain desirable qualities will make the right decisions.

    d. None of these are correct.

LO 2.3

14. List and define the seven basic principles of health care ethics.

Ethics Issues Making Ethical Decisions

Use your critical thinking skills to answer the questions that follow each ethics issue.

Ethics ISSUE 1:

Joyce Weathers is a 62-year-old patient with emphysema. Mrs. Weathers is a grandmother who has smoked a pack of cigarettes a day for more than 40 years. She enjoys smoking and does not want to quit. Her physician has become insistent that Mrs. Weathers quit. She tries, but each time she becomes nasty and irritable around her family. She lives with her daughter and two young grandchildren. The family members want her to quit, but it becomes very unpleasant at home when Mrs. Weathers tries to quit.

Discussion Questions

15. Using act-utilitarianism as a model, create a pain-avoided, pleasure-gained list to determine if Mrs. Weathers should continue smoking.

16. If your decision is that she should quit smoking, how can Mrs. Weathers's family help her?

Ethics ISSUE 2:

An eight-year-old girl is suffering from a rare form of cancer and is in need of a bone marrow transplant. Despite searches for the past year, no donor match has been located. The parents decide to have another child, hoping that the younger child will be a blood marrow match for their eight-year-old. The baby will be born in the next three months.

Discussion Question

17. Compare consequence-oriented decision making and duty-oriented decision making in this case. In your opinion, which method of decision making will lead to the best decision for everyone concerned, or are the methods equal in that both will lead to the optimum decision?

Ethics ISSUE 3:

Martha is the administrative assistant to Valerie, the practice manager in a five-physician practice. Salaries of staff are confidential. Since payroll is handled by an outside company, only the practice manager has knowledge of who makes what salary. Valerie has gone to lunch and left her door open. Several people have been in and out of Valerie's office dropping off reports or other information. Martha goes in the office to place a report on Valerie's desk and notices that a budget worksheet listing all staff salaries is in clear view. It would be easy to take a quick look, especially since Martha believes she is paid less than other employees with fewer responsibilities. Martha backs out of the office and locks Valerie's door without looking at the sheet. She thinks to herself, *If I should not know what everyone else is being paid, then no one else should either.*

Curtis is one of the employees who had left information on Valerie's desk before Martha closed the door. He also sees the budget sheet but does not stop to look at it. It did not occur to him to look at it, although it would have been great to know that he was being paid more than other employees. He puts his file down on Valerie's desk and thinks to himself, *I will warn Valerie that she needs to be more careful about what she leaves on her desk for anyone to see.*

Discussion Question

18. According to virtue ethics, who is more ethical—Martha, the one tempted to look but doesn't, or Curtis, who isn't even tempted to look? Defend your answer.

Case Studies

Use your critical thinking skills to answer the questions that follow each case study.

LO 2.3

Susan, a nursing student, is arguing with her friend Linda, also a nursing student, over the benefits of getting a flu shot.

"I'm not getting a flu shot this year," Linda declares. "I paid $14 for one last year, and I still got sick. I had a horrible sinus infection that kept me out of school for days."

"I remember, but that wasn't the flu," Susan argues. "Since we see so many people in the clinic—especially older people with weakened immune systems—don't you think we, of all people, should be immunized against the flu?"

The argument continues at length, with Linda finally raising her voice and stomping off.

19. In your opinion, is the question of whether or not the nursing students should get a flu vaccination an ethics question? Explain your answer.
20. If you decide that this is an ethics question, which theory of moral reasoning best applies?

Ethan is an orderly in a skilled nursing care facility. He is charged with supervising patients in the dining room on a day when two of his coworkers have called in sick, leaving the facility shorthanded. On this day, several patients seem more irritable than usual, and Ethan is kept busy preventing outbursts and calming them. He also worries about patients prone to choking episodes and finds himself feeling harried and stressed.

Wallace, an 80-year-old confined to a wheelchair, demands that Ethan help him back to his room. "It's a madhouse in here today," he shouts. Ethan knows he cannot leave his post and panics when Wallace heads for the door.

Ethan runs ahead of Wallace, shuts the double doors to the dining room, and locks them.

21. Has Ethan acted ethically? Explain your answer.
22. What would you do in a similar situation? Use steps one through five for ethical decision making to reach a solution. Describe how each step was used.
23. Do you believe your solution is more ethical than Ethan's? Why or why not?

Internet Activities

LO 2.3

Complete the activities and answer the questions that follow.

24. Locate the Web site for the organization representing the profession you plan to practice. Check the organization's code of ethics. Does the code conform to the seven principles of health care ethics? Explain your answer.
25. Visit the Web site for the National Center for Ethics in Health Care at www.ethics.va.gov/resources/ethicsresources.asp. Under the list of resource links, click on "Professionalism in Patient Care." What topics are listed under this link? How might these resources prove useful to you?

26. Visit Santa Clara University's Web site: www.scu.edu/ethics/practicing/decision/. Under "What is ethics?" list three things that, according to the site, ethics are *not*. Do you agree? Explain your answer. (If this URL is no longer available, do a Web search for "framework for thinking ethically." What was the number one result for this search, and how might you make use of the source?)

Resources

LO 2.1 and 2.3

Value Development Theories and the Seven Principles of Health Care Ethics

Edge, R., and J. Groves. *Ethics of Health Care: A Guide for Clinical Practice.* 3rd ed. New York: Thomson Delmar Learning, 2006.

Mappes, T., and D. Degrazia. *Biomedical Ethics.* 6th ed. Boston: McGraw-Hill, 2006.

LO 2.2

Value Choices Theories

Kohlberg, L. *The Psychology of Moral Development: Essays on Moral Development.* Vol. 2. San Francisco: Harper and Row, 1984.

Kohlberg, L., and R. A. Ryncarz. "Beyond Justice Reasoning: Moral Development and Consideration of a Seventh Stage." In *Higher Stages of Human Development: Perspectives on Adult Growth,* ed. C. N. Alexander and E. J. Langer. New York: Oxford University Press, 1990.

MacIntyre, Alasdair. *After Virtue.* Notre Dame: University of Indiana Press, 1984.

Mappes, T., and D. Degrazia. *Biomedical Ethics.* 6th ed. Boston: McGraw-Hill, 2006.

Power, F. C., A. Higgins, and L. Kohlberg. *Lawrence Kohlberg's Approach to Moral Education.* New York: Columbia University Press, 1989.

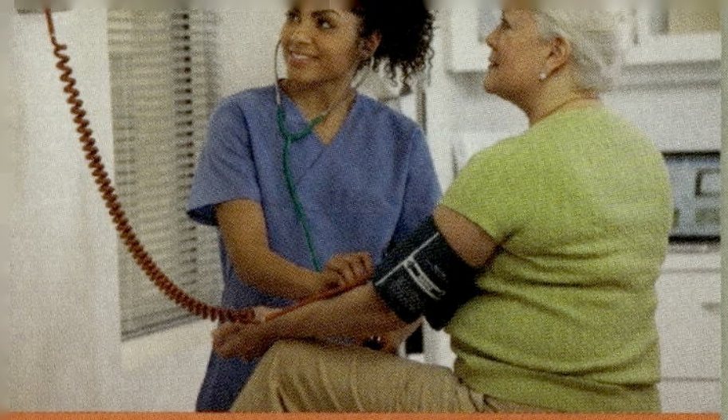

3

Working in Health Care

Key Terms

accountable care organization (ACO)
accreditation
certification
exclusive provider organization (EPO)
Health Care Education and Reconciliation Act (HCERA)
Health Insurance Portability and Accountability Act (HIPAA)
health maintenance organization (HMO)
health savings account (HSA)
independent practice association (IPA)
licensure
managed care
managed care organization (MCO)
medical boards
medical practice acts
medical services organization (MSO)
Patient Protection and Affordable Care Act (PPACA)
physician-hospital organization (PHO)
preferred provider organization/association (PPO/PPA)
primary care physician (PCP)
professional corporation
reciprocity
registration
scope of practice

LEARNING OUTCOMES

After studying this chapter, you should be able to:

LO 3.1 Define *licensure, certification, registration,* and *scope of practice* as they apply to requirements for individuals working in health care.

LO 3.2 Define *accreditation* as it applies to health care facilities, managed care organizations, and educational programs.

LO 3.3 Summarize the purpose and scope of authority for a state's medical practice acts and medical boards requirements.

LO 3.4 Explain the changing configuration of the business management aspect of medical practice.

LO 3.5 Distinguish between the different types of managed care organizations (MCOs).

LO 3.6 Discuss the major federal legislation enacted with the intention of improving the American health care system.

FROM THE PERSPECTIVE OF. . .

MELODY, A CERTIFIED NURSING ASSISTANT (CNA), works in a skilled nursing care facility caring for elderly patients. "I like the hands-on care," she says, "and I love just visiting with my patients. They come from all walks of life, and some of them have traveled all over the world."

The part of her job she dislikes the most, Melody adds, "is the demanding patients who want everything right now. Demanding relatives can also be unreasonable. A daughter will tell me, 'I want you to respond immediately whenever my mother calls for you.' They don't understand, or don't care, that I have several patients to look after."

Once, Melody recalls, several family members were visiting their elderly relative. "I walked in to check my patient, and one of his granddaughters asked me to get her a soda. There was a vending machine in the visitors' lounge, and I debated telling the woman I'm not a waitress and she could get her own drink. I didn't, though. I got her the drink, but I resented being asked to do it. I'm just a CNA, but I'm not there to wait on patients' relatives."

From Melody's perspective, her job did not include providing refreshments for patients' visitors.

From the demanding visitor's perspective, perhaps Melody's job is to serve all the needs of anyone in the patient's room.

3.1 Licensure, Certification, Registration, and Scope of Practice

Health care practitioners working in health care facilities today are, with few exceptions, licensed, registered, or certified to perform specific duties, depending on job classification and state requirements.

Licensure is a mandatory credentialing process established by law, usually at the state level. Licenses to practice are required in every state for all physicians, registered nurses, physician assistants, advanced registered nurse practitioners, dentists, pharmacists, psychologists, optometrists, physical and occupational therapists, dietitians, and many other health care practitioners. In most instances, as for the professions mentioned above, in order to obtain a license, courses of study or degree programs must be completed, followed by passing occupation-specific examinations. Individuals who do not have the required license are prohibited by law from practicing certain health care professions.

licensure
A mandatory credentialing process established by law, usually at the state level, that grants the right to practice certain skills and endeavors.

For those professions that require a state license, such as physician, registered nurse, physician assistant, advanced registered nurse practitioner, dentist, pharmacist, psychologist, optometrist, physical and occupational therapist, dietitian, and many other professions, **reciprocity** may be granted. This means that a state licensing authority will accept a person's valid license from another state as proof of competency without requiring reexamination.

reciprocity
The process by which a professional license obtained in one state may be accepted as valid in other states by prior agreement without reexamination.

If a state license is required and reciprocity is not granted when moving to another state, then the health care practitioner must apply to the state licensing authority to take required examinations to obtain a valid license to practice in the new state.

Endorsement is another process by which a license may be awarded based on individual credentials judged to meet licensing requirements in the new state of residence.

In some situations, physicians do not need a valid license to practice medicine in a specific state. These situations include the following:

- When responding to emergencies
- While establishing state residency requirements in order to obtain a license
- When employed by the U.S. armed forces, Public Health Service, Veterans Administration, or other federal facility
- When engaged solely in research and not treating patients

Physicians and other health care practitioners may be licensed in more than one state. Periodic license renewal is necessary; this usually requires simply paying a fee. However, many states require proof of continuing education units for license renewal.

LICENSE REVOCATION OR SUSPENSION

Licenses for health care professionals to practice can be revoked (canceled) or suspended (temporarily recalled) in certain circumstances.

An easy way to remember the most common reasons for loss of license to practice is the Federation of State Boards of Physical Therapy list titled "Ten Easy Ways to Lose Your License," which is applicable to most health care practitioner licenses:

- Sexual misconduct
- Substance abuse
- Professional discipline [for] criminal convictions or unprofessional conduct
- Fraud and misrepresentation
- Patient abuse
- Medication violations
- Unethical behavior
- Poor documentation or record keeping
- Unlicensed practice ("Forgetting" to renew a license is no defense.)

Source: Federation of State Boards of Physical Therapy list titled "Ten Easy Ways to Lose Your License."

Boundary violations could also be added to the above list. Such violations refer to scope of practice transgressions, where health care professionals have expanded duties they routinely perform in violation of duties they can lawfully perform under the license they hold. Such violations may also refer to licensed individuals lawfully performing the duties of their job description in one state or area, then moving to a new location and failing to learn what duties they can and cannot perform in the new work area. For example, a physical therapist assistant may have been allowed to use exercises he had developed for the elderly in one employment location, only to learn the same exercises must pass scrutiny in his new location before he receives permission from supervisory physical therapists to use them.

Personal or professional incapacity and defaulting on student loans should also be added to the list. Incapacity may be due to illness, injury, chronic alcoholism, drug abuse, senility, or other conditions that impair a health care practitioner's ability to practice. Failure to make payments on student loans (defaulting) may also cause loss of license—a fact many health care practitioners learn the hard way.

Certification is national in scope and is most often sponsored by a nongovernmental, private-sector group. Certification by a professional organization, usually through an examination, signifies that an applicant has attained a certain level of knowledge and skill. Because the process is voluntary, lack of certification does not prevent an employee from practicing the profession for which he or she is otherwise qualified. (In the opening scenario, Melody has chosen to fulfill requirements to become a *certified* nursing assistant. In her state, she could begin working as a nursing assistant without certification, but at a lower hourly wage.)

certification
A voluntary credentialing process whereby applicants who meet specific requirements may receive a certificate.

Registration is an entry in an official registry or record listing the names of persons in a certain occupation who have satisfied specific requirements. The list is usually made available to health care providers. One way to become registered is simply to add one's name to the list in the registry. Under this method of registration, unregistered persons are not prevented from working in a field for which they are otherwise qualified.

registration
A credentialing procedure whereby one's name is listed on a register as having paid a fee and/or met certain criteria within a profession.

A second way to become registered in a health occupation is to attain a certain level of education and/or pay a registration fee. Under this second method, when there are specific requirements for registration, unregistered individuals may be prevented from working in a field for which they are otherwise qualified.

Under no circumstances may persons claim to be licensed, certified, or registered if they are not. Table 3-1 below provides a summary.

Table 3-1 Types of Credentialing for Health Care Practitioners

	Licensure	Certification	Registration
Issuing agency	Governmental agency—usually the state	Nongovernmental agency—Usually a professional organization	Nongovernmental agency—Usually a professional organization
Process	Mandatory	Usually voluntary	Usually voluntary
To qualify	Education, experience, exam	Education, experience, exam	Usually training and experience-based, may require education and exam (e.g., registered health information technician, or RHIT)
Continuing education required?	Yes	Yes	Sometimes (e.g., RHIT requires continuing education)
Required for employment?	Yes	Sometimes but not always	Sometimes but not always
Major goal	Promote public safety	Employment advancement	Employment advancement

COURT CASE

Physician Loses License to Practice Medicine

A state Department of Health notified a physician who was the medical director for a pain clinic and supervised several advanced practice nurses that complaints had been filed against him and that his medical license was in jeopardy. The physician immediately surrendered his license to practice medicine to the state Board of Medical Examiners, believing that this would prevent a hearing before the board. The board was obligated to hear evidence substantiating the complaints against the physician, however, and his license to practice medicine was subsequently permanently revoked, based on findings that he:

- Failed to appear at his place of employment on numerous occasions but made no provision for a substitute physician.
- Did not review patient records when advanced practice nurses wrote prescriptions for controlled substances in his absence.
- Failed to develop or implement practice protocols and clinical guidelines, leaving the nurse practitioners he was supervising without guidance on the standard of care and without limitations or direction in diagnosing and prescribing to patients.

Source: *Wyttenback v. Board of Tennessee Medical Examiners*, No. M2014-02024-COA-R3-CV (Tenn. Ct. App. Mar. 15, 2016).

SCOPE OF PRACTICE

scope of practice
The determination of the duties/procedures that a person may or may not perform under the auspices of a specific health care professional's license.

For the purpose of protecting the public, licensure establishes a **scope of practice** for health care practitioners. Each state's laws, regulations, educational requirements, and licensing bodies for a health care practitioner determine the duties/procedures that person may and may not perform under the auspices of a specific license. Additionally, scope of practice for certified health care professionals such as medical assistants may be found in state laws, under the medical practice acts or administrative code sections. Professional associations for health care practitioners are a valuable resource for learning more about scope of practice for a specific profession.

Check Your Progress

1. Define *licensure, certification,* and *registration.*
2. How does licensure differ from registration or certification?
3. What provisions exist for licensed health care practitioners to transfer credentials to a new state?
4. Name three reasons that may be used to suspend or revoke a health care practitioner's license.
5. Define scope of practice.
6. Name five of the "Ten Easy Ways to Lose a License."

3.2 Accreditation

Unlike licensing, certification, and registration for those individuals practicing health care professions, **accreditation** does not refer to a qualification process for individuals. Instead, it refers to a process for officially authorizing, approving, and recognizing quality in health care education programs, facilities, managed care plans, and other health care organizations.

accreditation
Official authorization or approval for conforming to a specified standard for health care education programs, health care facilities, and managed care facilities.

Accreditation is usually voluntary. It represents health care facilities, organizations, and educational programs as credible, reputable, and dedicated to ongoing and continuous compliance with the highest standards.

At the time of an accreditation survey, health care entities must also demonstrate how they have maintained continuous compliance with standards for accreditation.

ACCREDITING AGENCIES FOR HOSPITALS AND OTHER PATIENT CARE FACILITIES

As part of the accreditation review process, professional accrediting agencies periodically conduct on-site surveys. Review committees for patient care facilities evaluate organizational structure; policies and procedures; compliance with federal, state, and local laws; leadership; patients' rights and responsibilities; fiscal operations; human resource management; provision of care; patient records; quality outcomes; performance improvement; infection control; and patient and employee safety.

The Joint Commission (TJC) is an independent, not-for-profit organization that accredits many types of health care organizations, including the following:

- General, psychiatric, children's, and rehabilitation hospitals
- Critical access hospitals
- Home care organizations, including those that provide home health services, personal care and support services, home infusion and other pharmacy services, durable medical equipment services, and hospice services
- Nursing homes and other long-term care facilities, including subacute care programs, dementia special care programs, and long-term care pharmacies
- Assisted living facilities
- Behavioral health care organizations
- Ambulatory care providers, such as outpatient surgery facilities, rehabilitation centers, infusion centers, and group practices, as well as office-based surgery
- Clinical laboratories, including independent or freestanding laboratories, blood transfusion and donor centers, and public health laboratories

To earn and maintain TJC accreditation, an organization must undergo an on-site survey by a TJC survey team at least every three years. Laboratories must be surveyed every two years.

In addition to The Joint Commission, other agencies that provide accreditation and establish standards for health care delivery include the following:

- National Committee for Quality Assurance (NCQA)
- Utilization Review Accreditation Commission (URAC)
- Accreditation Association for Ambulatory Health Care (AAAHC)

Each of the accrediting bodies has its own mission, activities, administering boards, and organizational histories, and each develops its own accreditation process and programs and sets its own accreditation standards.

A recognized accrediting agency for managed care plans is the National Committee for Quality Assurance (NCQA), an independent, nonprofit organization that evaluates and reports on the quality of the nation's managed care organizations. NCQA evaluates managed care programs in three ways:

1. Through on-site reviews of key clinical and administrative processes
2. Through the Healthcare Effectiveness Data and Information Set (HEDIS)—data used to measure performance in areas such as immunization and mammography screening rates
3. Through use of member satisfaction surveys

Participation in NCQA accreditation and certification programs is voluntary. At the NCQA Web site (www.ncqa.org/ReportCards), a person looking for quality medical facilities or health insurance plans can see rankings.

ACCREDITING AGENCIES FOR HEALTH CARE EDUCATION PROGRAMS

Accrediting agencies for health care education are national associations. An entire school may be accredited, or individual health care education programs (e.g., pharmacy education) may be accredited separately. It is important that an accrediting agency, such as the Commission on Accreditation of Allied Health Education Programs (CAAHEP), is recognized by the U.S. Department of Education and the Council on Higher Education Accreditation because some smaller accrediting agencies may be questionable. For this reason, a prospective student should research a program's or school's accreditation prior to enrollment.

Accrediting agencies for health care education programs evaluate the effectiveness of a program in terms of how well it prepares students to meet broad and specific professional standards. Do subjects offered incorporate laboratory sessions for practicing procedures required in certain job categories? Are a sufficient number of subjects and/or credit hours available for students to gain the knowledge necessary to pass licensing exams upon completion of the program? Are instructors and advisors available for additional assistance if students need help? Are students' concerns dealt with in a helpful and timely manner?

If the school where you are enrolled is accredited by a recognized regional or national accrediting agency, advantages for you include:

- Assurance of high-quality standards at your school and within your chosen program, based on the latest research and professional practice
- An opportunity for you to participate in federal and/or state financial aid programs

- A better chance that credits earned at your present school will be accepted at another institution if you transfer to another school or want to further your education
- Assurance that you can be considered for the necessary license or other recognized credential to practice your chosen field after graduation and successful completion of required examinations

Examples of recognized agencies for accrediting health care education programs include, but are not limited to, the following:

1. **Doctors:** The Liaison Committee on Medical Education (LCME) provides accreditation for medical schools granting a Medical Doctor (MD) degree. The Commission on Osteopathic College Accreditation (COCA) accredits medical schools granting the Doctor of Osteopathic Medicine (DO) degree.
2. **Nurses:** The Accreditation Commission for Education in Nursing (ACEN) accredits all types of nursing programs, including master's, baccalaureate, associate's, and diploma. The Commission on Collegiate Nursing Education (CCNE) accredits programs that offer only master's and baccalaureate nursing degrees. Specialty nursing programs such as nurse anesthetist and nurse midwifery have specific accreditation agencies.
3. **Pharmacy:** The Accreditation Council for Pharmacy Education evaluates professional degree programs in pharmacy up to the doctorate level.
4. **Allied Health Professionals:** The Commission on Accreditation of Allied Health Education Programs (CAAHEP) oversees the accreditation process of a variety of individual allied health educational programs. There are 28 different allied health professions under the CAAHEP umbrella. Examples include emergency medical technicians, anesthesiologist assistants, and respiratory therapists. Each profession has a specific accreditation process and review board. For example, medical assisting programs may be accredited by Medical Assisting Educational Review Board (MAERB). Additionally, the Accrediting Bureau of Health Education Schools (ABHES) does both institutional accreditation of schools of allied health and program-specific accreditation. Medical assisting programs may be accredited by ABHES or MAERB. Another example is the Commission on Accreditation for Health Informatics and Information Management Education (CAHIIM). The CAHIIM provides accreditation for programs that lead to the registered health information technician (RHIT) and registered health information administrator (RHIA).
5. **Physical Therapists:** The Commission on Accreditation in Physical Therapy Education (CAPTE) provides accreditation for both physical therapists and physical therapist assistants.
6. **Diet and Nutrition:** The Accreditation Council for Education in Nutrition and Dietetics provides accreditation for various nutrition and dietetics programs.

Tables 3-2 and 3-3 provide a summary of accreditation.

Table 3-2 Accreditation of Hospitals and Other Provider Agencies

Agency	Institutions Reviewed for Accreditation
The Joint Commission (TJC)	Hospitals • General hospitals • Psychiatric hospitals • Rehabilitation hospitals • Critical access hospitals Home care agencies Nursing homes Behavioral health facilities Ambulatory care facilities Clinical labs
The National Committee for Quality Assurance (NCQA)	Health plan organizations (HMOs and PPOs) Disease and case management plans Accountable care organizations (ACOs) Medical home organizations Wellness and health promotion plans
The Accreditation Association for Ambulatory Health Care (AAAHC)	Ambulatory surgery centers (ASCs) Community health centers Medical home organizations Endoscopy centers Office-based surgery centers College and university health centers Federally qualified health centers Urgent care centers Women's health centers A variety of other outpatient services

Table 3-3 Accreditation of Health Care Professions Educational Programs

Responsibility	Agencies
Oversight of all educational accrediting bodies in higher education	The U.S. Department of Education and the Council on Higher Education Accreditation (CHEA)
Oversight of specific health care career education programs	Organizations such as the Commission on Accreditation of Allied Health Education Programs (CAAHEP) and the Accrediting Bureau of Health Education Schools (ABHES)
Oversight of specific career education programs	**Physicians** Medical Doctor (MD)—Liaison Committee on Medical Education (LCME) Osteopathic Physicians (DO)—Commission on Osteopathic College Accreditation (COCA) **Nurses** All educational levels—Accreditation Commission for Education in Nursing (ACEN) Bachelor's and master's—Commission on Collegiate Nursing Education (CCNE) **Allied Health** Medical assisting—Medical Assisting Education Review Board (MAERB) or Accrediting Bureau of Health Education Schools (ABHES) Health information technician and Health information administrator—Commission on Accreditation for Health Informatics and Information Management Education (CAHIIM) **Physical Therapists and Physical Therapist Assistant** Commission on Accreditation in Physical Therapy Education (CAPTE) **Diet and Nutrition** The Accreditation Council for Education in Nutrition and Dietetics (ACEND)

Check Your Progress

7. Explain how licensure, registration, and certification for a health care practitioner differ from accreditation of a health care facility, managed care organization, or education program.
8. Accreditation is usually ______________________________.
9. Briefly state what qualities health care education program accrediting agencies evaluate.
10. Name four possible advantages for students enrolled in accredited health care education programs.

3.3 Medical Practice Acts and Medical Boards

In all 50 states, **medical practice acts** have been established by statute to govern the practice of medicine. Primary mandates of medical practice acts are to:

medical practice acts
State laws written for the express purpose of governing the practice of medicine.

1. Define what is meant by "practice of medicine" in each state.
2. Explain requirements and methods for licensure.
3. Provide for the establishment of medical licensing boards.
4. Establish grounds for suspension or revocation of license.
5. Give conditions for license renewal.

Medical practice acts were first passed in colonial times but were repealed in the 1800s, when citizens decided that the U.S. Constitution gave anyone the right to practice medicine. Quackery became rampant, and for the protection of the public, medical practice acts were reenacted.

Although laws are in place to protect consumers against medical quackery, even today unscrupulous people attempt to circumvent the law by hawking devices, potions, and treatments they say are "guaranteed" to cure any ailment or infirmity. Each state periodically revises its medical practice acts to keep them current with the times. Medical practice acts can be found in each state's code, which consists of laws for that state. Copies of state codes are available in most public libraries, in some university libraries, and on the Internet. (State codes as they apply to health care can be accessed electronically at official state Web sites under "medical practice acts.")

Each state's medical practice acts also mandate the establishment of **medical boards,** whose purpose is to protect the health, safety, and welfare of health care consumers through proper licensing and regulation of physicians and, in some jurisdictions, other health care practitioners. Board membership is composed of physicians and others who are, in most cases, appointed by the state's governor. Some boards act independently, exercising all licensing and disciplinary powers, while others are part of larger agencies such as departments of health. Funding for state medical boards comes from licensing and registration fees. Most boards include an executive officer, attorneys, and investigators. Some legal services may be provided by the state's office of the attorney general.

medical boards
Bodies established by the authority of each state's medical practice acts for the purpose of protecting the health, safety, and welfare of health care consumers through proper licensing and regulation of physicians and other health care practitioners.

Through licensing, each state medical board ensures that all health care practitioners who work in areas for which licensing is required have adequate and appropriate education and training and that they follow high standards of professional conduct while caring for patients. Applicants for license must generally:

- Provide proof of education and training.
- Provide details about their work history.
- Pass an examination designed to assess their knowledge and their ability to apply that knowledge and other concepts and principles important to ensure safe and effective patient care.
- Reveal information about their past medical history (including alcohol and drug abuse), arrests, and convictions.

Each state's medical practice acts also define unprofessional conduct for medical professionals. Laws vary from state to state, but examples of unprofessional conduct include:

- Physical abuse of a patient
- Inadequate record keeping
- Failure to recognize or act on common symptoms
- Prescribing drugs in excessive amounts or without legitimate reason
- Impaired ability to practice due to addiction or physical or mental illness
- Failure to meet continuing education requirements
- Performance of duties beyond the scope of a license
- Conviction of a felony
- Delegation of the practice of medicine to an unlicensed individual

COURT CASE

Supreme Court Decision Prevents Dental Board from Restricting Competition

North Carolina's State Board of Dental Examiners consists of eight members: six licensed, actively practicing dentists, one dental hygienist, and a consumer. In 2006, the board began issuing cease-and-desist letters to nondentists who were whitening teeth—a lucrative procedure for dentists. The nondentists offering teeth whitening generally charged much less than dentists offering the same service, and competition for the service had markedly increased. A member of the Board of Dental Examiners studied the issue, and the board subsequently persuaded the North Carolina Board of Cosmetic Art Examiners to warn cosmetologists against providing teeth whitening services. Additionally, the board sent letters to mall operators, stating that kiosk teeth whiteners were violating the Dental Practice Act and advising that the malls expel violators from their premises. As a result, nondentists stopped offering teeth whitening services in North Carolina.

In 2010, the Federal Trade Commission (FTC) filed an administrative complaint against the Board of Dental Examiners, charging that it had unreasonably restrained trade, in violation of the Sherman Antitrust Act. The FTC ordered the North Carolina Board of Dental Examiners to stop issuing cease-and-desist letters to nondentists offering teeth whitening services and to issue notices to all earlier recipients of the board's cease-and-desist orders advising them of the board's proper sphere of authority and saying, among other options, that the notice recipients had a right to seek declaratory rulings in state court.

The U.S. Supreme Court upheld the FTC's action.

Source: *North Carolina State Board of Dental Examiners v. Federal Trade Commission*, No. 13-534 (U.S. Feb. 25, 2015).

Minor disagreements and poor customer service do not fall under the heading of misconduct.

Other licensed health care professionals, such as registered nurses, pharmacists, physical therapists, dietitians, and some other licensed health care professionals, have a separate regulating act and governing board.

It is important to remember that while a variety of health care practitioners often work together as a team to provide medical care to patients, each individual is legally able to perform only those duties dictated by professional and statutory guidelines. Each health care practitioner is responsible for understanding the laws and rules pertaining to his or her job and for knowing requirements concerning renewal of licenses, recertification, and payment of fees for licensure, certification, and registration.

Fraud may, in some states, be considered unprofessional conduct, or it may be separately specified as grounds for revoking a health care professional's license. A health care professional could be considered guilty of fraud if "intent to deceive" can be shown. Acts generally classified as fraud include:

- Falsifying educational degrees, applications for licenses, licenses, or other credentials
- Billing a governmental agency for services not rendered
- Falsifying medical reports
- Falsely advertising or misrepresenting to a patient "secret cures" or special powers to cure an ailment

Revocations and suspensions of license are never automatic. A physician is always entitled to a written description of charges against him or her and a hearing before the appropriate state agency. If a hearing is held, the physician also has the right to counsel, the right to present evidence in his or her defense, the right to confront and question witnesses, and any other rights granted by state law. Decisions are usually subject to appeal through the state's court system.

An honest mistake or a single incident of alleged incompetence or negligence is not usually sufficient grounds for license revocation.

Check Your Progress

11. Define *medical practice acts.*
12. Where can you find the medical practice acts for your state?
13. What is the primary responsibility of state medical boards?
14. Health care professionals are licensed by the ______ in which they wish to practice.
15. Give at least three examples of unprofessional conduct as defined by a medical board.

3.4 Business Aspects of Medical Practice

Any organization established for the purpose of practicing medicine in exchange for fees for service is a business—and in today's world, health care is big business. The days have passed when there were two major classifications for outpatient health care management: sole proprietorship and group practice. Today, a physician or other licensed health care professional practicing alone (sole proprietorship) is not the norm, largely because providing health care services is complicated and expensive. Physicians, for example, are no longer the only medical professionals who independently bill for services. As any patient knows, instructions for follow-up care and bills for services can arrive separately from anesthetists, physical therapists, advanced registered nurse practitioners, and a host of additional providers. Plus, any health care practitioner or group seeking to open a practice needs staff members, both health care practitioners and health care practice management personnel, who are familiar with federal health care law, state and local health care regulations, employee management, case and utilization management, practice guidelines, disease management protocols, clinical reporting practices, and managed care protocol for reimbursement just in order to survive and profit financially. Increasingly, health care facilities also need employees familiar with health information technology because health care service facilities face government-imposed deadlines and rules for converting patient and practice records to electronic form. Such a business configuration requires extensive knowledge and funding.

Group practices, where health care professionals bind together to share the collective income, expenses, facilities, equipment, personnel, and patient records, are prevalent in the health care service industry. In fact, a health care business today is most likely a **professional corporation** consisting of many employees. A corporation is defined as *a body formed and authorized by law to act as a single person and legally endowed with specific rights and duties*. Corporation laws generally also provide that the incorporators and owners have limited liability in case lawsuits are filed.

professional corporation
A body formed and authorized by law to act as a single person.

Ownership of health care corporations may be traced to any number of sources, such as groups of physicians, health care professionals practicing the same medical specialty, groups of investors (e.g., Hospital Corporation of America, Ardent, Capella, and Cirrus Health), religious groups (e.g., Catholic or Jewish hospitals), state or local governments, university-affiliated medical schools, or insurance companies and managed care organizations (MCOs), where physicians and other health care practitioners are often salaried employees.

Clearly, providing health care services today is a complicated business requiring the expertise of specialized personnel. Reimbursement for services through managed care organizations is, in itself, a process requiring a degree of specialization.

3.5 Managed Care Organizations

managed care organization (MCO)
A corporation that links health care financing, administration, and service delivery.

Managed care organizations (MCOs) are corporations that link health care financing, administration, and service delivery. They pay for and deliver health care to subscribers for a set fee using a network of physicians and other health care providers. The network coordinates and refers patients to its health care providers and hospitals and monitors the amount and patterns of care delivered. The plans usually limit the services subscribers may receive under the plans. **Managed care** plans make agreed-upon payments to providers (hospitals or physicians) for providing health care services to health care subscribers. The payment from a managed care plan to providers may be one of several types, including contracted fee schedules, percentages of billed charges, capitation, and others. (*Capitation* is a set advance payment made to providers, based on the calculated cost of medical care of a specific population of subscribers.)

managed care
A system in which financing, administration, and delivery of health care are combined to provide medical services to subscribers for a prepaid fee.

Before managed care plans, private health insurance policies were traditionally written as third-party indemnity health insurance. *Third party* means that the insurance company reimburses health care practitioners for medical care provided to policyholders. Indemnity is coverage of the insured person against a potential loss of money from medical expenses for an illness or accident. Indemnity health insurance policies are fee-for-service and usually allow enrollees to see any doctor.

In an attempt to confront increasing health care costs—due in part to increasingly large awards in litigation, an aging population that requires more health care, the expensive technology used in modern-day medicine, and the impact of third-party payers for medical care—traditional fee-for-service health insurance companies now incorporate elements of managed care into their plans. (The impact of third-party payers is that there is little incentive to keep health care costs down when health care providers and recipients know that a third party—Medicare, Medicaid, other insurance—will pay.) Consequently, virtually all insured Americans have become familiar with such cost-containment/managed care measures as coinsurance, copayment fees, deductibles, formularies, and utilization review.

- *Coinsurance* refers to the amount of money insurance plan members must pay out of pocket, after the insurance plan pays its share. For example, a plan may agree to pay 80 percent of the cost for a surgical procedure, and the subscriber must pay the remaining 20 percent.
- *Copayment* fees are flat fees that insurance plan subscribers pay for certain medical services. For example, a subscriber might be required to make a $20 copayment for each visit to a physician office.
- *Deductible* amounts are specified by the insurance plan for each subscriber. For instance, the deductible for a single subscriber might be $500 a calendar year. In other words, the plan does not begin to pay benefits until the $500 deductible has been satisfied.
- *Formularies* are a plan's list of approved prescription medications for which it will reimburse subscribers.
- *Utilization review* is the method used by a health plan to measure the amount and appropriateness of health services used by its members.

HEALTH MAINTENANCE ORGANIZATIONS

Health maintenance organizations (HMOs) are one of several types of managed care organizations providing health care services to subscribers within the United States. HMOs and preferred provider organizations (PPOs) are the most common types of managed care plans. Under HMO

health maintenance organization (HMO)
A health plan that combines coverage of health care costs and delivery of health care for a specific payment.

plans, all health services are delivered and paid for through one organization. The two general types of HMOs are group model and staff model.

Group model HMOs contract with independent groups of physicians to provide coordinated care for large numbers of HMO patients for a fixed, per-member fee. They often provide medical care for members of several HMOs. Group model HMOs include prepaid group practices (PGPs). Physicians in PGPs are salaried employees of the HMO, usually practice in facilities provided by the HMO, and share in profits at the end of the year.

Staff model HMOs employ salaried physicians and other allied health professionals who provide care solely for members of one HMO. Subscribers to staff model HMOs can often see their doctors, get laboratory tests and X-rays, have prescriptions filled, and even order eyeglasses or contact lenses all in one location. Staff model HMOs also employ specialists or contract with outside specialists in some cases.

PREFERRED PROVIDER ORGANIZATIONS

preferred provider organization (PPO)
A network of independent physicians, hospitals, and other health care providers who contract with an insurance carrier to provide medical care at a discount rate to patients who are part of the insurer's plan. Also called **preferred provider association (PPA)**.

Preferred provider organizations (PPOs), also called **preferred provider associations (PPAs),** are managed care plans that contract with a network of doctors, hospitals, and other health care providers who provide services for set fees. Subscribers may choose their health provider from an approved list and must pay higher out-of-pocket costs for care provided by health care practitioners outside the PPO group.

PHYSICIAN-HOSPITAL ORGANIZATIONS

physician-hospital organization (PHO)
A health care plan in which physicians join with hospitals to provide a medical care delivery system and then contract for insurance with a commercial carrier or an HMO.

medical services organization
A physician group purchases a hospital, which then contracts with employers to provide full health care services.

Physician-hospital organizations (PHOs) are another type of managed care plan. PHOs are organizations that include physicians, hospitals, surgery centers, nursing homes, laboratories, and other medical service providers that contract with one or more HMOs, insurance plans, or directly with employers to provide health care services.

In some situations, a **medical services organization** may be formed with a physician group purchasing a hospital and then contracting with employers to provide full health care services.

OTHER VARIATIONS IN MANAGED CARE PLANS

exclusive provider organization (EPO)
A managed care plan that pays for health care services only within the plan's network of physicians, specialists, and hospitals (except in emergencies).

health savings account (HSA)
Offered to individuals covered by high-deductible health plans, these accounts let these individuals save money, tax free, to pay for medical expenses.

Managed care plans may also include the following identifying features:

- **Exclusive provider organization (EPO):** A managed care plan that pays for health care services only within the plan's network of physicians, specialists, and hospitals (except in emergencies).
- Health reimbursement arrangement or account (HRA): An employer-funded, tax-advantaged employer health benefit plan approved by the Internal Revenue Service (IRS) that reimburses employees for out-of-pocket medical expenses and individual health insurance premiums. There are no annual limits on the amounts employers may contribute to an HRA.
- **Health savings account (HSA):** Offered to individuals covered by high-deductible health plans. An HSA lets these individuals save

money, tax free, to pay for medical expenses. There are yearly limits on amounts one may contribute to an HSA.

- High-deductible health plan (HDHP): These plans have a higher deductible than other traditional insurance plans. For 2016, the deductible was $1,300 per person or $2,600 per family. Usually, employees select these plans in combination with an HSA or HRA.
- **Independent practice association (IPA):** An IPA is organized and owned by a network of independent physician practices to contract with employers and/or managed care organizations such as PPOs or HMOs.
- Open access plan: Under open access plans, subscribers may see any in-network health care provider without a referral. Both HMO and POS plans may offer open access features. However, the choice must be made from an approved directory of specialists or the member pays more of the associated cost.
- Point-of-service (POS) plan: The insured chooses a **primary care physician (PCP)** from a list of participating providers. The primary care physician may make referrals to other network providers when needed. Patients desiring to visit an out-of-network provider still need a referral, and there may be higher out-of-network charges.

independent practice association (IPA)
A type of HMO that contracts with groups of physicians who practice in their own offices and receive a per-member payment (capitation) from participating HMOs to provide a full range of health services for members.

primary care physician (PCP)
The physician responsible for directing all of a patient's medical care and determining whether the patient should be referred for specialty care.

The National Committee for Quality Assurance (NCQA), the accrediting agency mentioned earlier, has introduced a new concept in primary care called the patient-centered medical home (PCMH). The organization offers accreditation to qualifying primary care practices implementing PCMH and helps patients find those practices. The goal is to offer patients:

- Long-term partnerships between patients and clinicians, instead of patients being limited to sporadic, hurried visits
- Physician-led teams that will coordinate care, especially for illness prevention and chronic conditions
- An organization that will coordinate other clinicians' care and resources within the community, as needed
- Enhanced access, which will include expanded hours and online communication
- A role in decision making, ensuring informed choices and improved results
- Improved quality of care without ever denying care

An important added benefit, according to NCQA, is that insurers will pay for these services because they save more than they cost.

Managed care plans differ from one another in some respects, but all are designed to cut the cost of health care delivery. The impact of cost-cutting measures on the quality of health care remains a major point of contention. Advocates claim that managed care plans can deliver medical services more efficiently and at much less expense than traditional fee-for-service plans. Critics argue that necessary, quality medical services are often sacrificed for profit margins.

Check Your Progress

16. Briefly discuss how the business aspect of health care has changed over time.
17. Define *managed care.*
18. How does a point-of-service plan differ from an open access plan?
19. All managed care plans were designed to ____________.
20. Briefly define the concept *patient-centered medical home.*

3.6 Federal Legislation Improving the American Health Care System

HEALTH CARE QUALITY IMPROVEMENT ACT

In creating the Health Care Quality Improvement Act (HCQIA) of 1986, Congress found that "the increasing occurrence of medical malpractice and the need to improve the quality of medical care have become nationwide problems that warrant greater efforts than those that can be undertaken by any individual state." Accordingly, the act requires that professional peer review action be taken in some cases. It also limits the damages for professional review and protects from liability those who provide information to professional review bodies.

One of the most important provisions of the HCQIA was the establishment of the National Practitioner Data Bank (NPDB). Use of the NPDB was intended to improve the quality of medical care nationwide by encouraging effective professional peer review of physicians and dentists. Information that must be reported to the NPDB includes medical malpractice payments, adverse licensure actions, adverse clinical privilege actions, and adverse professional society membership actions. The NPDB is a resource to assist state licensing boards, hospitals, and other health care entities in investigating the qualifications of physicians, dentists, and other health care practitioners.

National Practitioner Data Bank queries are mandatory for physicians when they apply for privileges at a hospital and every two years for physicians already on the medical staff who wish to maintain their privileges. They are voluntary for hospitals conducting professional review, other health care entities with formal peer review programs, state licensing boards at any time, those who wish to self-query, and plaintiffs' attorneys under certain circumstances. The NPDB may not disclose information to a medical malpractice insurer, defense attorney, or member of the general public.

Health Insurance Portability and Accountability Act (HIPAA) of 1996
A federal statute that helps workers keep continuous health insurance coverage for themselves and their dependents when they change jobs, protects confidential medical information from unauthorized disclosure or use, and helps curb the rising cost of fraud and abuse.

HEALTH INSURANCE PORTABILITY AND ACCOUNTABILITY ACT

The **Health Insurance Portability and Accountability Act (HIPAA) of 1996** was an ambitious attempt by Congress to reform the American health care system. HIPAA helps workers keep continuous health insurance coverage for themselves and their dependents when they change jobs, but its many provisions go far beyond this mandate. The primary objectives of the law were to:

1. Improve the efficiency and effectiveness of the health care industry by:
   - Accelerating billing processes and reducing paperwork
   - Reducing health care billing fraud
   - Facilitating tracking of health information
   - Improving accuracy and reliability of shared data
   - Increasing access to computer networks within health care facilities
2. Help employees keep their health insurance coverage when transferring to another job.
3. Protect confidential medical information that identifies patients from unauthorized disclosure or use.

HIPAA also created the Healthcare Integrity and Protection Data Bank (HIPDB), but a provision of the 2010 Patient Protection and Affordable Care Act merged the HIPDB with the National Practitioner Data Bank. HIPDB is a national health care fraud and abuse data collection program for the reporting and disclosure of certain adverse actions taken against health care providers, suppliers, or practitioners. Data from the combined HIPDB and NPDB are available to federal and state government agencies and to health plans but are not available to the general public.

HIPAA requirements are discussed in more detail in Chapter 8.

PATIENT PROTECTION AND AFFORDABLE CARE ACT (PPACA)

The **Patient Protection and Affordable Care Act (PPACA,** also abbreviated **ACA)** became federal law in 2010. Additional changes to the health care system, primarily involving rules the ACA imposed on the insurance industry, became law as part of the **Health Care Education and Reconciliation Act (HCERA),** also enacted in 2010. The ACA was extensive in its regulation, but key features for clients paying for health plan coverage were as follows:

- Children under 19 can no longer be excluded from coverage due to preexisting conditions.
- Children under 26 can be covered by their parents' health plans.
- Insurers cannot cancel coverage because clients make simple mistakes in applying for insurance or in other correspondence.
- If a plan denies coverage, clients have the right to appeal.
- Health plan coverage must include certain recommended preventative health services.
- Clients can choose the primary care provider they want *from their plan's network* of participating providers.
- Clients can seek emergency services outside of their health plan's network.
- Lifetime dollar limits imposed by health care plans are eliminated.
- If a client can afford health insurance but chooses not to buy it, that person must pay a penalty, which is collected through federal tax forms.

Patient Protection and Affordable Care Act (PPACA)
A federal law enacted in 2010 to expand health insurance coverage and otherwise regulate the health insurance industry.

Health Care Education and Reconciliation Act (HCERA)
Also enacted in 2010, a federal law that added to regulations imposed on the insurance industry by PPACA.

The act also established a Health Insurance Marketplace, a resource where individuals, families, and small businesses can:

- Learn about their health coverage options.
- Compare health insurance plans based on costs, benefits, and other features.
- Choose a plan and enroll in coverage.

The Marketplace also provides information on programs that help people with low to moderate income and resources pay for coverage. This includes information on ways to save on the monthly premiums and out-of-pocket costs of coverage available through the Marketplace and information about other programs, including Medicaid and the Children's Health Insurance Program (CHIP). The Marketplace reportedly encourages competition among private health plans and is accessible through Web sites, call centers, and in-person assistance. In some states, the Marketplace is run by the state. An online federal government list of those states running a Health Insurance Marketplace is available at www.healthcare.gov/marketplace-in-your-state/. Individuals shopping for insurance in states without state-run plans can learn about possibilities for health insurance coverage for the current year at www.healthcare.gov.

accountable care organization (ACO)
A health care payment and delivery model that rewards doctors and hospitals for controlling costs and improving outcomes by allowing them to keep a portion of the savings if standards of quality are met.

Within its provisions, the ACA encouraged health care insurers to unite with health care providers to form **accountable care organizations (ACOs),** thus moving the health care system from the current fee-for-service base to a value-based system. The accountable care model emphasized preventive care, health care team coordination, electronic health records, treatment based on proof of effectiveness, and day or night access for patients. Those ACOs that met quality standards might also reward doctors and hospitals for controlling costs and improving patient outcomes by allowing them to keep a portion of savings.

COURT CASE Supreme Court Upholds Subsidies for Affordable Care Act

The case was filed on behalf of four Virginia residents on September 16, 2013. The plaintiffs brought the case because an IRS regulation implemented by the ACA subjects them to the act's individual mandate, which requires people to enroll in comprehensive health care coverage or pay a tax penalty. The plaintiffs did not want to purchase health care and objected to paying a tax penalty. On appeal of lower court decisions that upheld the mandate, the Supreme Court agreed to hear the case. In June 2015, the Court, by a 6-3 vote, upheld a crucial proponent of the ACA when it ruled that citizens of the 34 states that did not establish their own insurance marketplaces are eligible for federally subsidized premiums. The decision affected 5.4 million Americans. The challenge to the 2010 law actually focused on a section that said the subsidies were intended for people buying health care plans through an exchange "established by a state." Only 16 states opted for their own exchange. The Court concluded that the law's intent was to make insurance affordable for everyone and requiring broad participation was imperative to achieving that goal. "Congress passed the Affordable Care Act to improve health insurance markets, not to destroy them," the majority opinion concluded.

Source: *King v. Burwell,* 576 U.S. (2015).

According to Leavitt Partners, a health care consultancy business, in partnership with the Accountable Care Learning Collaborative, as of January 2016, there were 838 accountable care organizations active in all 50 states, translating to 28.3 million Americans covered by an ACO.

With the election of Donald Trump as President of the United States in November 2016, the continued implementation of provisions of the ACA were dependent upon the act remaining in force. In early 2017, shortly after taking office, President Trump, fulfilling a campaign promise to repeal the ACA, signed an Executive Order directing federal agencies to waive enforcement of large parts of the law—specifically those regulations that "impose a financial burden on a state, company, or individual." Visit www.hhs.gov/healthcare to determine which provisions have been implemented, postponed, or repealed to date.

As you begin your employment in the health care system, you must be aware of the requirements within your chosen profession for licensure, registration, or certification because the responsibility for satisfying those requirements lies with you. If your goal is to become a valued employee and a respected member of your chosen health care profession, it is also imperative that you understand how the health care business and the industry have changed and will continue to change as federal laws and reimbursement organizations keep pace.

Chapter Summary

Learning Outcome	Summary
LO 3.1 Define *licensure, certification, registration,* and *scope of practice* as they apply to requirements for individuals working in health care.	How do licensure, certification, and registration differ? • Licensure is a mandatory credentialing process established by law, usually at the state level. Licenses to practice are required in every state for all physicians and nurses and for many other health care practitioners as well. Individuals who do not have the required license are prohibited by law from practicing certain health care professions. • Certification is a voluntary credentialing process whereby applicants who meet specific requirements may receive a certificate. • Registration is an entry in an official registry or record listing the names of persons in a certain occupation who have satisfied specific requirements. What is scope of practice? • Scope of practice defines those acts individual health care practitioners can and cannot perform under the license they hold.
LO 3.2 Define *accreditation* as it applies to health care facilities, managed care organizations, and educational programs.	How does accreditation for health care facilities, managed care organizations, and educational programs differ from licensure, certification, and registration for health care practitioners? • Accreditation is the process for officially authorizing the health care entities mentioned above. • Organizations are accredited, whereas health care practitioners are either licensed, certified, or registered. Each state regulates the licensing process for individual health care occupations. How is accreditation achieved? • Recognized accreditation organizations survey the health care entity and look for relevant indicators of quality.
LO 3.3 Summarize the purpose and scope of authority for a state's medical practice acts and medical boards.	How are physicians licensed and regulated? • Each state's medical practice acts establish procedures for licensing physicians and regulating the practice of medicine within that state. • Other **licensed** health care professionals, such as registered nurses, physical therapists, and pharmacists, have individual regulations and governing boards.
LO 3.4 Explain the changing configuration of the business management aspects of medical practice.	How has the business of providing outpatient medical care changed over time? • Most medical practices are group practices. • Group practices include an ever-expanding number of corporations called managed care organizations (MCOs).
LO 3.5 Distinguish between the different types of managed care organizations (MCOs).	What are managed care organizations? • Corporations established to combine financing, administration, and delivery of health care on a fee-for-service or prepaid fee basis. What are some of the different types of managed care organizations? • Health maintenance organization (HMO): A health plan that combines coverage of health care costs and delivery of health care for a prepaid premium. • Individual (or independent) practice association (IPA): A type of HMO that contracts with groups of physicians who practice in their own offices and receive a per-member payment from participating HMOs to provide a full range of health services for members. • Preferred provider organization (PPO): A network of independent physicians, hospitals, and other health care providers who contract with an insurance carrier to provide medical care at a discount rate to patients who are part of the insurer's plan. • Physician-hospital organization (PHO): A health care plan in which physicians join with hospitals to provide a medical care delivery system and then contract for insurance with a commercial carrier or an HMO. • Exclusive provider organization (EPO): A managed care plan that pays for health care services only within the plan's network of physicians, specialists, and hospitals (except in emergencies).

- Health savings account (HSA): Offered to individuals covered by high-deductible health plans. An HSA lets these individuals save money, tax free, to pay for medical expenses. There are yearly limits on amounts one may contribute to an HSA.
- Health reimbursement arrangement or account (HRA): An IRS-approved, employer-funded, tax-advantaged employer health benefit plan that reimburses employees for out-of-pocket medical expenses and individual health insurance premiums. There are no annual limits on the amounts employers may contribute to an HRA.
- Medical service organization (MSO): A physician group purchases a hospital, which then contracts with employers to provide full health care services.

What are accountable care organizations?

- Accountable care organizations (ACOs) are health care payment and delivery models that can reward doctors and hospitals for controlling costs and improving patient outcomes by allowing them to keep a portion of what they save if standards of quality are met.
- Patient-centered medical homes (PCMH): A primary care concept that uses physician-led teams to coordinate patient care.

LO 3.6 Discuss the major federal legislation enacted with the intention of improving the American health care system.

What major federal legislation has affected health care insurance and payment fraud in the United States?

- Health Care Quality Improvement Act (HCQIA) of 1986: A federal statute passed to improve the quality of medical care nationwide.
- Health Insurance Portability and Accountability Act (HIPAA) of 1996: A federal statute that helps workers keep continuous health insurance coverage for themselves and their dependents when they change jobs, protects confidential medical information from unauthorized disclosure or use, and helps curb the rising cost of fraud and abuse.
- Patient Protection and Affordable Care Act (PPACA): A federal law enacted in 2010 to expand health insurance coverage and otherwise regulate the health insurance industry.
- Health Care Education and Reconciliation Act (HCERA): Also enacted in 2010, a federal law that added to regulations imposed on the insurance industry by PPACA.

Chapter 3 Review

Applying Knowledge

LO 3.1

Write "L" for licensure, "C" for certification, and "R" for registration in the space provided to indicate which is applicable in the following descriptions.

_____ 1. Involves a mandatory credentialing process established by law, usually at the state level.

_____ 2 Involves simply paying a fee.

_____ 3. Involves a voluntary credentialing process, usually national in scope, most often sponsored by a private-sector group.

_____ 4. Required of all physicians, dentists, and nurses in every state.

_____ 5. Consists simply of an entry in an official record.

_____ 6. To obtain, one must complete a course of study, followed by an occupation-specific examination.

7. Which of the following is mandatory for certain health professionals to practice in their field?
   a. Endorsements
   b. Reciprocity
   c. Licensure
   d. Certification

8. Licensure to practice medicine is done by

   a. Each individual state

   b. The federal government

   c. Local and state governments together

   d. The federal government and the local government

9. In which of the following situations may a physician practice without a license in a specific state?

   a. When responding to an emergency

   b. When employed by the United States armed forces

   c. When engaged solely in research and not treating patients

   d. All of the above

10. Which of the following processes lets a licensed health care practitioner transfer his or her license to a new state after moving without repeating an examination?

    a. Accreditation

    b. Registration

    c. Certification

    d. Reciprocity

11. A licensed advanced registered nurse practitioner might be accused of scope of practice violations if he

    a. Prescribes controlled substances without a supervising physician's knowledge or permission

    b. Fails to renew his license

    c. Advertises his services

    d. Commits a felony

LO 3.2

12. Which of the following is *not* true of accrediting agencies?

    a. They survey and evaluate the program or facility applying for accreditation.

    b. They never charge a fee.

    c. They exist for a wide range of health care entities.

    d. They check for continuing adherence to professional standards.

13. Which of the following indicates a health care facility, education program, or managed care organization is credible and maintains high standards?

    a. Licensure

    b. Registration

    c. Accreditation

    d. Certification

14. Which of the following is an advantage that might apply to individuals attending an accredited health care education program?

    a. Transfer of credits more easily accepted if one changes schools

    b. More likely to obtain a license after graduating

    c. More likely to be selected for a federal student aid program

    d. All of the above

15. Which of the following statements is *not* true of accreditation?

a. It is a voluntary process.

b. State law says it must be renewed every year.

c. Specific agencies are responsible for accrediting certain health education programs.

d. Accreditation reflects quality and is usually voluntary.

LO 3.3

16. Which of the following is *not* a purpose of medical practice acts?

a. To define what is meant by the practice of medicine in each state

b. To be sure physicians are adequately compensated for their services

c. To explain requirements and methods for licensure

d. To establish grounds for suspension or revocation of license

17. Each state's medical practice acts also provide for the establishment of

a. Health care teams

b. Hospital ethics committees

c. Medical boards

d. HMOs

18. Laws vary from state to state, but unprofessional conduct for medical professionals usually includes

a. Physical abuse of a patient

b. Inadequate record keeping

c. Failure to meet continuing education requirements

d. All of these are unprofessional conduct

19. Health care practitioners' actions generally classified as fraud include

a. Falsifying medical diplomas and other credentials

b. Falsifying medical reports

c. Promising a patient "secret cures" or other special ways to cure an ailment

d. All of these

20. The authority that governs the practice of medicine is called

a. Medical licensing act

b. Medical practice act

c. Occupational statute

d. Endorsement act

LO 3.4

21. Which of the following statements concerning health care practice management is *not* true?

a. The number of sole proprietorships is increasing.

b. Health care practices cannot, by law, operate as corporations.

c. Health care practices are businesses requiring a wide range of expertise.

d. No one can own a health care practice.

22. Which of the following health care practitioners can submit bills for their services on their own?
    a. Dietitians
    b. Advanced registered nurse practitioners
    c. Physicians
    d. All of the above
23. Which of the following statements is true?
    a. Insurance companies are forbidden by law to own medical facilities.
    b. A group of physicians cannot own a surgical center.
    c. A majority of health care practitioners now work for corporations.
    d. Hospitals must be owned by physicians.

LO 3.5

24. Which of the following best defines a managed care health plan?
    a. Preferred provider organization
    b. A corporation that pays for and delivers care to subscribers
    c. A sole proprietorship
    d. A group practice
25. What is a copayment?
    a. A percentage of the fee for services provided
    b. A set amount that each patient pays for each office visit
    c. The portion of the fee the physician must write off
    d. The portion of the fee that the insurance company pays
26. Under this type of plan, insured patients must designate a primary care physician (PCP).
    a. Point-of-service plan
    b. Open access plan
    c. Independent practice plan
    d. Health maintenance plan
27. When physicians, hospitals, and other health care providers contract with one or more HMOs or directly with employers to provide care, what is it called?
    a. A physician-hospital organization
    b. A preferred provider plan
    c. A health maintenance organization
    d. A fee-for-service plan
28. Under this type of plan, a patient may see providers outside the plan, but the patient pays a higher portion of the fees.
    a. Health maintenance plan
    b. Independent practitioner plan
    c. Preferred provider plan
    d. Primary care plan

LO 3.6

29. The National Practitioner Data Bank
    a. Is accessible to everyone
    b. Is accessible to other providers on a routine basis
    c. Is accessible only to hospitals and health care plans
    d. Is accessible only to the government agencies monitoring health care
30. Which federal law mandated that insurers carry children of an insured individual through age 26 and prohibited refusing to insure clients with preexisting conditions?
    a. HIPAA
    b. Health Care Quality Improvement Act
    c. Patient Protection and Affordable Care Act
    d. HMO
31. What recent federal law provides for the establishment of state-run insurance exchanges?
    a. Federal False Claims Act
    b. Health Insurance Portability and Accountability Act
    c. Patient Protection and Affordable Care Act
    d. Health Care Quality Improvement Act
32. Which of the following is *not* a stated goal of the Health Insurance Portability and Accountability Act?
    a. Ensure that every person has health insurance
    b. Improve the efficiency and effectiveness of the health care industry
    c. Help employees keep health insurance coverage when they transfer to another job
    d. Protect confidential medical information

Ethics Issues Working in Health Care

Use your critical thinking skills to answer the questions that follow each ethics issue.

Ethics ISSUE 1:

A young woman recently certified and employed as a medical assistant was well-groomed and knowledgeable when she appeared for her employment interview. Immediately after the woman began work, she changed her appearance markedly. During her first week on the job, she reported for work with bright blue streaks in her hair, which had been cut from shoulder length to very short. In addition, she now had an eyebrow stud, a nose stud, and a butterfly tattoo on her neck. The supervisor who had interviewed and hired the woman was appalled.

Discussion Questions

33. In your opinion, what should the supervisor do because she was obviously not pleased with the changes in her new hire?
34. Should the medical assistant have changed her appearance in this way?
35. Why or why not?
36. In the supervisor's place, what would you say to the medical assistant?

Ethics ISSUE 2:

A personable celebrity visits a physician in the medical center where you work. The celebrity travels frequently, and she has asked for an appointment with short notice. As the person responsible for scheduling appointments, you could easily use a trumped-up excuse to bump a patient at the desired day and time in order to accommodate the celebrity.

Discussion Questions

37. Would it be ethical for you to cancel a patient's appointment in order to accommodate the celebrity?
38. If the celebrity is a hospital patient, would it be ethical for the hospital administrator to drop in to be sure the celebrity is satisfied with her room and care?

Ethics ISSUE 3:

By law, health care practitioners can perform only those duties that are within their *scope of practice*—that is, those duties for which they are duly licensed, certified, registered, and competent.

Discussion Questions

39. You are a medical assistant in a clinic and a nurse asks for your assistance. She is way behind schedule, and she asks you to administer an intravenous drug push to a patient. You want to do what she asks, but is it ethical for you to comply?
40. As a student medical assistant, you have learned the correct technique for giving a shot, but you have never perfected the technique. You begin working in a clinic right after graduation, and your first assigned duty is to give a flu shot to an elderly patient, and you don't want to do it. Is it ethical for you to do it anyway? Would it be ethical for you to ask someone else to administer the shot?
41. As a new medical assistant, it takes you two attempts to successfully administer a flu shot to a young patient. You don't want to admit to the first failure, so you consider leaving the first unsuccessful attempt out of the medical record. Would this behavior be ethical?

Case Studies

LO 3.1

Use your critical thinking skills to answer the questions that follow each case study.

Physician assistants (PAs) are employed in physician offices throughout the United States. Although PAs provide direct patient care, they are under the supervision of a licensed physician. Duties include taking patients' medical histories, performing physical examinations, ordering diagnostic and therapeutic procedures, providing follow-up care, and teaching and counseling patients. In most states, PAs may write prescriptions. The PA may be the only health care practitioner a patient sees during his or her visit to the physician office. Therefore, patients often refer to a PA as "the doctor." Ned, a PA for five years, says the patients he sees often address him as "doctor."

Similarly, Marie, a long-time employee of a physician in private practice, is often called "the doctor's nurse." Although Marie has never had the training necessary to become a certified medical assistant or a registered nurse, she sometimes refers to herself as the "office nurse."

42. What legal and ethical considerations are evident in these situations?
43. Should Ned and Marie allow patients to call them "doctor" or "nurse," respectively? Why or why not?

Note: A health care practitioner is held to the standard of care practiced by a reasonably competent person of the same profession. A physician assistant using the title "doctor" and a medical assistant using the title "nurse" may be held to the standard of care of a physician and a nurse, respectively, and may be accused of practicing without the appropriate license.

LO 3.2

A source of potential problems for health care practitioners is advertising. Buying print ads, creating radio spots, or sponsoring Web sites are commonplace activities for today's health care practitioners, which may subject them to a different type of lawsuit.

For example, two New Jersey patients sued their physician over the Web site ads she ran for LASIK eye surgery. The patients claimed the doctor made false or misleading statements in her ads, leading them to believe she would provide all of their treatment. Instead, the patients said a physician who was not fully licensed provided their follow-up care. (This practice is generally medically acceptable.) The two patients sued the physician under their state's Consumer Fraud Act, an area of law from which physicians have traditionally been exempt. A trial court allowed the suit to proceed, but the state supreme court reversed that decision, preventing the patients from suing the physician for advertising fraud.

44. In your opinion, should health care practitioners be protected from consumer fraud suits over advertising? Explain your answer.

45. As a health care practitioner, would you advertise your services? Why or why not?

Internet Activities

LO 3.3 and LO 3.6

Complete the activities and answer the questions that follow.

46. Conduct a Web search for "Medical Practice Acts" followed by the name of your state. What types of information are available to you at this site?

47. Use the Internet to find two ethical issues affecting health care practitioners. Provide your instructor with a short list of links to more information about the ethical issues you have chosen. How will those issues affect your chosen health care profession?

48. Visit www.healthcare.gov/choose-a-plan/plan-types/. What actions are you invited to take? What are the "Three Things to Know" about choosing a health care plan?

Resources

LO 3.1

"Ten Easy Ways to Lose Your License": www.fsbpt.org/Licensees/EthicalConduct/TenEasyWaystoLose-YourLicense.aspx

LO 3.2

Accreditation:

www.ncbi.nlm.nih.gov/pubmed/11184667

www.jointcommission.org/achievethegoldseal.aspx

www.achc.org/getting-started/what-is-accreditation

www.caahep.org/

http://ope.ed.gov/accreditation/agencies.aspx

LO 3.3

American Association of Medical Assistants (List for state scope of practice laws): www.aama-ntl.org/employers/state-scope-of-practice-laws

LO 3.4

Health Insurance Marketplace:

www.healthcare.gov/glossary/health-insurance-marketplace-glossary/

www.healthcare.gov/screener

LO 3.5

Accountable care organizations: http://healthaffairs.org/blog/2016/04/21/accountable-care-organizations-in-2016-private-and-public-sector-growth-and-dispersion/

Health savings accounts: www.treasury.gov/resource-center/faqs/Taxes/Pages/Health-Savings-Accounts.aspx

Independent physician associations: www.aafp.org/about/policies/all/independent-physicianassoc.html

LO 3.6

Affordable Care Act:

www.hhs.gov/healthcare/about-the-law/index.html

https://marketplace.cms.gov/outreach-and-education/what-you-should-know-provider-networks.pdf

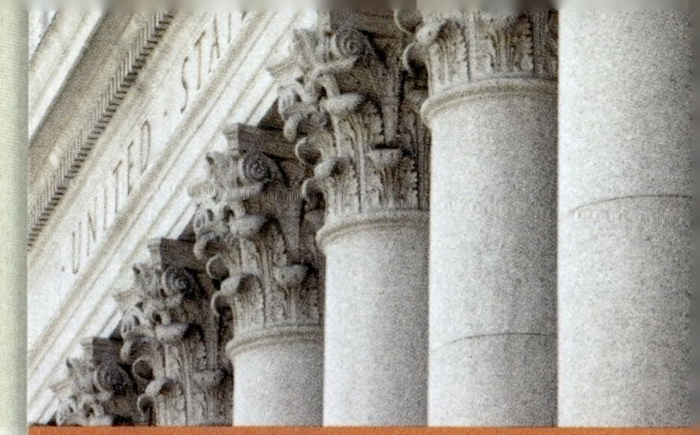

©Ryan McGinnis/Getty Images RF

4

Law, the Courts, and Contracts

LEARNING OUTCOMES

After studying this chapter, you should be able to:

LO 4.1 Discuss the basis of and primary sources of law.

LO 4.2 Identify the classifications of law.

LO 4.3 Define the concept of torts, and discuss how the tort of negligence affects health care.

LO 4.4 List the four essential elements of a contract, and differentiate between expressed contracts and implied contracts.

LO 4.5 Compare the contractual rights and responsibilities of physicians and patients.

Key Terms

administrative law
breach of contract
case law
civil law
common law
constitutional law
contract
criminal law
defendant
executive order
felony
jurisdiction
legal precedents
minor
misdemeanor
negligence
plaintiff
procedural law
prosecution
statute of frauds
statutory law
substantive law
tort
tortfeasor
void

FROM THE PERSPECTIVE OF. . .

CHRISTINE, A PATIENT BILLING SPECIALIST who works for a hospital in the Pacific Northwest, says "sometimes patients don't understand that what they are asking us to do is insurance fraud." When Babs, a hospital patient, was treated for breast cancer, her physician obtained her informed consent to use a new treatment that he had helped develop. A drug was injected into her breast that targeted for destruction just the small malignant tumor; no healthy tissue was destroyed. Babs's medical insurance company refused to pay for the procedure, claiming it was "experimental." The procedure was new, but Babs's physician had used it many times with success. "Can't you just say I had a traditional lumpectomy," Babs asked Christine, "so my insurance company will pay for it?"

"We had to explain to Babs that this would constitute insurance fraud, and we couldn't do it," Christine explains.

From Babs's perspective, she wanted her insurance company to help pay for the expensive procedure.

From Christine's perspective, lying about the procedure performed was not only illegal but also unethical.

4.1 The Basis and Primary Sources of Law

THE FEDERAL GOVERNMENT

Federal laws governing the administration of health care and all other national matters derive from powers and responsibilities delegated to the three branches of government by the U.S. Constitution. As you probably recall from basic government classes, the three branches of government are legislative, executive, and judicial. Here is a quick review of the three branches' composition and responsibilities.

The two houses of Congress—the Senate and the House of Representatives—make up the *legislative branch.* Each member of Congress is elected by the people of his or her state. The House of Representatives, with membership based on state populations, has 435 seats, while the Senate, with two members from each state, has 100 seats. Members of the House of Representatives are elected for two-year terms, and senators are elected for six-year terms. The primary duty of Congress is to write, debate, and pass bills, which are then passed on to the president for approval.

Other powers of Congress include:

- Making laws controlling trade between states and between the United States and other countries
- Making laws about taxes and borrowing money
- Approving the printing of money
- Declaring war on other countries

Functions specific to the House of Representatives include the following. Members of the House can:

- Introduce legislation that compels people to pay taxes.
- Decide if a government official should be put on trial before the Senate if he or she commits a crime against the country. (Such a trial is called *impeachment.*)

Functions specific to the Senate include the following. Senators can:

- Approve and disapprove any treaties the president makes.
- Approve or disapprove any people the president recommends for jobs, such as cabinet officers, Supreme Court justices, and ambassadors.
- Hold an impeachment trial for a government official who commits a crime against the country.

The president of the United States is the chief executive of the *executive branch* of government, which is responsible for administering the law. Through his or her ability to issue **executive orders,** the president has limited legislative powers. Executive orders become law without the prior approval of Congress. They are usually issued for one of three purposes: to create administrative agencies or change the practices of an existing agency, to enforce laws passed by Congress, or to make treaties with foreign powers.

executive order
A rule or regulation issued by the President of the United States that becomes law without the prior approval of Congress.

The U.S. Supreme Court heads the *judicial branch* of government, which also includes federal judges and courts in every state. The judicial branch interprets the law and oversees the enforcement of laws.

The division of powers and responsibilities among three branches of government ensures that a system of checks and balances will keep any one branch from assuming too much power (see Figure 4-1).

STATE GOVERNMENTS

State governments also have three branches: *legislative, executive,* and *judicial.* The number of state legislators a state may elect is based on the number of political districts in each state because citizens elect legislators from the various districts. Therefore, the number of members in state legislatures is not the same as the number of members in the U.S. Congress.

State legislative branches also consist of two chambers: the Senate and the House of Representatives. In some states, the House of Representatives is called the Assembly or General Assembly. Terms served may be the same as in the federal government—six years for senators and two years for representatives or assembly members—or they may differ.

The governor is the head of the state's executive branch. Each state has its own constitution, but state constitutions cannot conflict with the U.S. Constitution. Those responsibilities not delegated by the federal constitution are left to the states (see Table 4-1).

There are four types of law, distinguished according to their origin:

1. **Constitutional law** is based on a formal document that defines broad governmental powers. Federal constitutional law is based on the U.S. Constitution. State constitutional law derives from each state's constitution.

constitutional law
Law that derives from federal and state constitutions.

FIGURE 4-1 System of Checks and Balances

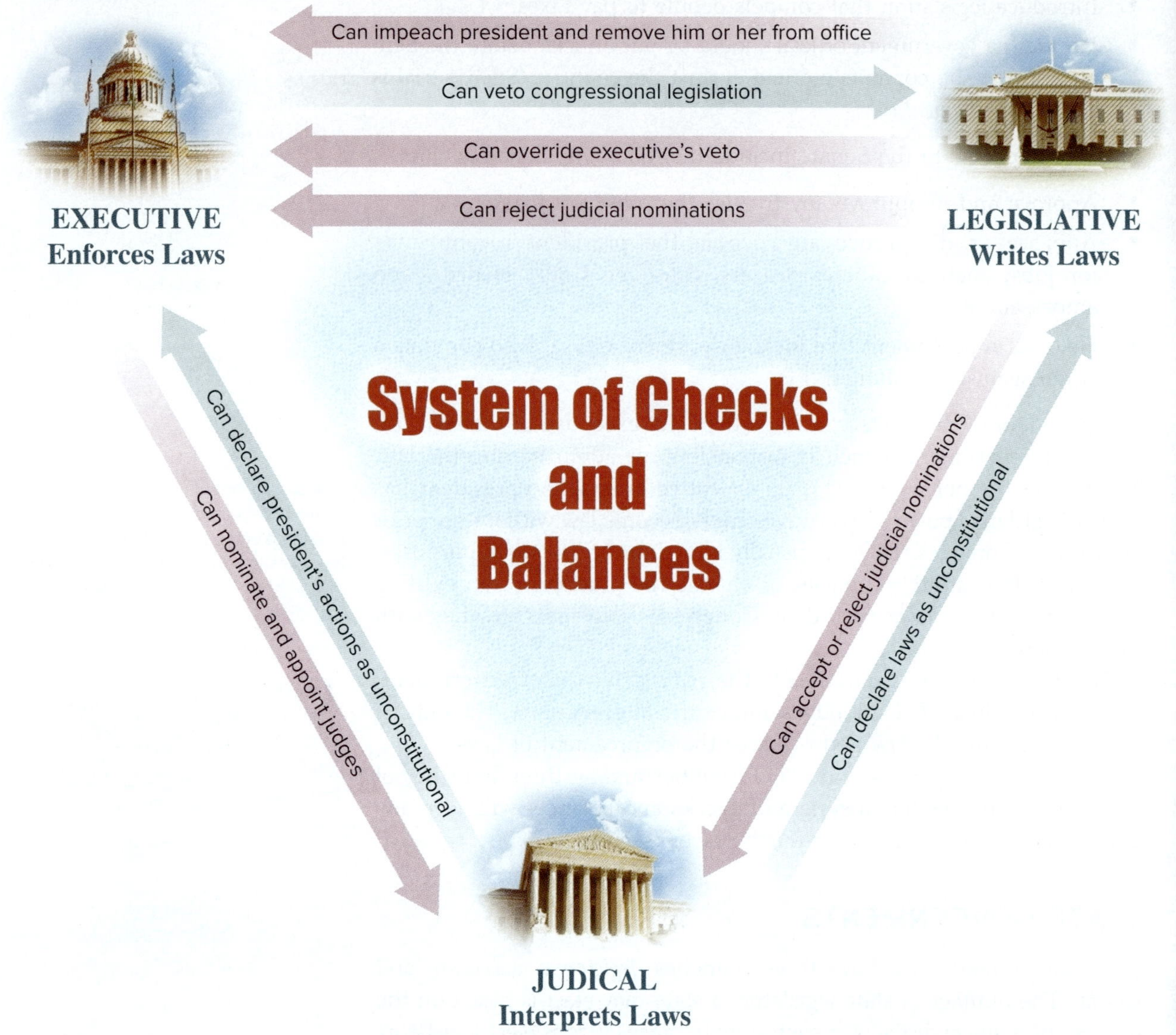

Table 4-1 Exclusive Powers of the National Government and State Governments

National Government	State Governments
Print money	Issue licenses
Regulate interstate (between states) and international trade	Regulate intrastate (within the state) businesses
Make treaties and conduct foreign policy	Conduct elections
Declare war	Establish local governments
Provide an army and navy	Ratify amendments to the Constitution
Establish post offices	Take measures for public health and safety
Make laws necessary and proper to carry out the above powers	May exert powers the Constitution does not delegate to the national government or prohibit the states from using

2. **Case law** is law set by legal precedent. Case law began with **common law.** In the early days in America, laws were derived from those originating in England, and they were often not written down. Matters of law were decided based on the customs and traditions of the people. Judges shared their decisions with other judges, and these decisions became common law.

   Later, court decisions were written down, and judges could then refer to past cases to help them make current decisions. These written cases were then used as **legal precedents.** When deciding cases with similar circumstances, judges were required to follow these earlier cases or legal precedents. Today, legal precedents are the rule of law, applying to future cases, even though they were not enacted by legislation. Precedents can be changed only by the court that originally decided a case or by a higher court.

case law
Law established through common law and legal precedent.

common law
The body of unwritten law developed in England, primarily from judicial decisions based on custom and tradition.

legal precedents
Decisions made by judges in various courts that become rule of law and apply to future cases, even though they were not enacted by legislation.

3. **Statutory law** refers to laws enacted by state or federal legislatures. Individual laws in this body of law are called statutes. (Laws passed by city governments are called municipal ordinances.) Statutes begin as bills at the federal or state levels. The bills may become laws, or the president or governors may veto them. Once passed, the laws may be amended, repealed, revised, or superseded by legislatures. The courts can review statutes for constitutionality, application, interpretation, and other legal questions (see Figure 4-2).

statutory law
Law passed by the U.S. Congress or state legislatures.

4. **Administrative law** includes statutes enacted to define specific powers and procedures when agencies are created. Administrative agencies are created by Congress, by the president, or by individual state legislatures. Regulations may be passed that pertain specifically to the functions of one agency, such as the Internal Revenue Service (IRS), Social Security Administration, or Occupational Safety and Health Administration (OSHA).

administrative law
Enabling statutes enacted to define powers and procedures when an agency is created.

Check Your Progress

Fill in the blanks or answer the following questions in the spaces provided.

1. Number the following two types of constitutions in the order in which they must be observed: state constitutions ______________ federal constitution ______________.
2. Which branch has exclusive authority to declare war on another country?
3. Which chamber of the U.S. Congress has exclusive authority to hold an impeachment trial?
4. What are the four types of law, based on their origin?
5. Which of the above types of law began with common law?
6. Briefly define *administrative law.*

FIGURE 4-2 How a Federal Bill Becomes a Law

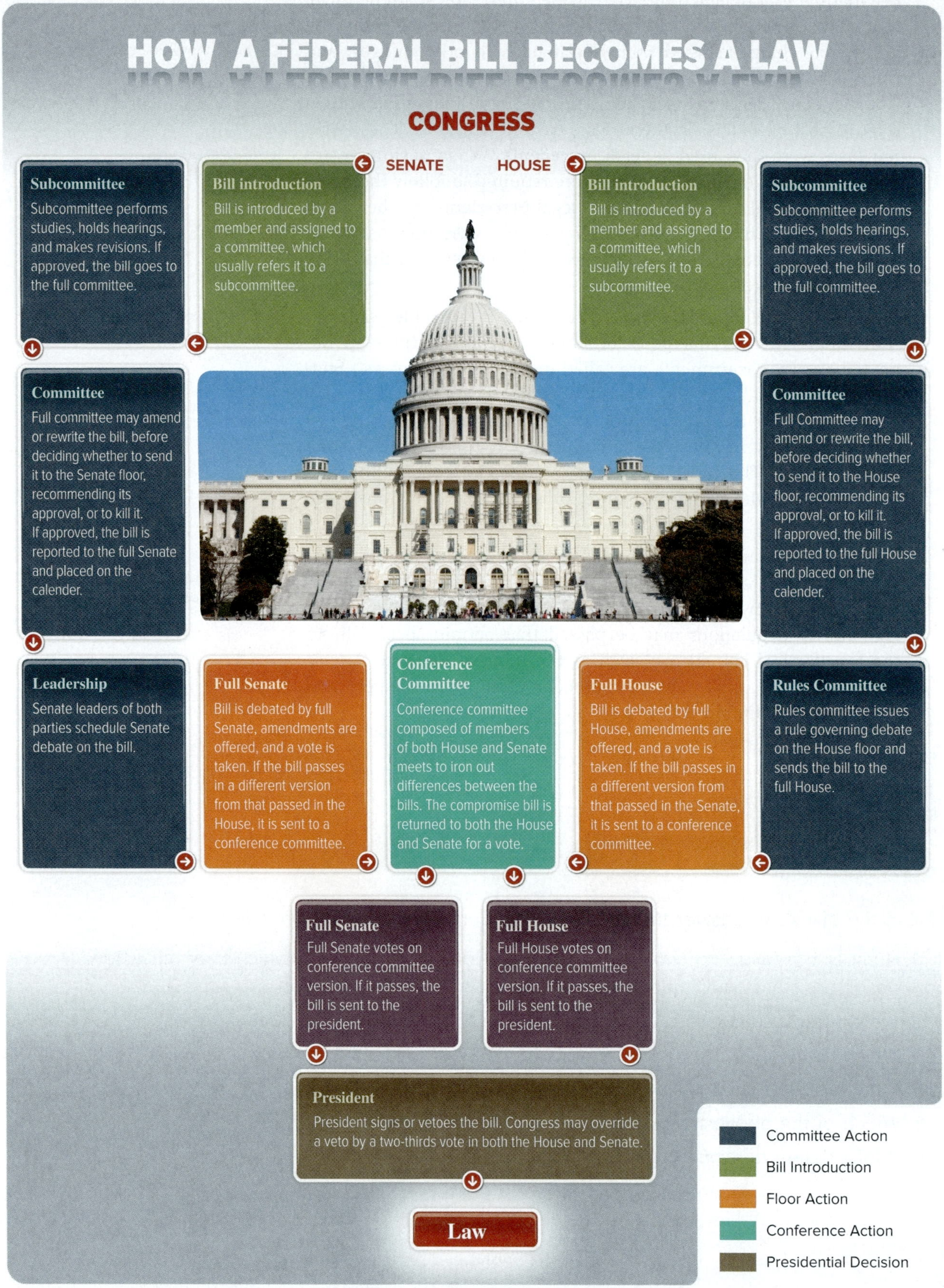

©Zack Frank/Shutterstock.com RF

4.2 Classifications of Law

After laws are created through constitutional, case, statutory, or administrative law, they are classified by type. Two broad types of law are substantive and procedural. **Substantive law** is the statutory or written law that defines and regulates legal rights and obligations. It defines the legal relationships between people or between people and the state, and is further classified as criminal, civil, military, and international law. Examples of substantive laws include the criminal laws that define murder, arson, and armed robbery as crimes and the civil laws that allow individuals to sue persons or entities.

substantive law
The statutory or written law that defines and regulates legal rights and obligations.

Procedural law defines the rules used to enforce substantive law. For example, laws that require law enforcement officers to read suspects their rights (the Miranda warning) and govern the arrest and trial process are procedural laws.

procedural law
Law that defines the rules used to enforce substantive law.

Criminal and civil laws are most likely to pertain to health care practitioners.

CRIMINAL LAW

A crime is an offense against the state or sovereignty, committed or omitted, in violation of a public law forbidding or commanding it. Therefore, the body of **criminal law** involves crimes against the state. When a state or federal criminal law is violated, the government brings criminal charges against the alleged offender (for example, *New York v. John Doe*).

criminal law
Law that involves crimes against the state.

State criminal laws prohibit such crimes as murder, burglary, robbery, arson, rape, larceny, mayhem (needless or willful damage or violence), and practicing medicine without a license. Federal criminal offenses include matters affecting national security (treason); crimes involving the country's borders; and illegal activities that cross state lines, such as kidnapping or hijacking.

A criminal act may be classified as a felony or a misdemeanor. A **felony** is a crime punishable by death or by imprisonment in a state or federal prison for more than one year. Felonies include abuse (child abuse, elder abuse, or domestic violence), arson, burglary, conspiracy, embezzlement, fraud, illegal drug dealing, grand larceny, manslaughter, mayhem, murder or attempted murder, rape, robbery, tax evasion, and practicing medicine without a license.

felony
An offense punishable by death or by imprisonment in a state or federal prison for more than one year.

Misdemeanors are less serious crimes than felonies. They are punishable by fines or by imprisonment in a facility other than a prison for one year or less. Examples of misdemeanors include some traffic violations, thefts under a certain dollar amount, attempted burglary, and disturbing the peace.

misdemeanor
Crime punishable by fine or by imprisonment in a facility other than a prison for less than one year.

Can Knowledge of a Crime Make You Guilty? Persons who commit crimes are, of course, the principals in criminal proceedings. However, those individuals who have knowledge of a crime may, in certain circumstances, also be subject to prosecution. An *accessory* is one who contributes to or aids in the commission of a crime—by a direct act, by an indirect act (such as encouragement), by watching and not giving aid, or by concealing the criminal's crime. For example, the person in charge of billing for health care services in a medical office may be an accessory to insurance fraud if he or she takes no action, even though he or she knows that some health care practitioners are billing for services not rendered.

CIVIL LAW

civil law
Law that involves wrongful acts against persons.

Criminal law involves crimes against the state; **civil law** does not involve crimes but instead involves wrongful acts against persons. Under civil law, a person can sue another person, a business, or the government. Civil disputes often arise over issues of contract violation, slander, libel, trespassing, product liability, or automobile accidents. Many civil suits involve family matters such as divorce, child support, and child custody. Court judgments in civil cases often require the payment of a sum of money to the injured party.

Check Your Progress

Fill in the blanks or answer the following questions in the spaces provided.

7. The written law that says murder is a crime is an example of ____________________ law.
8. The law that says a law enforcement officer must read a prisoner his or her rights is an example of which type of law?
9. One who contributes to or aids in the commission of a crime. ____________________
10. The laws that determine the rules for one person's suing of another are broadly classified as ____________________ law.
11. ____________________ law involves crimes against the state.
12. ____________________ law involves wrongful acts against persons.
13. Which two types of law are most likely to affect health care providers?
14. Under criminal law, practicing medicine without a license is classified as a(n) ____________________.
15. Which type of law does not involve crimes but may involve one person suing another?
16. Court judgments in lawsuits against health care practitioners most often include what as a penalty?

4.3 Tort Liability

tort
A civil wrong committed against a person or property, excluding breach of contract.

Civil law includes a general category of law known as torts. A **tort** is broadly defined as a civil wrong committed against a person or property, excluding breach of contract. The act, committed without just cause, may have caused physical injury, resulted in damage to someone's property, or deprived someone of his or her personal liberty and freedom. Torts may be intentional (willful) or unintentional (accidental).

INTENTIONAL TORTS

Some torts involve intentional misconduct. When one person intentionally harms another, the law allows the injured party to seek a remedy in a civil suit. The injured party can be financially compensated for any harm done by the **tortfeasor** (person guilty of committing a tort). If the conduct is judged to be malicious, punitive damages may also be awarded. Examples of intentional torts include the following:

tortfeasor
The person guilty of committing a tort.

Assault. The open threat of bodily harm to another or acting in such a way as to put another in the "reasonable apprehension of bodily harm."

Battery. An action that causes bodily harm to another. It is broadly defined as any bodily contact made without permission. Battery may or may not result from the threat of assault. In health care delivery, battery may be charged for any unauthorized touching of a patient, including such actions as suturing a wound, administering an injection, or performing a physical examination.

Defamation of Character. Involves damaging a person's reputation by making public statements that are both false and malicious. Defamation can take the form of libel or slander. Libel is expressing in published print, writing, pictures, or signed statements content that injures the reputation of another. Libel also includes reading statements aloud or broadcasting for the public to hear. Slander is speaking defamatory or damaging words intended to prejudice others against an individual in a manner that jeopardizes his or her reputation or means of livelihood.

False Imprisonment. The intentional, unlawful restraint or confinement of one person by another. The offense is treated as a crime in some states. Refusing to dismiss a patient from a health care facility on his or her request or preventing an employee or patient from leaving the facility might be seen as false imprisonment.

Fraud. Deceitful practices in depriving or attempting to deprive another of his or her rights. Health care practitioners might be accused of fraud for promising patients "miracle cures" or for accepting fees from patients for using mystical or spiritual powers to heal.

Invasion of Privacy. An intrusion into a person's seclusion or private affairs, public disclosure of private facts about a person, false publicity about a person, or use of a person's name or likeness without permission. Improper use or breaching the confidentiality of medical records may be seen as invasion of privacy.

Intentional torts may also be crimes. Therefore, some civil wrongs may also be prosecuted as criminal acts in separate court actions. See Table 4-2 for a summary of intentional torts.

UNINTENTIONAL TORTS

The more common torts within the health care delivery system are those committed unintentionally. Unintentional torts are acts that are not intended to cause harm but are committed unreasonably or with a disregard for the consequences. In legal terms, this constitutes **negligence.**

negligence
An unintentional tort alleged when one may have performed or failed to perform an act that a reasonable person would or would not have done in similar circumstances.

Table 4-2 Intentional Torts

Tort	Description
Assault	Threatening to strike or harm with a weapon or physical movement, resulting in fear
Battery	Unlawful, unprivileged touching of another person
Trespass	Wrongful injury to or interference with the property of another
Nuisance	Anything that interferes with the enjoyment of life or property
Interference with contractual relations	Intentionally causing one person not to enter into or to break a contract with another
Deceit	False statement or deceptive practice done with intent to injure another
Conversion	Unauthorized taking or borrowing of personal property of another for the use of the taker
False imprisonment (false arrest)	Unlawful restraint of a person, whether in prison or otherwise
Defamation	Wrongful act of injuring another's reputation by making false statements
Invasion of privacy	Interference with a person's right to be left alone
Misuse of legal procedure	Bringing legal action with malice and without probable cause
Infliction of emotional distress	Intentionally or recklessly causing emotional or mental suffering to another
Fraud	Dishonest or deceitful practices in depriving, or attempting to deprive, another of his or her rights

Negligence is charged when a health care practitioner fails to exercise ordinary care and a patient is injured. The accused may have performed an act or failed to perform an act that a reasonable person, in similar circumstances, would or would not have performed. "Didn't intend to do it" or "should have known better" best describes a negligent act. Under principles of negligence, civil liability exists only in cases in which the act is judicially determined to be wrongful. A health care practitioner, for example, is not necessarily liable for a poor-quality outcome in delivering health care. He or she becomes liable only when his or her conduct is determined to be malpractice, the negligent delivery of professional services.

Negligence and defenses to liability suits are discussed in detail in Chapter 5.

Medical negligence cases may be brought against individual physicians or other health care professionals, as well as against hospitals, outpatient surgical centers, nursing homes, or any institution that provides health care. When evaluating a case for institutional negligence, the organization is held to the same standard of care as an individual health care provider. The question is what would/should a reasonably careful hospital or other institution do under similar circumstances? Often both the individual provider and the institution are sued, as is illustrated in the two court cases below.

There are two different ways a hospital can face liability under medical malpractice. A hospital can be held liable for the medical negligence conducted by its agents or employees, or it can be held liable for its own institutional negligence. According to legal experts, a hospital owes its patients a duty to exercise a reasonable degree of care when dealing with an apparent risk.

COURT CASE University Sued for Negligence

A 50-year-old woman was taken to the local hospital with symptoms of right shoulder pain, limited range of motion of her right upper extremity, a cough, and a fever. Blood tests were ordered, and the doctors discharged the patient the next day without knowing the results.

Several days later, she was taken to a second local hospital with similar symptoms and again discharged. The results of the blood tests were not known to the second hospital.

When the doctors at the first hospital learned of the blood test results, they did not contact the patient. These blood tests revealed an infection. At the third visit to the second hospital, the true cause of her condition, an epidural abscess, was found. However, by then she had developed slurred speech, acute renal failure, and progressive paraplegia. These problems were not reversible, and the patient was totally disabled at age 50.

The patient and her family sued the resident physicians and the University of Cincinnati because it was operating the program that placed medical residents in the various local hospitals. It was a resident at the first hospital who failed to notify the patient of the results of her blood test. The Court of Claims approved a settlement against the University of Cincinnati for $2.3 million. The Ohio Court of Appeals upheld the settlement.

Source: *Adae v. State*, 2013-Ohio-23. No. 12AP-406 (Ct. of Cl. No. 2007-08228) January 2013.

COURT CASE A Simple Hernia Surgery

A 62-year-old female patient was scheduled for simple laparoscopic hernia surgery. Her surgeon had done more than 200 of the same procedures with no problems. While in the operating room, a resident physician came in to assist in what was a routine procedure. The surgeon asked the resident physician if he had ever used a bladeless optical trocar before. The resident physician said he had used the instrument before. However, when he began using the trocar, it was evident that he was not familiar with the instrument, and the surgeon resumed control of the surgery. The surgeon looked for any perforations but did not see any.

Thirty-six hours later, it was apparent that the patient's colon had been cut and she had a serious infection. Emergency surgery was done. The patient spent 34 days in the intensive care unit and a total of 70 days in the hospital, had six more surgeries, and amassed $1 million in medical bills. The patient now sits in a scooter and can only eat foods that can be easily digested. A jury awarded the patient and her husband a total of $12 million to be paid by both the hospital and the physicians.

Source: *Vivian Gagliano and Philip Gagliano v. Danbury Hospital*, Joseph Gordon and Venkata Bodavula 2014 Jury Verdicts LEXIS 4589.

Various types of evidence are useful in establishing a hospital's standard of care, including expert testimony, existing federal and state laws, hospital bylaws, custom and community practice, and accreditation standards. And while expert testimony is typically required in medical malpractice cases, sometimes institutional negligence can be established without expert testimony.

THE COURT SYSTEM

The type of court that tries a case depends on the state or federal law that was allegedly violated. The federal court system, with some exceptions, hears cases involving federal matters. State court systems are independent of one another, and each system has its own rules and regulations. Generally, state courts decide cases involving matters occurring within their own state borders.

jurisdiction
The power of a court to hear and decide a case before it.

Federal Courts **Jurisdiction** is the power of a court to hear and decide a case before it. In most common law systems, jurisdiction is conceptually divided between jurisdiction over the subject matter of a case and jurisdiction over the person of the litigants. Examples of cases over which federal courts have jurisdiction include federal crimes, federal antitrust law, bankruptcy, patents, copyrights, trademarks, suits against the United States, and areas of admiralty law (pertaining to the sea).

State Courts Each state has its own court system, but the general structure is the same in all states. The bottom tier consists of local courts. The next highest tier is trial courts, followed by appellate courts, and then the state supreme court. As with the federal court system, there are also special state courts with jurisdiction in certain kinds of cases.

Figure 4-3 shows the various federal and state court systems in the United States.

plaintiff
The person bringing charges in a lawsuit.

prosecution
The government as plaintiff in a criminal case.

defendant
The person or party against whom criminal or civil charges are brought in a lawsuit.

Players in the Court Scene When criminal and civil cases go to court, a complaining party–the **plaintiff**–must show that he or she was wronged or injured. The government–the **prosecution**–is the plaintiff in criminal cases. A private individual is the plaintiff in civil cases. The **defendant,** who is charged with an offense, must dispute the complaint.

Officers of the court are responsible for carrying out courtroom duties:

- *Judges* are elected or appointed to preside over the court and in most states must be licensed attorneys. They rule on points of law about trial procedure, presentation of evidence, and all laws that apply to the case. If there is no jury, the judge determines the facts in the case. Judges hand down sentences after a verdict is rendered.
- *Attorneys* represent plaintiffs and defendants, presenting evidence so that the jury or the judge can reach a verdict.
- *Court clerks* keep court records and seals, enter court orders and judgments into the record, and keep the papers of the court.
- *Bailiffs* keep order in the courtroom and may remove disruptive persons from the court at the judge's request.
- *Court reporters* make a running account of all court proceedings, using a stenotype machine that types shorthand symbols onto a tape.
- *Juries* are most often selected from lists of registered voters. Six or twelve jurors are chosen to hear the evidence presented in court and render a verdict.

Check Your Progress

Fill in the blanks to accurately complete the following statements.

17. The highest tier of federal courts consists of ______________.
18. A lawsuit brought by a patient against a health care practitioner would be heard first in a(n) ______________ court.
19. Torts are wrongs committed against ______________.
20. The two broad types of torts include ______________ and ______________.
21. The type of tort most likely to concern health care practitioners is ______________.

FIGURE 4-3 Court Systems in the United States

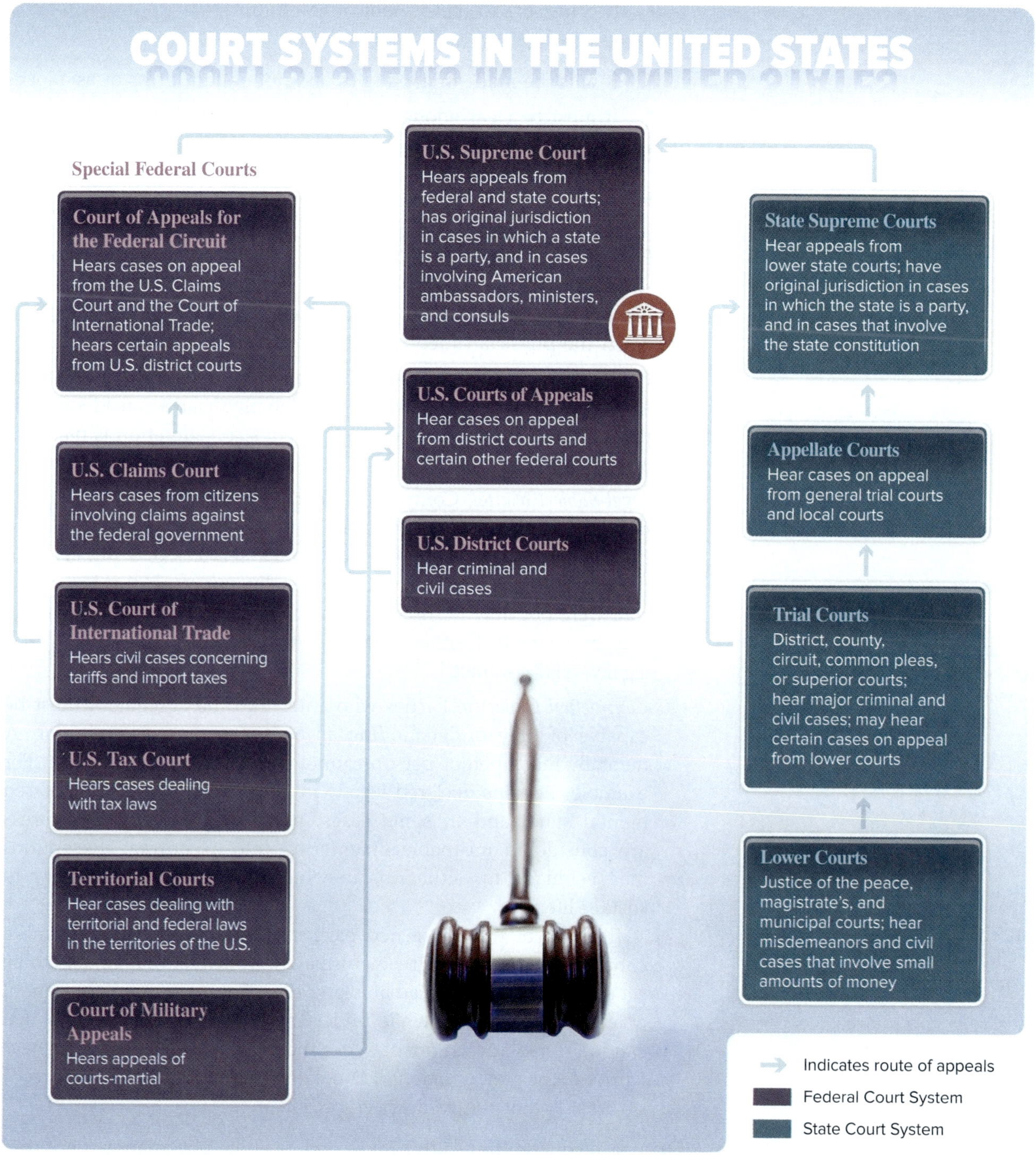

©Michael Grimm/Getty Images RF

4.4 Contracts

A **contract** is a voluntary agreement between two parties in which specific promises are made for a consideration. The elements of a contract are important to health care practitioners because health care delivery takes place under various types of contracts. To be legally binding, four elements must be present in a contract.

contract
A voluntary agreement between two parties in which specific promises are made for a consideration.

1. *Agreement.* One party makes an offer, and another party accepts it. Certain conditions pertain to the offer:
   - It can relate to the present or the future.
   - It must be communicated.
   - It must be made in good faith and not under duress or as a joke.
   - It must be clear enough to be understood by both parties.
   - It must define what both parties will do if the offer is accepted.

   For example, a physician offers his or her services to the public by obtaining a license to practice medicine and opening for business. Patients accept the physician's offer by scheduling appointments, submitting to physical examinations, and allowing the physician to prescribe or perform medical treatment. The contract is complete when the physician's fee is paid.
2. *Consideration.* Something of value is bargained for as part of the agreement. In the previous example, the physician's consideration is providing his or her services; the patient's consideration is payment of the physician's fee.
3. *Legal Subject Matter.* Contracts are not valid and enforceable in court unless they are for legal services or purposes. For example, a contract entered into by a patient to pay for services of a physician in private practice would be **void** (not legally enforceable) if the physician were not duly licensed to practice medicine. **Breach of contract** may be charged if either party fails to comply with the terms of a legally valid contract.
4. *Contractual Capacity.* Parties who enter into the agreement must be capable of fully understanding all of its terms and conditions. A mentally incompetent person cannot enter into a legal contract. For example, persons declared legally insane, persons in a drug-altered mental state, and in some cases, persons under extreme duress are considered incapable of entering into a contract. Exceptions may be made for situations in which a contract is necessary to sustain life.

   If either of the concerned parties is incompetent at the time a contract is made, the agreement may be voidable, that is, able to be set aside or to be validated at a later date. Say, for example, a patient enters into a contract while under the effects of a medication that can interfere with judgment. After the effects of the medication have worn off, the patient may say, "No, I don't want the contract enforced" or "Yes, I want the contract enforced."

void
Without legal force or effect.

breach of contract
Failure of either party to comply with the terms of a legally valid contract.

Of special concern to health care providers is the physician–patient contract as applied to minors. Because of the risk of being accused of battery or assault, health care practitioners cannot treat a minor without the consent of a responsible parent or legal guardian, except in cases where minors suffer a life-threatening emergency or have been legally determined to be mature. A **minor** is defined as anyone under the age of majority, which is 18 in most states and 21 in some jurisdictions. See Chapter 11 for a more extensive discussion of minors and the administration of medical services.

minor
Anyone under the age of majority: 18 years in most states, 21 years in some jurisdictions.

Types of Contracts

The two main types of contracts are expressed contracts and implied contracts. Expressed contracts are explicitly stated in written or spoken words. Implied contracts are unspoken; their terms result from actions of the involved parties.

EXPRESSED CONTRACTS

An expressed contract may be written or oral, but all terms of the contract are explicitly stated. In the medical office, some contracts, to be legally valid, must be in writing. In each state, the **statute of frauds,** derived from the Statute for the Prevention of Frauds and Perjuries formulated in England in 1677, states which contracts must be in writing to be enforced.

statute of frauds
State legislation governing written contracts.

Termination of Contracts The contract between a physician and a patient is usually terminated (ended) when all treatment has been completed and the bill has been paid. Situations may arise, however, in which premature termination of the contract takes place, as in the following situations:

Failure to Pay for Services. A physician may stop treatment of a patient and end the physician–patient relationship if the patient habitually does not pay or fails to make satisfactory arrangements to pay for medical services, but only if adequate notice is given to the patient.

Failure to Keep Scheduled Appointments. To protect the physician from charges of abandonment, all missed appointments should be noted on the patient's chart.

Failure to Follow the Physician's Instructions. It makes no difference whether the failure is due to a patient's willfulness or negligence.

A Patient Seeks the Services of Another Physician. Whenever a patient acknowledges, orally or in writing, that he or she will seek medical care from another physician, the medical office employee should document this on the patient's chart and then send a letter to the patient verifying the termination. A copy of the letter should be filed with the patient's records. Seeking a second opinion, however, does not necessarily terminate the physician–patient relationship.

A patient may terminate a physician–patient relationship at any time. After a physician agrees to treat a patient, however, his or her responsibilities to the patient continue until the relationship is properly terminated. If a physician suddenly withdraws from treatment while the patient is still in need of medical care, fails to visit a hospitalized patient, or otherwise abandons the patient without arranging for substitute care, he or she may be charged with abandonment. Depending on the circumstances, the physician may also be charged with breach of contract and/or negligence.

To properly terminate the physician–patient relationship, the physician must give the patient formal written notice that he or she is withdrawing from the case. The physician should also note any need for the patient to receive continued medical care. In addition, the patient must be given time to find another physician. The notice of discharge of withdrawal should be sent by certified mail, return receipt requested, and a copy should be filed with the patient's records. Figure 4-4 illustrates a notice of termination.

Managed care plans *may* restrict a physician from terminating patient care without the approval of the managed care plan.

Laws Governing Payment of Fees at Fulfillment of Contract

Certain federal and state laws govern the payment of fees when contracts have been fulfilled. For example, a type of contract often used in the medical office that falls under the Statute of Frauds, which is state law governing written contracts, is the third-party payer contract. Insurance policies are also third-party payer contracts, but as used here, the term means agreements by a third party to pay for services rendered to another. Such contracts must be in writing to be enforced and should

FIGURE 4-4 Physician's Letter of Dismissal for Nonpayment

Health & wellness Center

Date ____________________

William Smith
1212 Economy Drive
Dallas, Texas
75001

Certified Mail # ____________________

Dear William Smith,

This letter is to inform you that I will no longer be your physician and will stop providing medical care to you effective 30 days from the date you receive this letter.

I will continue to provide routine and emergency medical care to you for 30 days while you seek another physician.

I suggest you consult the local physician referral service, your county medical society, or the yellow pages of your telephone book as soon as possible so that you may find another physician who will assume responsibility for your care.

I will be pleased to assist the physician of your choice by sending him or her a copy of your medical records.

Sincerely,

____
(Physician Signature)

Department of ____________________

be signed before health care services are rendered. For example, suppose Susan becomes ill while visiting her aunt in a distant city, and the aunt makes an appointment for Susan to see her physician. The aunt tells the medical office assistant, "I will pay Susan's bill." The medical office assistant may ask Susan's aunt to sign a third-party payer contract.

Not all financial arrangements that require written contracts fall under the Statute of Frauds. Others are governed by Regulation Z or Regulation M of the Consumer Protection Act of 1968, also known as the Truth-in-Lending Act. Regulation Z applies to each individual or business that offers or extends consumer credit if four conditions are met:

1. The credit is offered to consumers.
2. Credit is offered on a regular basis.
3. The credit is subject to a finance charge (interest) or must be paid in more than four installments according to a written agreement.
4. The credit is primarily for personal, family, or household purposes. Regulation M applies only if credit is extended to businesses or for commercial or agricultural purposes.

For example, Regulation Z of the Consumer Protection Act applies in a health care setting such as the following: A patient and a physician make a bilateral payment agreement (one in which both parties are mutually affected) that medical fees will be paid in four or more installments or will include finance charges. (It is legal and ethical for physicians to levy finance charges, as long as this is made clear to the patient before the charges are incurred.) This agreement must be in writing and must contain the following information:

- Fees for services
- Amount of any down payment
- The date each payment is due
- The date of the final payment
- The amount of each payment
- Any interest charges to be made

The patient signs the agreement and is given a copy. A second copy is filed with the patient's records.

For agreements falling under Regulation Z of the Truth-in-Lending Act, the medical office must supply the patient with a written disclosure statement (see Figure 4-5). The primary purpose of this legislation is to protect consumers from fraudulent or deceptive hidden finance charges levied by creditors, but creditors can also use it to collect outstanding debts.

The federal Fair Debt Collection Practices Act (FDCPA) of 1978 requires debt collectors and creditors to treat debtors fairly. It ensures fair treatment by prohibiting certain methods of debt collection. Debt collection practices prohibited by the act include harassment, misrepresentation, threats, disseminating false information about the debtor, and engaging in unfair or illegal practices in attempting to collect a debt. Personal, family, and household debts are covered under the act. This includes money owed for the purchase of an automobile, medical care, and charge accounts.

FIGURE 4-5
Truth-in-Lending Payment Agreement

Bruce Whiting, MD
310 Madison Avenue,
Anderson, Indiana 46027

I agree to pay $ ______________ per week/month on my account balance of $__________.

Payments are due by the __________ of each____________ and will begin____________.
(week/month) (date)

Interest will/will not be changed on the outstanding balance (see Truth-in-Lending form below for rate of interest).

I agree that if payments are not made in the full amount stated above or if payments are not received on time, the entire account balance will be considered delinquent and will be due and payable immediately.

I agree to be responsible for any reasonable collection costs or attorney fees incurred in collecting a delinquent account.

Date ______________________ Signature ______________________

This disclosure is in compliance with the Truth-in-Lending Act.

Patient's Name ______________________ Address ______________________

Responsible Party (if other than patient) ______________________ City, State, Zip Code ______________________

1. Cash price (Medical and/or Surgical Fee)
   Less cash down payment (Advance) ______________________
2. Unpaid balance of cash price ______________________
3. Amount financed ______________________
4. Finance charge ______________________
5. Total of payments (3 + 4) ______________________
6. Deferred payment price (1 + 4) ______________________
7. Annual percentage rate ______________________

The "Total of payments" shown above is payable to Bruce Whiting, MD, at the address shown above in ______ monthly installments of $______ the first installment being payable ____________ (date) and all subsequent installments are due on the same day of each consecutive month until paid in full.

Date ______________________ Signature ______________________

IMPLIED CONTRACTS

Implied contracts are those in which the conduct of the parties, rather than expressed words, creates the contract. Most contracts in the medical office are implied. For example, suppose a patient comes to a clinic complaining of a sore throat and asks to see a physician. The physician does not literally say to the patient, "I offer to treat your condition," but by making his or her services available, he or she has made an offer to treat. A patient does not state to the physician, "I accept your offer to provide medical care." Acceptance is implied by the patient's actions in allowing the physician to examine him or her and prescribe treatment. The physician's consideration is providing services. The patient's consideration is payment of the physician's fee. The contract is valid if both parties understand the offer, both are competent, and the services provided are legal.

A physician who provides emergency treatment to a patient in a situation not covered by a special arrangement, such as in an emergency room, is limited to providing treatment at the site of the emergency. In such a situation, an implied limited contract between the physician and the patient is created, based on the patient's implied request for and consent to emergency treatment. The patient's promise to pay for the physician's services is also implied. In this case, the physician's obligation for care does not extend to treatment after the emergency situation has been resolved.

PHYSICIAN–PATIENT CONTRACTS AND MANAGED CARE

Managed care plans have added a third element to the physician–patient contract. Physicians still have contracts with their patients, but they may also have contracted with managed care programs to deliver medical services. If a physician terminates his or her contractual relationship with a managed care plan, this does not mean he or she cannot continue to see patients insured with the plan. It simply means the managed care plan will no longer pay for the subscriber's visits to this physician.

All insurance providers, including managed care plans, have access to patients' medical records for purposes of utilization review, inpatient stay review, case management review, and quality management. Insurance providers also check enrollees' medical records to monitor care and to identify ways of preventing illness and disease.

Check Your Progress

22. List the four elements present in a legally valid contract, and give an example of each.
23. Tell whether each of the following examples involves an expressed or an implied contract:
    ______ A man agrees to buy his friend's car and seals the deal with a handshake.
    ______ A medical center outpatient agrees to undergo a colonoscopy.
    ______ A patient in a physician's office agrees to a physical examination.
    ______ A physician treats a patient for a broken leg in a hospital emergency room.
24. List three federal laws governing collections in the medical office.
25. Briefly explain how managed care has impacted physician–patient contracts.

4.5 Physicians' and Patients' Rights and Responsibilities

PHYSICIANS

A physician has the right, after agreeing to accept an individual as his or her patient, to make reasonable limitations on the relationship. The physician is under no legal obligation to treat patients who may wish to exceed those limitations. Under the provisions of the physician–patient contract, both parties have certain rights and responsibilities. A physician has the right to:

- Set up practice within the boundaries of his or her license to practice medicine. A specialist, for instance, does not have to practice outside the area of specialty and, in fact, would be severely criticized for doing so, except in an emergency in which no other physician were available.
- Set up an office wherever he or she chooses and establish office hours.
- Specialize.
- Decide which services he or she will provide and how those services will be provided.

While practicing within the context of an implied contract with the patient, the physician is not bound to:

- Treat every patient who seeks medical care. The physician is free to use his or her own discretion–with one exception. If a physician is hired specifically to treat patients in one area or locale, such as a hospital emergency room, he or she must treat every patient who comes to that locale.
- Restore the patient to his or her original state of health. The fact that a patient grows progressively worse while under a physician's care and shows improvement when care is withdrawn does not necessarily constitute liability.
- Possess the highest skills possible within the profession or the maximum education attainable.
- Effect a recovery with every patient. The physician who fails to heal a patient cannot be condemned for lack of skill.
- Be familiar with the various reactions of patients to anesthetics or drugs of any kind. However, the physician is bound to note any allergic or adverse reactions to medications reported by the patient before treatment is administered.
- Be as skilled as a specialist if he or she is a general practitioner.
- Make a correct diagnosis in every case.
- Be free from mistakes of judgment in difficult cases.
- Display infallibility of judgment.
- Continue services after being discharged by the patient or by some responsible person, even if harm should come to the patient.
- Guarantee the successful result of any treatment or operation. In fact, guarantees of "cures" may constitute fraud on the part of the physician.

Under an implied contract with the patient, the physician has the obligation to:

- Use due care, skill, judgment, and diligence in treating patients, which other physicians of the same practice usually exercise in similar locations and under similar circumstances.
- Stay informed about the best methods of diagnosis and treatment.
- Perform to the best of his or her ability, whether or not he or she is to receive a fee.
- Exercise his or her best professional judgment in all cases, particularly those in which considerable doubt is involved.
- Consider the established, customary treatment administered by members of the medical profession in similar cases.

- Abstain from performing experiments on a patient without first securing the patient's complete understanding and approval.
- Provide proper instructions for a patient's care to the person responsible for such care, so that proper treatment will be administered to the patient in the doctor's absence.
- Furnish complete information and instructions to the patient about diagnosis, options and methods of treatment, and fees for services.
- Take every precaution to prevent the spread of contagious disease.
- Advise patients against needless or unwise operations.

PATIENTS

In the United States, patients generally have the right to choose the physician they will see, although some managed care plans may limit choices. As a guide to other patients' rights, the American Hospital Association (AHA) created a Patients' Bill of Rights in 1973, which was used extensively throughout the health care system. A variety of attempts were made to make the AHA Bill of Rights a federal law, but none succeeded. In 2003, the AHA dropped the Bill of Rights and created a brochure entitled "Patient Care Partnership: Understanding Expectations, Rights and Responsibilities" ©American Hospital Association. This brochure is written for a patient's hospital visit but could apply to a variety of health care visits. The partnership encourages high quality care, a clean and safe environment, patient involvement in their care, protection of patient privacy, and help with leaving the hospital as well as billing claims.

Creating a national legal patients' bill of rights has been elusive. A number of states have enacted statutes that reflect a patients' bill of rights. Additionally, the Patient Protection and Affordable Care Act (PPACA) provides a series of protections for consumers when dealing with their insurance companies and has been referred to as a bill of rights. Chapter 8 explores PPACA in more detail.

Patients also have the right to terminate a physician's services if they wish. Terminating a physician's services extends to the right of hospitalized patients to leave before their physicians have discharged them or to leave *against medical advice (AMA).*

According to the Agency for Healthcare Research and Quality (AHRQ), the federal agency charged with improving the quality, safety, efficiency, and effectiveness of health care for all Americans, in any one year, approximately 0.8 percent to 2.2 percent of patients in hospitals are discharged against medical advice.

According to the AHRQ, three types of patients are most likely to leave the hospital against doctors' orders:

1. Those who are worried about paying the medical bills
2. Those with alcohol or substance abuse problems
3. Those who have had a previous discharge against medical advice

The best medical results depend on hospitalized patients staying until discharged by physicians, of course, but everyone who has been hospitalized knows the stay can be inconvenient and stressful. How much schoolwork will you have to make up? Will your employer dock wages for the time missed? Who will check your house or apartment, take care of your children, water the plants, or feed the pets? And if you don't have health insurance, who will pay the medical bills?

To protect against liability for any medical consequences resulting from early discharge, the patient's insistence on leaving should be charted, and a form such as the one illustrated in Figure 4-6 should be signed and filed with the patient's medical record.

The patient also has certain implied duties to:

- Follow any instructions given by the physician and cooperate as much as possible.
- Give all relevant information to the physician to reach a correct diagnosis. If an incorrect diagnosis is made because the patient fails to give the physician the proper information, the physician is not liable.
- Follow the physician's orders for treatment, provided the treatment is similar to that administered by members of the system or school of medicine to which the physician belongs. If a patient willfully or negligently fails to follow the physician's instructions, that patient has little legal recourse.
- Pay the fees charged for services rendered.

FIGURE 4-6
Form for Patient Discharged against Medical Advice

Health & wellness Center

William Smith
1212 Economy Drive
Dallas, Texas
75001

Date ____________ Time ____________ A.M. / P.M.

____
Signature of Party Leaving Against Medical Advice

WITNESS: IF PARTY DEMANDING DISCHARGE IS OTHER THAN PATIENT:

____________________ ____________________
Signature of Witness Signature of Party

Relationship ____________________

INSTRUCTIONS: This demand for discharge should be signed by the patient or authorized party if he/she insists on leaving the Wellness Medical Center against medical advice. If the patient or authorized party not only demands to leave but also refuses to sign this form the following should be completed: ____________________
(Name of Party Demanding Discharge)
has not only demanded discharge but also has refused to sign this form documenting his/her demand.

Date ____________ Time ____________ A.M. / P.M.

____
Signature of Person Receiving Demand

Check Your Progress

Cross out the incorrect responses to complete the following statements that pertain to express or implied contracts between physicians and patients, and payment of contract fees.

26. A physician is/is not obligated to effect a recovery with every patient.
27. A physician is/is not obligated to use due care, skill, and diligence in treating each patient.
28. A physician is/is not obligated to note allergic or adverse reactions to medications reported by a specific patient.
29. A patient is/is not obligated to give all relevant information to the physician to help him or her reach a correct diagnosis.
30. A patient is/is not obligated to take part in all research relevant to his or her medical condition.
31. A patient can/cannot leave the hospital against medical advice.
32. A patient is/is not responsible for paying medical bills if the outcome of treatment is unsatisfactory.
33. A Patients' Bill of Rights was/was not enacted to give patients more rights under the law.

Chapter Summary

Learning Outcome	Summary
LO 4.1 Discuss the basis and primary sources of law.	What is the basis of law in the United States? • Federal statutes • State statutes • Municipal ordinances • Constitutional law: Law that derives from federal and state constitutions. • Case law: Law established through common law and legal precedent. • Common law: The body of unwritten law developed in England, primarily from judicial decisions based on custom and tradition.

LO 4.2 Identify the classifications of law.	How are laws classified?
	• Substantive: The statutory or written law that defines and regulates legal rights and obligations.
	    • Criminal law involves crimes against the state.
	        • A felony is a criminal offense punishable by death or by imprisonment in a state or federal prison for more than one year.
	        • A misdemeanor is a crime punishable by fine or imprisonment in a facility other than a prison for less than one year.
	    • Civil law does not involve crimes but instead involves wrongful acts against persons. Under civil law, a person can sue another person, a business, or the government.
	• Procedural: Law that defines the rules used to enforce substantive law.

LO 4.3 Define the concept of torts, and discuss how the tort of negligence affects health care.	What are torts, and how do they affect health care practitioners?
	• A tort is a civil wrong committed against a person or property, excluding breach of contract.
	    • Intentional torts involve intentional misconduct.
	    • Unintentional torts are acts that are not intended to cause harm but are committed unreasonably or with a disregard for the consequences. In legal terms, this constitutes negligence, a charge most often alleged against health care practitioners.

LO 4.4 List the four essential elements of a contract, and differentiate between expressed contracts and implied contracts.	What is a contract, and what are its essential elements?
	• A contract is a voluntary agreement between two parties in which specific promises are made for a consideration. It includes:
	    • The agreement: One party makes an offer, and another party accepts it.
	    • The consideration: Something of value is bargained for as part of the agreement.
	    • Legal subject matter: Contracts are not valid and enforceable in court unless they are for legal services or purposes.
	    • Contractual capacity: Parties who enter into the agreement must be capable of fully understanding all of its terms and conditions.
	How do expressed contracts differ from implied contracts?
	• Expressed contracts are spoken or written in precise terms.
	• Implied contracts are not spoken or written in precise terms but are understood.

LO 4.5 Compare the contractual rights and responsibilities of both physicians and patients.	What are the contractual rights and responsibilities of both physicians and patients? A physician has the right to: • Set up practice within the boundaries of his or her license to practice medicine. A specialist, for instance, does not have to practice outside the area of specialty and, in fact, would be severely criticized for doing so, except in an emergency in which no other physician were available. • Set up an office wherever he or she chooses and establish office hours. • Specialize. • Decide which services he or she will provide and how those services will be provided.

The physician has the obligation to:

- Use due care, skill, judgment, and diligence in treating patients.
- Stay informed about the best methods of diagnosis and treatment.
- Perform to the best of his or her ability.
- Exercise his or her best professional judgment in all cases.
- Consider the established, customary treatment administered by members of the medical profession in similar cases.
- Abstain from performing experiments on a patient without first securing the patient's complete understanding and approval.
- Provide proper instructions for a patient's care to the person responsible for such care.
- Furnish complete information and instructions to the patient about diagnosis, options and methods of treatment, and fees for services.
- Take every precaution to prevent the spread of contagious disease.
- Advise patients against needless or unwise operations.

Patients have the right to:

- Receive considerate and respectful care.
- Receive complete current information concerning his or her diagnosis, treatment, and prognosis.
- Receive information necessary to give informed consent prior to the start of any procedure and/or treatment.
- Refuse treatment to the extent permitted by law.
- Receive every consideration of his or her privacy.
- Be assured of confidentiality.
- Obtain reasonable responses to requests for services.
- Obtain information about his or her health care.
- Know whether treatment is experimental, and be free to refuse to participate in research projects.
- Expect reasonable continuity of care.
- Examine his or her bill and have it explained.
- Know which hospital rules and regulations apply to patient conduct.
- Terminate the physician–patient contract, which includes leaving a hospital or refusing treatment against medical advice.

Patients are obligated to:

- Follow any instructions given by the physician and cooperate as much as possible.
- Give all relevant information to the physician to reach a correct diagnosis. If an incorrect diagnosis is made because the patient fails to give the physician the proper information, the physician is not liable.
- Follow the physician's orders for treatment, provided the treatment is similar to that administered by members of the system or school of medicine to which the physician belongs. If a patient willfully or negligently fails to follow the physician's instructions, that patient has little legal recourse.
- Pay the fees charged for services rendered.

Chapter 4 Review

Applying Knowledge

LO 4.1

1. List and define three functions a state government *can* assume.
2. Which governmental functions are reserved strictly for the federal government?
3. Define *common law.*
4. Define *administrative law.*
5. Decisions made by judges in the various courts and used as a guide for future decisions are called what?

LO 4.2

6. Substantive law
   a. Defines the legal relationships between people or between people and the state
   b. Is never written down
   c. Is a type of common law
   d. Is created solely by executive order
7. Procedural law
   a. Is the same as substantive law
   b. Defines the rules used to enforce substantive law
   c. Applies only to criminal law
   d. Does not involve penalties for violations
8. Criminal law
   a. Includes financial payment for violations but never jail time
   b. Never involves health care practitioners
   c. Involves crimes against the state
   d. Allows violators to be tried in civil court
9. Civil law
   a. Includes felonies and misdemeanors
   b. Is the area of law most likely to affect health care practitioners
   c. Does not involve court cases
   d. Involves crimes against the state
10. A civil offense
    a. Is never unethical
    b. Never involves lawsuits
    c. May involve a family matter
    d. Never applies to health care practitioners
11. *Jurisdiction* refers to
    a. The city in which a felony occurs
    b. The fines levied for civil offenses

c. Crimes against people

d. The court that has the authority to hear and decide a case

LO 4.3

12. Define *tort.*

 a. A tort is a specific type of felony.

 b. A tort is a civil wrong committed against a person or property.

 c. Tort is another term for breach of contract.

 d. A tort is none of the above.

13. What is a tortfeasor?

 a. It is the attorney who represents a client in civil court.

 b. It is a person who commits a felony.

 c. It is the person who commits a tort.

 d. It refers to a court's specific jurisdiction.

14. Negligence is

 a. An intentional tort

 b. The same as assault

 c. A criminal matter

 d. An unintentional tort

15. Intentional torts

 a. Include negligence

 b. Always involve jail time when successfully prosecuted

 c. Include assault, battery, and defamation

 d. Are always felonies

16. If a physician examines a patient without consent, he or she could be charged with which of the following offenses?

 a. Breach of contract

 b. Kidnapping

 c. Battery

 d. Defamation of character

LO 4.4

17. A contract

 a. Is breached only if all parties agree

 b. Is valid only if parties on both sides are competent

 c. Can never be broken

 d. Is valid if an illegal act is involved

18. For what are health care practitioners legally liable?

 a. For all unsatisfactory medical outcomes

 b. For actions of their employees, performed in the course of employment

c. For actions of their employees away from work

d. For actions of their coworkers, performed on the job

19. What is the *consideration* of a contract?

a. The fee, if any, that will be charged

b. Something of value bargained for

c. The terms of the agreement

d. None of these

20. A contract may be voidable if

a. One party leaves town

b. One party decides to cancel the contract

c. One party is a minor

d. One party engages in an illegal act

21. Under what circumstances may breach of contract be charged?

a. If either party fails to fulfill the terms of a valid contract

b. If one party becomes angry with the other

c. If the contract was invalid from the beginning

d. None of these

22. The Statute of Frauds

a. Is federal legislation governing health practitioners accused of fraud

b. Covers both expressed and implied contracts

c. Is state legislation governing written contracts

d. Must be revised every 10 years

23. Third-party payer contracts

a. May be implied

b. Are legally invalid

c. Promise, in writing, that a third party will pay a patient's medical bill

d. Are never used in the medical office

24. Regulation Z of the Consumer Protection Act of 1968 requires that certain financial arrangements be in writing and include

a. Proof of ability to pay a debt

b. A finance charge

c. A minimum of 10 installment payments

d. Proof that the arrangement is for business purposes

25. Which of the following is an example of an implied limited contract?

a. A physician in a medical clinic examines a new patient.

b. A physical therapist meets regularly with a patient and administers range of motion exercises.

c. A dental hygienist cleans a patient's teeth.

d. A physician at the scene provides emergency care to a car accident victim.

LO 4.5

Answer the following questions in the spaces provided.

26. List 10 items to which a physician is *not* bound contractually in the context of an implied physician–patient contract.
27. List 10 items to which a physician is obligated in an implied physician–patient contract.
28. List four responsibilities borne by the patient as implied duties.
29. Is there a federal law that is considered a Patients' Bill of Rights? If not, are there documents that provide an outline for some patients' rights?
30. What are the primary reasons that a patient may leave the hospital against physician orders?

Ethics Issues Law, the Courts, and Contracts

Use your critical thinking skills to answer the questions that follow each ethics issue.

Ethics ISSUE 1:

Advertising by health care providers used to be considered inappropriate and unprofessional. However, now advertising by health care providers is commonplace and accepted by the various professional organizations, as long as there are no false or misleading statements.

Discussion Questions

31. A dentist advertises that he specializes in creating "dazzling smiles." In your opinion, is this an ethical advertisement? Explain your answer.
32. A chiropractor advertises "miracle" treatments to alleviate back pain. In your opinion, is this an ethical advertisement? Explain your answer.
33. Many health care providers advertise on television and online. Do you find these advertisements effective? Have you ever followed up to obtain care as a result of seeing the ad? Describe your experience.
34. What advantages and disadvantages for health care practitioners can you see to the ads?

Ethics ISSUE 2:

Providing proper instructions for a patient's care to the patient or person responsible for the patient is an important aspect of a provider's responsibility. In areas of the country where many different languages may be spoken, this may be a challenge if the providers and staff speak only English. It is also a challenge if the patient or responsible party is unable to read or write.

Discussion Question

35. How would the providers and staff provide written instructions for their patients who do not speak English or if they speak English but are unable to read?

Ethics ISSUE 3:

While in private practice, physicians may determine that they will not accept certain new patients because of their inability to pay or because they have an insurance plan with a poor reimbursement policy.

Discussion Question

36. Should all physicians be required to accept a certain number of patients who cannot pay their bills? In other words, should physicians be required to do a certain amount of charity care? Explain your answer.

Ethics ISSUE 4:

The first objective and the primary goal of every code of ethics and ethics guideline for health care practitioners is the *welfare of the patient.*

Discussion Question

37. A nursing assistant working under the supervision of a registered nurse in a hospital has witnessed several occasions when the RN behaves abusively to elderly patients. What should the nursing assistant do? Are there any possible legal liabilities for the nursing assistant?

Case Studies

Use your critical thinking skills to answer the questions that follow each case study.

LO 4.3 and LO 4.5

An internist had a 54-year-old obese patient who smoked and had a stressful job. After he died of a heart attack, an autopsy revealed that the overweight man had coronary artery disease. The patient's family sued the physician for negligence and won a $3.5 million judgment against the internist. During jury deliberations, some jurors who heard testimony in the case argued that the physician did everything possible to try to help the patient, but others maintained that he could have done more.

38. In your opinion, was the internist negligent for not referring this patient to a cardiologist, as the patient's wife claimed in court? Why or why not?

39. In your opinion, does this case show that people need to take more personal responsibility for their health? Explain your answer.

LO 4.4

Dan, a medical office assistant in a busy clinic, is a sympathetic and understanding employee. Therefore, when an elderly patient complained to him that she "felt terrible most of the time," Dan consoled her. "Don't worry, Mrs. Smith," he told the woman. "Dr. Jones will make you feel better in no time."

40. Has Dan, acting as Dr. Jones's agent, created an implied contract with Mrs. Smith? Explain your answer.

41. If Dan has created an implied contract, can Mrs. Smith sue Dr. Jones if he fails to fulfill the "terms" of the contract? Explain your answer.

42. How might you respond to a patient under similar circumstances?

LO 4.5

43. Does a patient have the legal right to leave the hospital, even though his or her physician believes treatment is incomplete? What procedure should be followed if a patient leaves a hospital against medical advice?

44. Does a patient have the right to know if medical treatment is experimental and to refuse to participate in such treatment? Explain your answer.

Internet Activities

LO 4.1 and LO 4.2

Complete the activities and answer the questions that follow.

45. Does your state have a statutory Patients' Bill of Rights? Where in the statutes is it found? If your state does not have a statutory Patients' Bill of Rights, find a state that does.
46. Locate the Web site for the Agency for Healthcare Research and Quality (AHRQ). Who sponsors this Web site? What is its purpose? Find at least two important studies about health care access and summarize the cases.

Resources

LO 4.1, 4.2, 4.3, and 4.4

Kubasek, Nancy, et al. *Dynamic Business Law.* New York: McGraw-Hill, 2009.

Liuzzo, Anthony L. *Essentials of Business Law.* New York: McGraw-Hill, 2010.

Mitchell, Joyce, and Lee Haroun. *Introduction to Health Care.* New York: Delmar, 2002.

LO 4.5

Patients' Bill of Rights: www.aha.org/advocacy-issues/communicatingpts/pt-care-partnership.shtml

Against Medical Advice: www.ncbi.nlm.nih.gov/pmc/articles/PMC2664598/ and https://psnet.ahrq.gov/webmm/case/96

PART TWO

Legal Issues for Working Health Care Practitioners

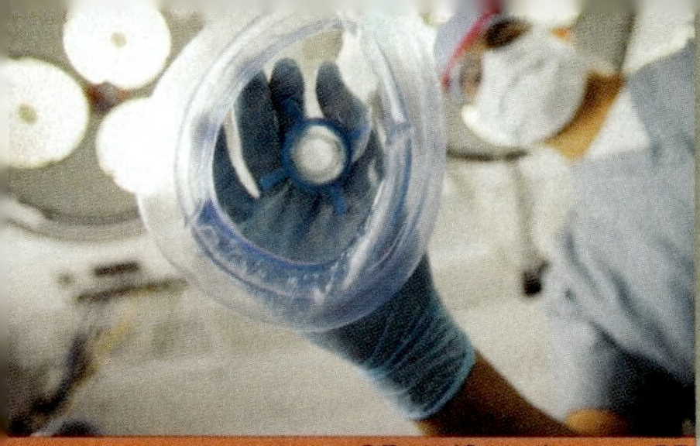

©Fuse/Getty Images RF

5

Professional Liability and Medical Malpractice

Key Terms

alternative dispute resolution (ADR)
confidentiality
damages
deposition
duty of care
interrogatory
law of agency
liable
malfeasance
misfeasance
nonfeasance
privacy
privileged communication
reasonable person standard
res ipsa loquitur
respondeat superior
standard of care
subpoena
subpoena *duces tecum*
summons
testimony
wrongful death statutes

LEARNING OUTCOMES

After studying this chapter, you should be able to:

LO 5.1 Define *liability, law of agency,* and *respondeat superior.*

LO 5.2 Describe the reasonable person standard, standard of care, and duty of care.

LO 5.3 Briefly outline the responsibilities of health care practitioners concerning privacy, confidentiality, and privileged communication.

LO 5.4 Explain the four elements necessary to prove negligence (the four Ds).

LO 5.5 Outline the phases of a lawsuit.

LO 5.6 Discuss patient safety standards as related to medical malpractice prevention.

LO 5.7 Identify when the use of alternative dispute resolution in resolving medical malpractice claims is most effective.

FROM THE PERSPECTIVE OF. . .

TINA, A MEDICAL RECORDS SUPERVISOR in a small-town medical clinic, always spends a lot of time with new employees reviewing the importance of confidentiality. One of her real-life lessons is about the new employee, Samantha, who accidentally and innocently violated confidentiality, causing the clinic where she worked to be sued.

Samantha saw one of her high school friends in the hallway of the clinic. The friend told Samantha that she was pregnant. A week later, Samantha saw her friend's mother in the local grocery store and congratulated her on becoming a grandmother. What Samantha did not know was that her friend was not planning to continue the pregnancy and had told no one that she was pregnant. The clinic was sued for violating confidentiality. Tina's strong advice to all employees has since become: "What you learn in this clinic *stays* in this clinic."

From Tina's perspective, even remarks that seem innocent and harmless, if spoken outside the health care workplace, can violate privacy and create liability for employers and employees.

From the perspective of new employees, Samantha's experience is a lesson well-learned.

From the perspective of Samantha, who did not think twice before she spoke, what she thought were innocent remarks created a distressing and damaging situation. Samantha's career in health care was over before it had begun.

5.1 Liability

The **law of agency,** sometimes referred to simply as agency, refers to the common law situation in business where the principal (employer) authorizes an agent (employee) to deal with a third person (the customer, supplier, or other third party) on the principal's behalf. While all competent adults are **liable,** or legally responsible for their actions, both on and off the job, agency has held that employers are vicariously liable for the acts of their employees performed as part of their employment. Even if an employer was not present when an employee performed certain acts and even if the employer had no intention to cause harm, he or she can be held liable for an employee's acts.

Agency may be expressed or implied. If agency is expressed, a written contract exists, naming the employee as the employer's agent. If agency is implied, both parties have agreed, although not explicitly in writing, that the employee will act on the employer's behalf. In the health care environment, agency is most often implied. Health care practitioners act as their employers' agents when they schedule patient appointments; speak with patients, their families, and representatives; help with or perform patient exams; order supplies for the workplace; file insurance claims; and so on.

Agency often comes up in personal injury cases when an injured plaintiff sues both a defendant and the defendant's employer under the rule of ***respondeat superior***, which means "Let the master answer." When an agency relationship exists, the principal (employer/master) is

law of agency
The law that governs the relationship between a principal and his or her agent.

liable
Legally responsible or obligated.

respondeat superior
Literally, "Let the master answer." A doctrine under which an employer is legally liable for the acts of his or her employees, if such acts were performed within the scope of the employees' duties.

responsible for any injuries his agent (employee) causes while dealing with the third person (plaintiff). Injuries claimed may be physical, emotional, and financial.

For a lawsuit to succeed under *respondeat superior*, the injured plaintiff must prove:

1. The injury to the plaintiff occurred while the employee was actually working for the employer.
2. The injury was caused by something the employee would ordinarily do while working for the employer.
3. The employer benefited in some way, however small or indirect, from the action the employee was performing when the injury occurred.

Employers have general liability for:

Employment Buildings and Grounds. Adequate upkeep helps ensure that employees and third parties are not injured on the premises. Employers must provide protection against theft, fire, and burglary in the building and must take all precautions to ensure that business records are protected. Employers must have theft, fire, and liability insurance to cover the workplace.

Automobiles. If employees must use their own or the employer's automobile in the performance of their daily work (for example, to drop off or pick up mail or supplies), the employer must be adequately insured for liability in the event of an accident.

Employee Safety. Employers must provide a reasonably comfortable and safe work environment for employees. State (and, in some instances, federal) regulations apply, but they vary from state to state. Employers should check with the state agency governing safety in the workplace, with workers' compensation laws, and with state medical societies to determine safety rules, rights, and responsibilities. A general safety procedure book for medical office workers should include guidelines for the handling of hazardous laboratory wastes and materials.

COURT CASE Patient Sues Hospital over Nurse's Statements

A man entered a hospital in Billings, Montana, for the purpose of having a blood clot removed from his leg. The patient alleged that the medical personnel intentionally injured him during the procedure, and he charged assault and battery. The assault and battery charges were dismissed, but the patient filed additional charges that an unidentified nurse on staff at the hospital told him the blood clot in his leg had been removed when, in fact, it had not. The patient also claimed that the nurse had slandered him when she told the patient's sister that he was "out of his mind" and should be committed to a mental hospital. The patient also alleged the hospital was responsible for the nurse's actions under the doctrine of *respondeat superior.* The nurse was never named in the patient's lawsuit, and the court found that her alleged statement was not part of her expected duties as an employee of the hospital, so the hospital could not be held liable. The court also held that the nurse had expressed a personal opinion, and as such, it did not fall under the state's liable laws. The hospital was granted summary judgment, and the action was dismissed.

Source: *Kerr v. St. Vincent Healthcare*, District. Court, D Montana 2016.

5.2 Standard of Care and Duty of Care

Standard of care refers to the level of performance expected of a health care practitioner in carrying out his or her professional duties. **Duty of care** is the obligation of health care workers to patients and, in some cases, nonpatients. Physicians have a duty of care to patients with whom they have established a physician–patient relationship, but they may also be held to a duty of care toward people who are not patients, such as the patient's family members, former patients, and even office personnel. Generally, if actions or omissions within the scope of a health care

standard of care
The level of performance expected of a health care practitioner in carrying out his or her professional duties.

duty of care
The legal obligation of health care workers to patients and, sometimes, nonpatients.

LANDMARK COURT CASE

Therapists Found Guilty of Failure to Warn

In October 1969, Prosenjit Poddar, a foreign student from Bengal, India, killed Tatiana Tarasoff. Two months before, Poddar had confided his intention to kill Tarasoff to Dr. Lawrence Moore, a psychologist employed by the Cowell Memorial Hospital at the University of California, Berkeley. Poddar told Moore he would kill Tarasoff after she returned from spending the summer in Brazil.

Acting on this information, Moore notified the campus police, who briefly detained Poddar but determined that Poddar was rational and released him. Upon Poddar's release, Moore's superior, Dr. Harvey Powelson, directed that all of the letters and notes Moore had written while counseling Poddar be destroyed and no further action be taken to detain Poddar in the future.

Soon thereafter, Poddar convinced Tarasoff's brother to share an apartment with him near Tarasoff's residence. When she returned from Brazil, Poddar went to Tarasoff's home and killed her. Tarasoff had not been warned of the possible danger Poddar posed.

Tarasoff's parents sued, arguing that the psychologist had a duty to warn them of Poddar's danger to their daughter and that the campus police negligently released Poddar without notifying them of their daughter's grave danger. They also argued that the police failed to confine Poddar under the Lanterman-Petris-Short Act, a California law designed to protect mentally ill and mentally disabled persons from certain abuses and to guarantee and protect the public interest.

The defendants argued that there was no duty of care toward Tatiana Tarasoff and that, as employees of the state, they had governmental immunity. The trial court granted the defendants' motion to dismiss. On the plaintiffs' appeal, the court affirmed dismissals against defendant police on all claims, stating there was no duty to plaintiffs. Dismissals against the defendant therapists were also upheld, holding they were protected by governmental immunity. Plaintiffs appealed to the Supreme Court of California.

The Supreme Court allowed the plaintiffs to amend their appeal to state that the therapists failed to warn Tarasoff (rather than her parents, as in the original complaint).

The Supreme Court of California heard the case based on the question "Did defendant therapists have a duty to warn Tatiana Tarasoff?"

Yes, the court determined. It was found that the defendant therapists should have determined that Poddar presented a serious danger to Tarasoff and that they failed to exercise reasonable care to protect her from that danger (i.e., when a therapist determines that a patient poses a danger to another individual, he or she is obligated to use reasonable care to protect that individual). Therefore, defendant therapists breached their duty of care to Tatiana Tarasoff and were negligent by not warning her of the possible danger posed by Poddar.

Prosenjit Poddar was later convicted of second-degree murder, but the conviction was appealed and overturned, based on the decision that the jury was inadequately informed. No second trial was held, and Poddar was released on the condition that he return to India.

Source: *Tarasoff v. Regents of University of California,* 17 Cal.3d 425, 131 Cal. Rptr. 14, 551 P.2d 334 (1976).

practitioner's job could cause harm to someone, that person is owed a duty of care.

For example, medical facility custodians are nonpatients to whom a duty of care is owed. Various drugs, equipment, and supplies are used and discarded daily in a medical facility. Procedures for the proper disposal of drugs and potentially hazardous materials should be detailed in a facility's safety manual, so that employees who handle these materials do not accidentally prick themselves with used needles or otherwise injure themselves.

In some instances, depending on the situation and state law, physicians may have a duty under standard of care to warn nonpatients of danger, as in the case of a psychiatric patient who threatens harm to others or in the case of a patient with a communicable disease.

reasonable person standard
That standard of behavior that judges a person's actions in a situation according to what a reasonable person would or would not do under similar circumstances.

We are responsible for our actions (or our failure to act) under the **reasonable person standard.** That is, we may be charged with negligence if someone is injured because we failed to perform an act that a reasonable person, in similar circumstances, would perform or if we committed an act that a reasonable person would not commit. Professionals—individuals who are specially trained to perform specific tasks—are held to a higher standard of care than nonprofessionals (laypersons). If a patient is injured because a health care professional failed to exercise the care and expertise that under the circumstances could reasonably be expected of a professional with similar experience and training, then that professional may be liable for negligence.

PHYSICIANS

A physician in general practice is expected to conform to the standards of other general practitioners in his or her own or a comparable community. A specialist is held to a higher standard of care than that expected of a general practitioner. The standard of care for a specialist is generally the same as that for like specialists, wherever they practice. Similarly, any health care practitioner—nurse, phlebotomist, dental assistant, physician assistant—is expected to conform to the standards of like practitioners in his or her own or a comparable community.

Courts have generally held that informal consultations among physicians do not create a physician–patient relationship and thus do not create a duty of care, as discussed in the classic case, "Consultation Did Not Establish a Duty of Care" in this section.

GUIDELINES FOR PHYSICIANS AND OTHER HEALTH CARE PRACTITIONERS

The following guidelines can help all health care practitioners stay within the scope of their practices and operate within the law and the policies of any employing health care facility. All are addressed at length throughout the text.

- Practice within the scope of your training and capabilities.
- Use the professional title commensurate with your education and experience.
- Maintain confidentiality.
- Prepare and maintain health records.

- Document accurately.
- Use appropriate legal and ethical guidelines when releasing information.
- Follow an employer's established policies dealing with the health care contract.
- Follow legal guidelines and maintain awareness of health care legislation and regulations.
- Maintain and dispose of regulated substances in compliance with government guidelines.
- Follow established risk management and safety procedures.
- Meet the requirements for professional credentialing.
- Help develop and maintain personnel, policy, and procedure manuals.

Laws clearly dictate what a member of a health care profession can and cannot do on the job. However, in addition to knowing the law, a health care practitioner should know what policies and procedures apply specifically to his or her place of employment. Policy and procedure manuals that clearly define a health care practitioner's responsibilities can serve as a valuable guide and as evidence that policies and procedures are in writing if legal suits should arise.

LANDMARK COURT CASE

Consultation Did Not Establish a Duty of Care

The doctrine that informal physician consultations do not create a physician–patient relationship was established in 1973 in the California decision *Ranier v. Grossman*. Morton Grossman was a professor of gastroenterology who often lectured physicians at their hospitals, then offered to review their cases with them. After one such lecture, a physician presented the X-rays and medical history for a patient who suffered from ulcerative colitis. Grossman advised surgery without examining the patient. The surgery was subsequently performed, and the patient sued, claiming that the surgery had been unnecessary. Grossman was cited as a codefendant in the patient's lawsuit. An appeals court upheld summary judgment in Grossman's favor, holding that he had no duty to the patient because he had no direct contact with her and had no control over her treating physicians.

Source: *Rainer v. Grossman*, 107 Cal. Rptr. 469, 31 Cal. App. 3d 539 (1973).

Check Your Progress

1. Define *law of agency*.
2. Define *respondeat superior*.
3. What three elements must be met for a lawsuit to be filed under *respondeat superior*?
4. ______________________ refers to the level of performance expected of health care practitioners in carrying out their professional duties.
5. ______________________ refers to the legal obligation of health care workers to patients and, sometimes, nonpatients.
6. ______________________ refers to the standard of behavior that judges a person's actions in a situation according to the actions of others considered "reasonable."

5.3 Privacy, Confidentiality, and Privileged Communication

privacy
Freedom from unauthorized intrusion.

confidentiality
The act of holding information in confidence, not to be released to unauthorized individuals.

privileged communication
Information held confidential within a protected relationship.

Not only do physicians and other health care professionals owe a duty of care to patients, but it is also their ethical and legal duty to safeguard a patient's **privacy** and maintain **confidentiality.**

Privileged communication refers to information held confidential within a protected relationship. Attorney–client and physician–patient are examples of relationships in which the law, under certain circumstances, protects the holder of information from forced disclosure on the witness stand. Privileged communication statutes vary from state to state, but in most states, patients may sue a physician or any other health care practitioner for breach of confidence if the holder released protected information and damage to the patient resulted. In many states, breach of confidence is grounds for revocation of a physician's license.

Because health care procedures and facilities present numerous opportunities for a breach of confidentiality (as was the case with Samantha in the chapter's opening scenario), health care practitioners must make every effort to safeguard each patient's privacy. Privacy, confidentiality, and privileged communication are such important subjects for health care practitioners that they are discussed separately in Chapter 8.

The following suggestions for maintaining confidentiality of patient health care records can serve as a guide for all health care practitioners who may be asked to provide or release patient information:

- Do not disclose any information about a patient to a third party without signed consent. This extends to insurance companies, attorneys, and curious neighbors, and it includes acknowledging whether or not the person in question is a patient.
- Do not decide confidentiality on the basis of whether or not you approve of or agree with the views or morals of the patient.
- Do not reveal financial information about a patient because this is also confidential. For instance, be discreet when revealing a patient's account balance so that others in the vicinity do not overhear.
- When talking on the telephone with a patient, do not use the patient's name if others in the room might overhear.
- Use caution in giving the results of medical tests to patients over the telephone to prevent others in the medical office from overhearing. Furthermore, when leaving a message on voice mail or at a patient's place of employment, simply ask the patient to return a call regarding a recent visit or appointment on a specific date. No mention should be made of the nature of the call. It is inadvisable to leave a message with a receptionist or coworker on an answering machine for the patient to call an oncologist, an obstetrician-gynecologist, and so forth. If test results are abnormal, usually the physician speaks directly to the patient, and an appointment is made to discuss the results.
- Do not leave patient information of any kind where other patients or visitors can see it. Confidentiality protocol must be duly noted in the facility's procedures manual, and new employees must learn it.

- If a patient is unwilling to release privileged information, the information should not be released. Exceptions include legally required disclosures, such as those ordered by subpoena; those dictated by statute to protect public health or welfare; or those considered necessary to protect the welfare of a patient or a third party.

Confidentiality may be waived under the following circumstances:

- Sometimes when a third party requests a medical examination, such as for employment, and that party pays the physician's fee
- Generally when a patient sues a physician for malpractice and patient records are subpoenaed
- When a waiver has been signed by the patient allowing the release of information (see Figure 5-1)

I authorize:

Name of person or institution ____________________
(Provider of information)

Street address ____________________

City, state, Zip code ____________________

To release medical information to:

Name of person or institution ____________________
(Recipient of information)

Street address ____________________

City, state, Zip code ____________________

Attention ____________________

Nature of information to be disclosed:

☐ Clinical notes pertaining to evaluation and treatment ____________________

☐ Other, please specify ____________________

Purpose of disclosure:

☐ Continuing medical care ____________________

☐ Second opinion ____________________

☐ Other, please specify ____________________

This authorization will automatically expire one year from the date of signature, unless specified otherwise ____________________

This consent may be revoked at any time by sending written notice to the above-named provider of information. Any release of information made prior to the revocation of this complaint, authorization is not a breach of confidentiality. Disclosed information may be reviewed by contacting the provider of information.

Patient's name ____________________

Signature of patient or legal guardian ____________________ Date ____________________

Complete address ____________________

Relationship, if not the patient ____________________ Patient's date of birth ____________________

Specific consent for release of information protected by state or federal law

Iowa law (and in some cases federal law) provides spacial confidentiality protection to information relating to substance abuse, mental health, and HIV-related testing. In order for information to be released on this subject matter, this specific authorization and the above authorization must be signed:

I authorize release of information relating to:

☐ Substance abuse (alcohol/drug abuse)

Signature of patient or legal guardian ____________________ Date ____________________

☐ Mental health (includes psychological testing and mental health counseling)

Signature of patient or legal guardian ____________________ Date ____________________

☐ HIV-related information (AIDS-related testing)

Signature of patient or legal guardian ____________________ Date ____________________

Date Information is sent ____________________

Sent by (name) ____________________

To the recipient of this information: This information has been disclosed to you from records protected by federal confidentiality rules. The federal rules prohibit you from making further disclosure without additional consent.

FIGURE 5-1
Consent to Release Information

Check Your Progress

7. Define *privileged communications.*
8. Is breach of confidentiality an offense for which a health care provider may be sued? Explain your answer.

5.4 The Tort of Negligence

The unintentional tort of negligence is the basis for professional malpractice claims and is the most common liability in medicine. When health care practitioners are sued for medical malpractice, the term generally means any deviation from the accepted medical standard of care that causes injury to a patient.

Hospitals have also been found guilty of negligence. Under the theory of corporate liability, hospitals have been found to have an independent duty to patients, including a duty to grant privileges only to competent doctors, to supervise the overall medical treatment of patients, and to review the competence of staff physicians.

All medical professional liability claims are classified in one of three ways, based on the root word *feasance,* which means "the performance of an act."

malfeasance
The performance of a totally wrongful and unlawful act.

Malfeasance. The performance of a totally wrongful and unlawful act. For example, in the absence of the employing physician, a medical assistant determines that a patient needs a prescription drug and dispenses the wrong drug from the physician's supply. Medical assistants are not licensed to practice medicine, and the wrong drug was dispensed, so the act was totally wrongful and unlawful and could be called malfeasance.

misfeasance
The performance of a lawful act in an illegal or improper manner.

Misfeasance. The performance of a lawful act in an illegal or improper manner. Suppose a physician orders his or her nurse-employee to change a sterile dressing on a patient's burned hand. The nurse changes the dressing but does not use sterile technique, and the patient's burn becomes infected. The nurse is legally authorized to carry out the physician's instructions in dressing the patient's hand but violated proper procedure in carrying out the physician's order.

nonfeasance
The failure to act when one should.

Nonfeasance. The failure to act when one should. For example, a newly certified emergency medical technician (EMT) is first on the scene of a traffic accident. An injured motorist stops breathing and appears to be in cardiac arrest. The EMT, though trained in cardiopulmonary resuscitation, "freezes" and does nothing. The patient dies. In failing to act, the EMT could be guilty of nonfeasance.

Four elements must be present in a given situation to prove that a health care professional is guilty of negligence. Sometimes called the "four Ds of negligence," these elements include:

- *Duty*–The person charged with negligence owed a duty of care to the accuser.
- *Dereliction*–The health care provider breached the duty of care to the patient.

- *Damage*–The health care provider's dereliction of duty caused *injury* to the patient. (Depending on the outcome of malpractice trials, monetary awards to plaintiffs may be court-ordered as compensation for proven injuries. These awards are referred to as damages.)
- *Direct Cause*–The breach of the duty of care to the patient was a direct cause of the patient's injury.

In this chapter's opening scenario, how does Samantha's act illustrate the four Ds? In your opinion, does her act illustrate malfeasance, misfeasance, or nonfeasance?

When a plaintiff sues a health care practitioner (defendant) for negligence, the burden of proof is on the plaintiff. That is, it is up to the accuser's attorney to present evidence of the four Ds.

State statutes must be consulted for restrictions that apply to actions against health care providers. Some states limit damage awards or mandate procedural rules that must be followed in medical malpractice claims. In some states, for example, medical review panels must screen claims before they are brought to court. The panel examines the facts and then issues a finding of "malpractice" or "no malpractice." Such panels are generally composed of physicians with expertise in the medical specialty in question and sometimes include a neutral attorney.

COURT CASE

Appellate Court Allows Negligence Case to Proceed

In 2009, a woman went to an ambulatory surgery center for an endoscopic ultrasound. A registered nurse tried to start an intravenous line on the patient's right wrist prior to the scheduled procedure. The patient experienced immediate pain, in response to which the nurse allegedly exclaimed, "Oops. I slipped. . . . I haven't done that in 20 years." The nurse left the patient's bedside "visibly upset," returning with someone the patient believed to be a supervisor, who successfully inserted the IV line. Following the failed IV insertion, the patient experienced pain, swelling, bruising, and a loss of strength in her right wrist. According to the patient's treating orthopedist, her condition was most likely the result of an "irritation of the superficial radial nerve."

The patient started a medical malpractice and negligence action against the nurse, seeking to recover for the injury allegedly sustained as the result of the failed IV attempt. In a deposition, the nurse said she didn't recall the incident but was "reasonably sure" she had followed standard procedure for inserting an IV line. She also said if it was true that she erred in starting the IV line, she "would have charted the mistake." Because there was no error recorded in the patient's medical record, she continued, "it didn't exist." The nurse moved for summary judgment to dismiss the claim, which the court denied and an appellate court affirmed, allowing the suit to proceed.

(As of mid-2016, no final resolution was published.)

Source: *Weeks v St. Peter's Hosp.*, 128 AD3d 1159, 1160 [2015].

Check Your Progress

9. Distinguish between *malfeasance*, *misfeasance*, and *nonfeasance*.
10. Define the four Ds of negligence.

RES IPSA LOQUITUR

res ipsa loquitur
"The thing speaks for itself"; also known as the doctrine of common knowledge. A situation that is so obviously negligent that no expert witnesses need be called.

Res ipsa loquitur is Latin for "the thing speaks for itself." It is also known as the doctrine of common knowledge. It means that the mistake is so obvious—such as leaving a sponge or surgical instrument inside a patient after surgery or operating on the wrong body part—that negligence is obvious. The defendant in such a case may argue that the event was an inevitable accident and had nothing to do with his or her responsibility of control or supervision. Traditionally, expert witnesses did not have to be called to testify in a medical malpractice lawsuit alleging *res ipsa loquitur,* but courts have made exceptions in many cases and allowed expert witness testimony. Judicial consideration of this doctrine varies. Generally, for *res ipsa loquitur* to apply, three conditions must exist:

1. The act of negligence must obviously be under the defendant's control.
2. The patient must not have contributed to the act.
3. It must be apparent that the patient would not have been injured if reasonable care had been used.

Cases that fall under the doctrine of *res ipsa loquitur* include:

- Unintentionally leaving foreign bodies, such as sponges or instruments, inside a patient's body during surgery
- Accidentally burning or otherwise injuring a patient while he or she is anesthetized
- Damaging healthy tissue during an operation
- Causing an infection by the use of unsterilized instruments

COURT CASE

Res Ipsa Loquitur Case Results in Damage Award

In 2001, a registered nurse had a hysterectomy at a Kentucky Medical Center. The patient's doctor performed the surgery, with the medical center providing operating room facilities and the surgical support staff. In the years following the 2001 surgery, the patient began experiencing intestinal and digestive problems, pain, and other serious physical symptoms indicating that something was wrong in her abdomen. In 2005, a CT scan revealed the presence of a surgical sponge in the patient's abdomen. The sponge was surgically removed the next day. The surgery required a trisection of the patient's small intestines and disclosed an infection in the area where the sponge was located.

Appellants filed a timely action alleging that the sponge left in the patient's abdomen was caused by the negligence of the doctor who performed the surgery in 2001 and three of the medical center's operating room nurses. The first trial ended in a damage award of $861,178.08 for the plaintiff. The suit progressed through several appeals and a second trial, where evidentiary issues were confronted, but the damage award was allowed to stand.

Source: *Savage v. Three Rivers Medical Center*, 390 SW 3d 104 Supreme Court 2012

Table 5-1 Damage Awards

Types of Damages	Purpose	Considered by Court	Award
General compensatory	To compensate for injuries or losses due to violation of patient's rights	Physical disability? Loss of earnings? Mental anguish? Loss of service of spouse or child? Losses to date? Future losses?	Specified by court. Dollar value need not be proved; loss must be proved.
Special compensatory	To compensate for losses not directly caused by the wrong	Additional medical expenses?	Specified by court. Dollar value and loss must be proved.
Consequential	To compensate for losses caused indirectly by a product defect	Loss covered by product warranty? Personal injury?	No limit on damages if personal injuries
Punitive	To punish the offender	How serious was the breach of conduct? How much can the defendant afford to pay?	In some cases, the amount of damages is set by law.
Nominal	To recognize that rights of the patient were violated, though no actual loss was proved	Legal rights of the patient violated? Actual loss proved?	Token award, usually $1

DAMAGE AWARDS AND MEDICAL MALPRACTICE INSURANCE

When a defendant is found guilty of a tort—such as negligence, breach of contract, libel, or slander—the plaintiff is awarded compensation based on the extent of his or her injuries, loss of income, damage to reputation, or other harm that can be proved. This monetary compensation is called **damages.** Table 5-1 explains the various types of damages and how the court determines them.

damages
Court-ordered monetary awards to patients, given as a result of legally recognized injuries to patients

Physicians and many other professional health care providers carry liability insurance, which pays damage awards in the event of a negligence or malpractice suit up to the limits of the policy (see Table 5-2 for survey of 4,000 physicians in 2015).

Medical groups maintain that high damage awards in tort cases have led to a malpractice insurance crisis for physicians, especially those in high-risk specialties such as obstetrics-gynecology, orthopedic surgery, and general surgery. Recent studies and news articles have reported that doctors in some states are participating in walkouts and demonstrations, relocating to states where caps have been legislated on medical malpractice damage awards, limiting procedures, performing additional patient tests to cover all liability bases, and even leaving the profession. Furthermore, some hospitals have shut down or threatened to shut down trauma centers, and long-term care facilities have closed.

In an attempt to address rapidly rising premiums for medical malpractice insurance, some states have placed caps on damage awards in medical malpractice cases. Attorney organizations, however, insist that damage caps are unfair to injured patients.

The issue is an important one for both health care practitioners and patients and is not likely to be settled

Table 5-2 Medical Specialties Most Likely to Be Sued

In a survey of 4,000 physicians surveyed by Medscape in 2015, the following specialties said they had been sued:

Ob/Gyn/Women's health	85%
Surgery	83%
Orthopedics	79%
Radiology	72%
Anesthesiology	58%
Internal medicine/Family medicine	46%
Oncology	34%

Source: *Medscape Malpractice Report 2015*: "Why Most Doctors Get Sued" www.medscape.com/features/slideshow/public/malpractice-report-2015.

uniformly across the country. As a future or present health care practitioner, you should stay informed on the issues of medical malpractice insurance and tort reform and form your own opinion.

WRONGFUL DEATH STATUTES

wrongful death statutes
State statutes that allow a person's beneficiaries to collect for loss to the estate of the deceased for future earnings when a death is judged to have been due to negligence.

Most states have enacted **wrongful death statutes** that allow a patient's beneficiaries to collect from a health care practitioner for loss to the patient's estate of future earnings when a patient's death is judged to have been due to negligence of health care practitioners. In most states, a cap has been placed on the amount of damages that can be recovered in a civil action for wrongful death.

The state may also prosecute a health care practitioner under criminal statutes for the wrongful death of a patient.

Check Your Progress

11. What is the legal basis for professional malpractice claims?
12. Name two types of cases that fall under the doctrine of *res ipsa loquitur.*
13. For what purpose are special compensatory damages awarded? Punitive damages?
14. When a patient's death is judged to have been due to negligence of health care practitioners, a suit may be brought by the deceased patient's beneficiaries under ______________.
15. What have some states done to address rapidly rising premiums for medical malpractice insurance?

5.5 Elements of a Lawsuit

As indicated in Chapter 4, the type of court that hears a case depends on the offense or complaint. In civil malpractice or negligence cases, the party bringing the action (plaintiff) must prove the case by presenting to a judge or jury evidence that is more convincing than that of the opposing side (defendant).

PRETRIAL SCREENING BEFORE A LAWSUIT

Before a lawsuit is actually filed, informal screenings, or *pretrial screenings,* may be held by a neutral party to assess the relative strengths of each party's case and determine whether the situation merits going to trial. Such screenings are a way to discourage cases that are not based on merit and save costs to both parties. One reason this is particularly well suited to the medical field is the fact that approximately 70 percent of medical malpractice cases are dismissed by a judge during summary judgment as meritless. However, there are high costs associated with defending a lawsuit, even to the point of dismissal—typical costs at this stage range between $24,000 and $90,000—and pretrial screenings allow both parties to avoid these costs and to avoid the stress inherent in experiencing a lawsuit.

Pretrial screenings are helpful for a second reason as well: They can help educate plaintiffs that there may not be sufficient grounds for a successful lawsuit. One reason for the high number of meritless claims of medical malpractice is that plaintiffs are often confused about what does and does not constitute negligence. For instance, the practice of medicine, particularly surgery, carries inherent risk. Complications such as infection, bleeding, pain, and death are inevitable no matter how well trained or conscientious the surgeons and other medical professionals. For the patient, however, complications after any surgery or medical procedure may trigger the desire for some form of remedy. In some cases, the remedy sought may be as simple as an explanation or an apology, but because medical professionals often fear explanations or apologies will indicate guilt, they move first to defend themselves against the perception that they erred. When combined with an injured patient's distress, the result is sometimes a lawsuit.

Approximately half of all states require pretrial screening before plaintiffs (parties bringing the action) pursue medical malpractice litigation against defendants (accused parties) in civil court.

After pretrial screening, a case may or may not proceed to medical malpractice litigation.

PHASES OF A LAWSUIT

The typical malpractice or negligence lawsuit proceeds as follows:

1. A patient feels he or she has been injured.
2. The patient seeks the advice of an attorney.
3. If the attorney believes the case has merit, he or she then requests copies of the patient's medical records. The attorney reviews the medical records and the appropriate standard of care to ascertain merits of the case. In some states, before proceeding to a lawsuit, the attorney must obtain an expert witness report stating that the standard of care has been violated. An affidavit to that effect must then be submitted. An affidavit is a sworn statement in writing made under oath. It may also be a declaration before an authorized officer of the court.

Pleading Phase

4. The plaintiff's (injured patient's) attorney files a complaint with the clerk of the court. In this document, the plaintiff states his or her version of the situation and the amount of money sought from the defendant (the practitioner being sued) for the plaintiff's injury.
5. A **summons** is issued by the clerk of the court and is delivered with a copy of the complaint to the defendant, directing him or her to respond to the charges. If the defendant does not respond within the specified time limit, he or she can lose the case by default.
6. The defendant's attorney files an answer to the summons, and a copy of it is sent to the plaintiff. In this document, the defendant

summons
A written notification issued by the clerk of the court and delivered with a copy of the complaint to the defendant in a lawsuit, directing him or her to respond to the charges brought in a court of law.

presents his or her version of the case, either admitting or denying the charges. The defendant may also file a counterclaim or a cross-complaint.

7. If a cross-complaint is made, the plaintiff files a reply.

Interrogatory or Pretrial Discovery Phase

8. The court sets a trial date.
9. Pretrial motions may be made and decided. For example, the defendant may request that the lawsuit be dismissed, the plaintiff may amend the original complaint, or either side may request a change of venue (ask that the trial be held in another place).
10. Discovery procedures may be used to uncover evidence that will support the charges when the case comes to court. A court order called a **subpoena** may be issued commanding the presence of the physician or a medical facility employee in court or requiring that a **deposition** be taken. A deposition is sworn testimony given and recorded outside the courtroom during the pretrial phase of a case. (See the following section entitled "Witness Testimony.")

    An **interrogatory** may be requested instead of or in addition to a deposition. This is a written set of questions requiring written answers from a plaintiff or defendant under oath.

    The subpoena commanding a witness to appear in court and to bring certain medical records is called a **subpoena *duces tecum***. Failure to obey a subpoena may result in contempt-of-court charges. Contempt of court is willful disobedience to or open disrespect of a court, judge, or legislative body. It is punishable by fines or imprisonment.
11. A pretrial conference may be called by the judge scheduled to hear the case. During this conference, the judge discusses the issues in the case with the opposing attorneys. This helps avoid surprises and delays after the trial starts and may lead to an out-of-court settlement. (*Note:* At any point after the complaint is filed before the case comes to trial, an out-of-court settlement may be reached.)

subpoena
A legal document requiring the recipient to appear as a witness in court or to give a deposition.

deposition
Sworn testimony given and recorded outside the courtroom during the pretrial phase of a case.

interrogatory
A written set of questions requiring written answers from a plaintiff or defendant under oath.

subpoena *duces tecum*
A legal document requiring the recipient to bring certain written records to court to be used as evidence in a lawsuit.

Trial Phase

12. The jury is selected (if one is to be used), and the trial begins.
13. Opening *statements* are made by the lawyers for the plaintiff and the defendant, summarizing what each will prove during the trial.
14. Witnesses are called to testify for both sides. They may be cross-examined by opposing attorneys.
15. Each attorney makes closing *arguments* that the evidence presented supports his or her version of the case. No new evidence may be presented during summation.
16. The judge gives instructions to the jury (if one was chosen), and the jury retires to deliberate.
17. The jury reaches a verdict.
18. The final judgment is handed down by the court. The judge bases his or her decision for judgment on the jury's verdict.

Appeals Phase

19. Posttrial motions may be filed.
20. An appeal may be made for the case to be reviewed by a higher court if the evidence indicates that errors may have been made or if there was injustice or impropriety in the trial court proceedings. During an appeal, the judge has the option of affirming, reversing, or modifying a decision. A judgment is final only when all options for appeal have been exercised.

WITNESS TESTIMONY

An estimated 9 out of 10 lawsuits are settled out of court, but health care practitioners are often asked to give testimony. Testimony may be given in court on the witness stand, or it may be given in an attorney's conference room in a pretrial proceeding called a deposition. (See the earlier section entitled "Interrogatory or Pretrial Discovery Phase.") Depositions are of two types:

1. Discovery depositions.
2. Depositions in lieu of trial.

Discovery depositions cover material that will most likely be examined again when the witness testifies in court. Because there will be an opportunity for the opposing attorney to question the witness a second time in court, the deposition need not cover every possible question.

Both before a deposition and before in-court testimony, the witness is sworn to tell the truth and then is questioned by attorneys representing both sides. During courtroom testimony, however, a judge is present to rule on objections raised by the attorneys. When an objection is raised, the witness should stop speaking until the judge either *sustains* or *overrules* the objection. If the objection is sustained, the witness need not answer the question. If the objection is overruled, the witness must answer. If in doubt about whether an objection to a question was sustained or overruled, the witness may ask the judge whether a question should be answered. During a deposition, witnesses should take the attorney's advice regarding questions that should be answered.

Depositions in lieu of trial are used instead of the witness's in-person testimony in court. Because the opposing attorney has one opportunity to question the witness, questions are thorough, and the witness should carefully consider his or her answers.

Sometimes depositions in lieu of trial are videotaped, to be played in the courtroom during the trial. Witnesses whose depositions will be videotaped should be informed in advance, so they can dress as though they were appearing in court in person.

Witnesses may offer two kinds of **testimony:** fact and expert. Health care practitioners or laypersons may offer *fact testimony,* and this type of testimony concerns only those facts the witness has observed. For example, regarding testimony in a medical malpractice case, medical assistants, LPNs/LVNs, and registered nurses may testify about how many times a patient saw the physician, the patient's appearance during a particular visit, or similar observations. If asked to give fact testimony, a health care practitioner's powers of observation and memory are more important than his or her professional qualifications. A health care practitioner giving fact testimony is not allowed to give his or her opinion on the facts.

testimony
Statements sworn to under oath by witnesses testifying in court and giving depositions.

Only experts in a particular field have the education, skills, knowledge, and experience to give *expert testimony.* In medical negligence lawsuits, physicians are usually called as expert witnesses to testify to the standard of care regarding the matter in question. Expert witnesses may, and usually do, give their opinions on the facts. If the defendant/physician is a specialist, the expert witness generally practices or teaches in the same specialty. Acceptable expert witnesses are not coworkers, friends, or acquaintances of the defendant. It is ethical and acceptable for expert witnesses to set and accept a fee commensurate with time taken from regular employment and time spent preparing their expert testimony.

COURTROOM CONDUCT

Most health care practitioners will never have to appear in court. If you should be asked to appear, however, the following suggestions can help:

- Attend court proceedings as required. If you were subpoenaed but fail to appear, you could be charged with contempt of court. (If either the plaintiff or the defendant fails to appear, that person forfeits the case.)
- Find out in advance when and where you are to appear, and do not be late for scheduled hearings.
- Bring the required documents to court, and present them only when requested to do so.
- Before testifying, refresh your memory concerning all the facts observed about the matter in question, such as dates, times, words spoken, and circumstances.
- When testifying, speak slowly, use layperson's terms instead of medical terms whenever possible, and do not lose your temper or attempt to be humorous.
- Answer all questions in a straightforward manner, even if the answers appear to help the opposing side.
- Answer only the question asked, no more and no less.
- Because you are testifying about what you recall, be careful of broad generalizations, such as "That is all that took place." A better answer might be, "As I recall, that is what took place."
- Your attorney may help you prepare your testimony, but do not discuss your testimony with other witnesses or others outside the courtroom. Answer truthfully if asked whether you discussed your testimony with counsel.
- Appear well groomed, and dress in clean, conservative clothing.

Check Your Progress

16. Of what use might pretrial screenings be in preventing medical malpractice lawsuits?
17. How does a *deposition* differ from an *interrogatory?*
18. At what point in a lawsuit is the court's judgment handed down? When is the judgment final?
19. What is the purpose of a subpoena *duces tecum?*
20. Name the four phases of a typical medical professional liability lawsuit. Describe how someone practicing your chosen profession might be involved in each phase.

5.6 Patient Safety Standards

Avoiding medical mistakes and safeguarding patients while they are being examined or treated are vital issues for health care practitioners, both to ensure excellent patient care and to avoid issues of medical malpractice liability.

While conscientious health care practitioners do their best to avoid making mistakes, they are human, and mistakes do occur. The legal and ethical response when health care mistakes are made is to report the mistake to attending physicians and supervisors and on the patient's medical record, and to tell the patient he or she has been harmed. In fact, health care practitioners and health care facilities that try to cover up mistakes are most likely to be sued, and failing to disclose mistakes could cause such facilities to lose their Joint Commission accreditation.

The Joint Commission publishes patient safety goals for hospitals, ambulatory care, behavioral care, home care, and critical access hospital care. The following safety goals for hospital care were published online in 2016:

1. Identify patients correctly. Use at least two ways to identify a patient, such as the patient's name and date of birth.
2. Make sure patients receiving blood transfusions get the correct blood.
3. Get important test results to the right staff person on time.
4. Before a procedure, label all medicines in all containers–syringes, cups, and basins–located in the area where medicines and supplies are set up.
5. Find out what medicines the patient is taking. Take extra care with patients who take blood-thinning medications. Compare all medicines the patient has been taking to new medicines given to the patient. Are there contraindications? Make sure the patient knows which medicines to take when they are at home. Tell the patient it is important to bring their up-to-date list of medicines every time they visit a doctor. Record and pass along correct information about a patient's medicines.
6. Check alarms on all medical equipment and make sure that they can be heard and are responded to on time.
7. Use the Centers for Disease Control and Prevention or the World Health Organization guidelines for hand cleaning. Set and disseminate goals for improving hand cleaning.
8. Use proven guidelines to prevent:
   a. Infections that are difficult to treat
   b. Blood infections from central lines
   c. Infection after surgery
   d. Infections of the urinary tract caused by catheters.
9. Find out which patients are most likely to commit suicide, and be sure others treating such a patient are aware.

10. Make sure the correct surgery is done on the correct patient and at the correct place on the patient's body.
    a. Mark the correct place on the patient's body where the surgery is to be done.
    b. Pause before the patient's surgery to make sure that no mistakes are being made. It helps if the surgeon calls out, "We are performing ___________ on the ___________ of patient, ___________, birth date _________________."

Source: www.jointcommission.org/assets/1/6/2016_NPSG_HAP_ER.pdf.

Additional guides for patient safety are available at this site, and the exact language of the goals is available at www.jointcommission.org.

In many health care facilities, The Joint Commission guidelines for patient safety are used as checklists before surgeries and other procedures. Even so, egregious errors have occurred:

- At a Rhode Island hospital, a third-year resident failed to mark which side of a patient's brain was to have a surgical procedure, and a surgeon operated on the wrong side.
- At the same Rhode Island hospital, a surgeon began an operation on the wrong side of a patient's brain, and a surgical nurse who knew the surgeon was making a mistake allowed him to complete a scalp incision before speaking up. (When a third incident occurred involving surgery in the wrong area, an $80,000 fine was reportedly levied against the hospital.)
- A woman undergoing surgical removal of an eye woke enough during surgery to feel pain and hear conversation but was unable to move. The surgeon and a nurse finally realized the patient's condition and ordered more anesthesia. The patient continued to be severally traumatized by the experience long after the surgery.
- An electrical cauterizing tool ignited an alcohol solution on a patient's face, causing second- and third-degree burns.
- A man who had thoracic surgery in a Pittsburgh hospital suffered continual pain for several months after the surgery until a chest X-ray revealed the presence of surgical forceps in his chest.
- A 17-year-old died after receiving a heart and double-lung organ transplant—from a donor with an incompatible blood type.
- A 70-year-old died after surgery in which physicians removed a healthy kidney instead of the diseased kidney.

While these horrible mistakes are not commonplace, they illustrate the absolute importance of placing the patient's safety first, which involves using patient safety lists as guidelines before and during any patient procedure.

5.7 Alternative Dispute Resolution

alternative dispute resolution (ADR)
Settlement of civil disputes between parties using neutral mediators or arbitrators without going to court.

Alternative dispute resolution (ADR) consists of techniques for resolving civil disputes without going to court. As court calendars have become overcrowded in recent years, ADR has become increasingly popular. Several alternative methods of settling legal disputes are possible, including mediation, arbitration, med-arb, and neutral or case evaluation.

Some states require mediation and/or arbitration for certain civil cases, while in other states, alternative dispute resolution methods are voluntary. *Mediation* is an ADR method in which a neutral third party listens to both sides of the argument and then helps resolve the dispute. The mediator does not have the authority to impose a solution on the parties involved.

Arbitration is a method of settling disputes in which the opposing parties agree to abide by the decision of an arbitrator. An arbitrator is either selected directly by the disputing parties or chosen in one of the following two ways:

1. Under the terms of a written contract, an arbitrator is chosen by the court or by the American Arbitration Association.
2. If no contract exists, each of the two involved parties selects an arbitrator, and the two arbitrators select a third.

Arbitration may be *binding*, in which the two parties agree to accept the decision of the arbitrator in lieu of going to trial, or *nonbinding*, in which the disagreeing parties may choose to go to trial if neither party likes the arbitrator's decision.

In an informal proceeding, each side presents evidence and witnesses. In the alternative dispute resolution method called med-arb, the mediator resolves the dispute if the two parties are unable to reach agreement after mediation.

Some states allow a fourth type of mediation called neutral evaluation or case evaluation, in which each party in the dispute presents his or her side to a neutral evaluator. After listening to both sides of the argument, the evaluator then gives an opinion on the strengths and weaknesses of each party's evidence and about how the dispute could be resolved. The evaluator is often an expert in the subject matter of the dispute. Although the evaluator's opinion is not binding, the parties typically use it as a basis for trying to negotiate a resolution of the dispute. Neutral evaluation is useful in cases where there are many technical issues or when the only unresolved issue is the amount of damages to be paid.

Advocates of alternative dispute resolution claim that these methods are faster and less costly than court adjudication. Critics claim that medical malpractice cases are best decided when all the factual information is brought out, as in pretrial judicial discovery procedures. Critics also argue that selecting arbitrators acceptable to both parties can take weeks, months, even years and that attorneys' fees and damage awards can be as costly as in court-tried cases.

ADR FOR SETTLING MEDICAL MALPRACTICE CLAIMS

As the costs of health care and medical malpractice insurance and litigation continue to rise, alternative dispute resolution has become a recommended method of settling cases alleging medical negligence. As mentioned earlier under "Pretrial Screening," sometimes medical professionals are reluctant to offer apologies and explanations to injured patients because of the fear that they will be used against them in court. However, 35 states have passed some form of "I'm Sorry" legislation that allows physicians to offer some form of confidential and inadmissible (in a court) apology to the patient. The laws differ with states, with some outlining conditions that must be followed.

Recent studies have found that mediation, which does not require the presence of attorneys, is an especially effective way to resolve medical negligence disputes. Not only is the process time-efficient for all involved—with issues resolved in hours or a few days, as opposed to litigation times that can stretch to years—parties on both sides have found satisfaction in being able to speak for themselves, expressing frustrations and concerns that often result in the implementation of new patient safety policies, better ways of training personnel, improved informed consent requirements, or more explicit and understanding methods of explaining medical procedures and health care institutional policies.

Other advantages of the use of ADR in resolving medical malpractice claims include:

- The use of a more qualified decision maker who might better understand the medical terms and procedures necessary to testimony than a jury of lay persons unfamiliar with medical jargon.
- Reduces expenses of settling a claim. Sometimes damages awarded in court are insufficient to cover the plaintiff's cost in follow-up medical care or the legal fees incurred in pursuing a lawsuit; whereas damages arrived at in ADR may be more realistic.
- Reduces the trauma associated with two parties facing off in court, where medical professionals feel persecuted as criminals, and injured parties feel neglected and ignored.
- Improves the quality of experts used in both sides of the argument because they are not usually paid "medical testimony professionals," as they may be in a court of law.
- Reduces the number of frivolous medical malpractice claims because, once both sides are heard, the potential plaintiff may decide that proceeding with a lawsuit is unnecessary.
- Preserves relationships and reputations because ADR procedures are confidential and not part of public record as in lawsuits.

Professional liability and medical malpractice are major concerns for all health care practitioners. However, the individual who is aware of the risks and how to avoid them, and practices competently within the law and within his or her scope of practice, can enjoy a long, successful, and satisfying career without ever facing malpractice charges.

Check Your Progress

21. What national organization recommends safety checklists for a variety of health care settings?
22. How can patient safety checklists prevent medical malpractice charges?
23. Name two precautions to take when preparing a patient for surgery that will help prevent injury to the patient.
24. Define *binding* arbitration as opposed to *nonbinding* arbitration.
25. Identify at least three advantages of ADR.

Chapter Summary

Learning Outcome	Summary
LO 5.1 Define *liability, law of agency,* and *respondeat superior.*	What is liability? • One's legal responsibility for one's action. What is law of agency? • The common law situation in business in which employees act as agents for their employers in dealing with third parties on behalf of the employers. • Agency makes employers vicariously responsible for the acts of their employees while the employees are working on behalf of the employers. What is *respondeat superior?* • A legal remedy derived from the law of agency that is most often used in personal injury lawsuits. • It makes employers equally liable for employees charged with injuring a third party. What must the injured plaintiff prove for a lawsuit to succeed under *respondeat superior?* • The injury to the plaintiff occurred while the employee was actually working for the employer. • The injury was caused by something the employee would ordinarily do while working for the employer. • The employer benefited in some way, however small or indirect, from the action the employee was performing when the injury occurred. What are the three areas of general liability for which an employer is responsible? • The building and grounds • Automobiles used as a part of the employees' duties • Employee safety
LO 5.2 Describe the reasonable person standard, standard of care, and duty of care.	What are the differences among the reasonable person standard, standard of care, and duty of care? • Under the reasonable person standard, individuals may be charged with negligence if someone is injured because he or she failed to perform an act that a reasonable person in similar circumstances would perform or if he or she committed an act that a reasonable person would not commit. • Standard of care is the level of performance expected of a health care practitioner in carrying out his or her professional duties. • Duty of care is the legal obligation of health care workers to patients and, sometimes, nonpatients.
LO 5.3 Briefly outline the responsibilities of health care practitioners concerning privacy, confidentiality, and privileged communication.	What are the responsibilities of health care practitioners concerning privacy, confidentiality, and privileged communication? • Health care practitioners have a legal and ethical obligation to safeguard a patient's privacy and maintain confidentiality, which is the act of holding information in confidence, not to be released to unauthorized individuals. • Privileged communication refers to information held confidential within a protected relationship, such as the physician–patient relationship, and patients may sue for breach of confidence if protected information is released and results in damage to the patient.
LO 5.4 Explain the four elements necessary to prove negligence (the four Ds).	What are the four Ds of negligence? • *Duty*—The person charged with negligence owed a duty of care to the accuser. • *Dereliction*—The health care provider breached the duty of care to the patient. • *Direct cause*—The breach of the duty of care to the patient was a direct cause of the patient's injury. • *Damages*—There is a legally recognizable injury to the patient. Under what circumstances might a *res ipsa loquitor* (the thing speaks for itself) lawsuit prevail? • If the error that caused a person's injury is so obvious that only negligence could have caused it.

LO 5.5 Outline the phases of a lawsuit.	What is pretrial screening? • A review of an alleged medical negligence issue by a neutral, qualified evaluator. What are the phases of a lawsuit? • Pleading phase • Interrogatory or pretrial discovery phase • Trial phase • Appeals phase What is the difference between testimony by deposition and interrogatory testimony? • A deposition is sworn testimony given and recorded outside the courtroom during the pretrial phase of a case. An interrogatory is a written set of questions requiring written answers from a plaintiff or defendant under oath.
LO 5.6 Discuss patient safety standards as related to medical malpractice prevention.	What relationship exists between The Joint Commission and prevention of medical malpractice lawsuits? • Extensive lists for double-checking patient identify, ordered procedures, and other factors before surgery is performed. • The Joint Commission issues patient safety lists for hospital care, ambulatory surgery, ambulatory care, behavioral care, home care, and critical access hospital care.
LO 5.7 Identify the use of alternative dispute resolution in resolving medical malpractice claims.	What types of ADR might be used? • Arbitration, mediation, med-arb, and neutral or case evaluation What are the apparent advantages of ADR? • Faster, less costly, less formal, less damaging to relationships and reputations What are the advantages of ADR for medical malpractice cases? • The use of a more qualified decision maker • Reduces expenses of settling a claim • Reduces the trauma associated with two parties facing off in court • Improves the quality of experts used in both sides of the argument • Reduces the number of frivolous medical malpractice claims • Preserves relations and reputations

Chapter 5 Review

Applying Knowledge

LO 5.1

1. Briefly define *liable.*
2. Briefly explain the relationship between the law of agency and *respondeat superior.*
3. Employers have general liability for which three areas?

LO 5.2

4. According to the reasonable person standard as discussed in this chapter, in which of the following situations might a person be charged with negligence?
   a. A woman is injured when she steps in front of a car, and no one prevents the accident.
   b. A bystander does not intervene when a man with a gun robs another person on the street.
   c. A nurse fails to document her administration of a patient's medicine, and another nurse unknowingly administers a second dose, which constitutes an injurious overdose for the patient.
   d. A motorist stops to aid victims of a car accident.

5. A lab technician fails to use an alcohol swab on the draw site before drawing blood from a patient. However, the technician uses all other standards of care when drawing the blood. To what standard of care could the lab technician be held?

   a. Any reasonable person

   b. A nurse

   c. Any lab technician

   d. A physician

6. In the previous situation, to whom is a duty of care owed?

   a. No duty of care is owed because no health care relationship was established.

   b. A duty of care is owed to the lab technician.

   c. A duty of care is owed to the patient.

   d. None of these

7. Which of the following statements is true of standard of care?

   a. Titles are not important if appropriate care is administered.

   b. If a certified nursing assistant is able to perform the duties of a nurse, he or she should be legally and ethically allowed to use the title "nurse."

   c. If one uses the title "nurse," one can be held to the standard of care of a nurse.

   d. Standard of care has no legal implications.

8. A physician assistant is seeing a patient in an assisted living facility. Her patient clearly has the flu. She treats the patient and then advises the facility's nursing director of the communicable disease. This is an example of:

   a. Reasonable person standard

   b. Standard of care

   c. Privacy standard

   d. Duty of care

9. To establish a standard of care in a trial, __________ is(are) required.

LO 5.3

10. In which of the following situations has patient privacy been violated?

    a. A female patient is ushered into a medical clinic examination room, and a male phlebotomist draws a blood sample.

    b. A medical assistant knocks, then enters an exam room to take a patient's blood pressure.

    c. A physician performs a physical examination.

    d. In the presence of other patients in a clinic waiting room, a medical assistant tells a patient that her pregnancy test was positive.

LO 5.4

11. What is the basis for most medical malpractice claims?

    a. Practicing medicine without a license

    b. Missed diagnoses

    c. Negligence

    d. Assault

12. A patient falls on a hospital's slippery tile floor and injures herself. Assuming that patient safety procedures were lax, what undesirable occurrence could result for the hospital?

    a. The patient could leave without paying his or her bill.

    b. The patient could become angry and refuse further treatment.

    c. The patient could sue the hospital.

    d. The patient could decide never to use the hospital's services again.

13.–16. Name the four Ds of negligence.

17. *Res ipsa loquitur* is the doctrine of ____________________.

18. When a patient sues a physician for negligence, who has the burden of proof in court?

    a. The plaintiff

    b. The defendant

    c. The judge

    d. The jury

19. What purpose do expert witnesses serve in a medical negligence lawsuit?

    a. They testify that the person accused is of good character.

    b. They testify about the medical care given to the patient.

    c. They testify that the accuser is of good character.

    d. None of these

20. The doctrine of *res ipsa loquitur* might be applied in which of the following?

    a. A surgeon operates on a patient's foot, but it is the wrong foot.

    b. A woman's front teeth are knocked out while she is under anesthesia for surgery on her toe.

    c. A woman is anesthetized for a tubal ligation but receives a hysterectomy.

    d. All of these

Match the following statements with the correct terms by writing the appropriate letter in the space provided. A letter may be used more than once.

_____ 21. Monetary compensation awarded to a plaintiff to compensate for injuries or losses due to violation of the plaintiff's rights.

_____ 22. The defendant must pay, but the dollar value of the violation need not be proved.

_____ 23. The defendant must pay, the dollar value need not be proved, but the loss must be proved.

_____ 24. Money is awarded the plaintiff, recognizing a wrong, but the amount is nominal.

_____ 25. Money awarded is intended to punish the defendant.

a. Punitive damages

b. Special compensatory damages

c. Consequential damages

d. General compensatory damages

e. Nominal damages

LO 5.5

26. A written notification to appear in court to defend against a lawsuit is called a(n) __________.

27. A court order for an individual to appear in court is called a(n) __________.

28. An order to bring certain records to court is called a(n) __________.

29. Define the term *deposition.* __________

30. Who is most likely to give factual testimony in a trial?

a. A person who was present during certain events and can tell what happened

b. An expert who knows how certain medical treatments should be performed

c. A witness who was not present during disputed events but can determine if they might have occurred as indicated by other testimony

d. None of these

31. Which of the following legal actions may be taken if you are subpoenaed to appear in court as a witness or to give a deposition and you fail to appear?

a. You can immediately be jailed.

b. No action will be taken.

c. You may be charged with contempt of court.

d. You are asked to come in at a more convenient time.

32. What is the result if you are the plaintiff or the defendant in a lawsuit and you fail to appear in court?

a. The case can be lost by default.

b. No action is taken.

c. You can immediately be jailed.

d. You are asked to reschedule a court date.

33. A jury is selected in the __________ phase of a lawsuit.

34. A plea is made for the case to be reviewed by the higher court in the __________ phase of a lawsuit.

35. In the __________ phase of a lawsuit, subpoenas are issued.

36. A pretrial conference may be called in the __________ phase of a lawsuit.

37. Attorneys make opening and closing statements in the __________ phase of a lawsuit.

38. Witnesses are called to testify in the __________ phase of a lawsuit.

39. A deposition is taken in the __________ phase of a lawsuit.

LO 5.6

40. Which of the following penalties could ensue if a health care facility has a large number of patient safety violations?

a. The facility could lose its accreditation.

b. Fines could be levied.

c. Medical practice claims could increase.

d. All of the above.

41. Which of the following is recommended by The Joint Commission as a safe and reliable way of checking a patient's identity before surgery?

a. Ask the patient to spell her last name.

b. Ask the patient her name *and* birth date, and check for accuracy of both on her ID band.

c. Ask a relative of the patient to vouch for his identity.

d. Ask the patient's physician to identify the patient.

LO 5.7

42. Which of the following statements best defines *alternative dispute resolution?*

a. A specific kind of court case

b. Dismissal of a court case

c. Refusal to allow expert witnesses in a court case

d. Settlement of civil disputes between parties using neutral mediators or arbitrators without going to court

43. How is *mediation* best defined?

a. Attorneys on opposing sides reach a decision out of court.

b. A suit is dismissed for lack of grounds.

c. A neutral third party listens to both sides of the argument and then helps resolve the dispute.

d. None of these

44. Which of the following is an advantage for settling a medical malpractice dispute through ADR?

a. Damage awards are greater.

b. No time is lost in deliberation.

c. Attorneys are always the mediators.

d. Relationships and reputations can remain intact.

Ethics Issues Professional Liability and Medical Malpractice

Use your critical thinking skills to answer the questions that follow each ethics issue.

Ethics ISSUE 1:

As citizens and as professionals with special training and experience, health care practitioners are ethically obligated to assist in the administration of justice. If a patient who has a legal claim requests a health care practitioner's assistance, he or she should furnish medical evidence, with the patient's consent, to secure the patient's legal rights.

Medical experts should have recent and substantive experience in the area in which they testify and should limit testimony to their sphere of medical expertise.

Discussion Questions

45. An orthopedic surgeon who has been retired from practice for 15 years and is a friend of the plaintiff's has been called to testify in the plaintiff's suit alleging damage to his hip joint sustained in a car accident. In your opinion, is it ethical for the physician described previously to testify? Explain your answer.

46. In your opinion, is it ever ethical for a health care practitioner to testify against another health care practitioner in a medical malpractice lawsuit? Explain your answer.

47. As a health care practitioner, do you consider it ethical to charge for your services to testify as an expert witness? Explain your answer.

48. Are there circumstances in which you might consider it unethical to charge for your services as an expert witness? Explain your answer.

Ethics ISSUE 2:

Health care practitioners are ethically bound to respect the patient's dignity and to make a positive effort to secure a comfortable and considerate atmosphere for the patient in such ways as providing appropriate gowns and drapes, private facilities for undressing, and clear explanations for procedures.

Discussion Questions

49. An adolescent male patient is visibly uncomfortable as a female physician begins a physical examination. What actions might the physician and/or her attending certified medical assistant take to make the patient more comfortable?

50. A hospital patient who is mentally disabled becomes extremely agitated and violent. She disrobes and runs through the hallways. Nurses and other employees are unable to calm the woman, and security officers arrive. Other patients and employees in the area stand around watching the woman as the officers attempt to subdue her. As a health care practitioner in the immediate vicinity, what, if anything, might you do to protect the woman's privacy?

51. A nurse who is at the end of a 12-hour shift misreads drug labels and administers the wrong medication to the patient. What should she do?

52. Are there legal implications in the previous example? Explain your answer, detailing any preventative measures that could have been taken to avoid them.

Case Studies

Use your critical thinking skills to answer the questions that follow each case study.

LO 5.1 and LO 5.2

A 33-year-old male swallows 30 antidepressants and tells his wife, "I want to die." She takes him to the local hospital's emergency department, where he is treated and released that same evening. In the hospital parking lot, he pushes a security guard and is arrested and taken into custody. In the county jail, a nurse places the man on suicide watch. The following evening, while the man is still in custody, a psychologist speaks to him for five minutes, then releases him from suicide watch. The man is returned to his cell, and two hours later, he hangs himself.

53. Does the emergency department have liability for discharging a suicidal patient without further treatment?

54. Does the psychologist have liability for releasing the patient from suicide watch after a five-minute consultation?

55. The psychologist is an "independent contractor" of the jail. Is the county liable for his actions?

LO 5.2

A woman gave birth in the back seat of a taxicab while en route to the hospital. To what standard of care would each of the following individuals be held?

56. The taxicab driver who comforted the mother

57. A registered nurse, also a passenger in the cab, who assisted the mother

58. A physician in general practice who was a passenger in the cab with the expectant mother and assisted the birth taking place in the cab

59. A police officer who stopped the cab for speeding, observed the situation, and assisted with the birth

A woman trained in cardiopulmonary resuscitation (CPR) worked as the office manager for an insurance business. When her coworker at the next desk had a heart attack and fell to the floor, the office manager began CPR and shouted for others in the room to dial 911. The department supervisor came running and told the office manager to stop CPR. She reluctantly obeyed. Emergency medical technicians arrived, but the heart attack victim died.

60. The victim's husband sued the supervisor, the office manager, and the employees' parent organization for failure to render medical assistance. In a finding for the defendants, an appeals court ruled there was "no duty of care" for the employees to render assistance. Despite this court's ruling, in a similar situation, would you have acted as the CPR-trained office manager did? Explain your answer.

LO 5.4

During an endoscopic retrograde cholangiopancreatography (ERCP) (a gallbladder X-ray that requires injection of a dye), an inexperienced nurse injected the dye too forcefully and caused the patient to develop pancreatitis (inflammation of the pancreas) and suffer other debilitating injuries.

61. The patient sued and won. Refer to the four Ds of negligence to explain the court's decision.

Internet Activities

LO 5.1 and LO 5.6

Complete the activities and answer the questions that follow.

62. Visit the Web site of the Healthcare Providers Service Organization at www.hpso.com/individuals/professional-liability/why-do-i-need-coverage.

    Watch the videos under 1 and 2. Discuss whether or not you would consider personal liability insurance for the health care profession you plan to practice.

63. Visit this Web site for The Joint Commission: www.jointcommission.org/speakup.aspx

    What is the "Speak Up" patient safety program?

Resources

LO 5.1

Law of agency: www.rotlaw.com/legal-library/what-is-the-law-of-agency/

Melvin, Sean. *The Legal Environment of Business*. New York: McGraw-Hill, 2010.

LO 5.2

Duty of care: http://legal-dictionary.thefreedictionary.com/duty+of+care

Standard of care: http://legal-dictionary.thefreedictionary.com/standard+of+care

Reasonable person standard: http://medical-dictionary.thefreedictionary.com/reasonable+person+standard

LO 5.4

The four Ds of negligence: https://emrnews.com/the-four-ds-of-negligence/

LO 5.6

Patient safety: www.jointcommission.org/assets/1/6/2016_NPSG_HAP_ER.pdf

The Joint Commission: www.jointcommission.org

Medical mistakes: www.cnn.com/2012/06/09/health/medical-mistakes/

LO 5.7

Alternative dispute resolution types and benefits: www.courts.ca.gov/3074.htm

Alternative dispute resolution strategies in medical malpractice: http://scholarship.law.duke.edu/cgi/viewcontent.cgi?article=1295&context=alr

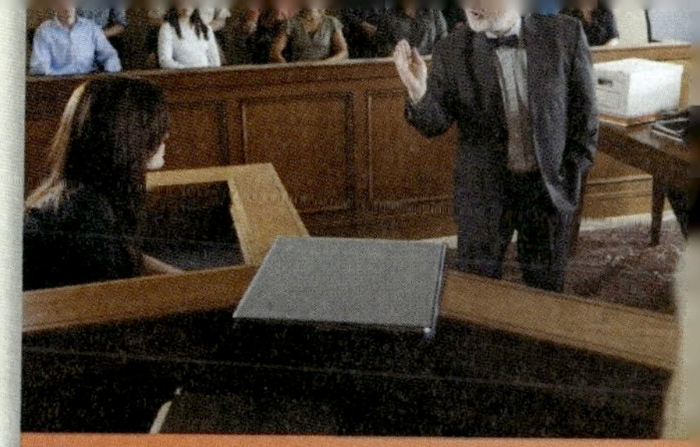

©RichLegg/E+/Getty Images RF

Defenses to Liability Suits

6

Key Terms

affirmative defenses
assumption of risk
claims-made insurance
comparative negligence
contributory negligence
denial
emergency
liability insurance
occurrence insurance
prior acts insurance coverage
quality improvement (QI) or quality assurance (QA)
release of tortfeasor
res judicata
risk management
self-insurance coverage
statute of limitations
tail coverage
technical defenses

LEARNING OUTCOMES

After studying this chapter, you should be able to:

LO 6.1 Define the 4 Cs, relating them to workplace precautions that help to prevent medical malpractice lawsuits.

LO 6.2 Describe the various defenses to professional liability suits.

LO 6.3 Explain the purpose of quality improvement and risk management within a health care facility.

LO 6.4 Identify five different types of medical liability insurance.

FROM THE PERSPECTIVE OF. . .

DARYL, AS AN EMERGENCY MEDICAL TECHNICIAN (EMT), has encountered a number of "difficult" patients. For example, called to a residence by a man who had accidentally cut his wrist while slicing bread, he and his new partner, Joann, found the man bleeding profusely and nearly hysterical.

"Don't touch me!" he screamed when the two EMTs began their assessment of his injuries.

Joann, startled, pulled back and removed her hand from the man's uninjured wrist. Daryl, however, proceeded calmly and carefully, but with determination.

"We're here to help you," Daryl replied in a level voice, making eye contact with the man. "We need to get that bleeding stopped; then we can get you the help you need." As he spoke, Daryl gently applied pressure to the man's bleeding wound and motioned for Joann to begin the assessment of the injured man's vital signs.

The man, agitated and sweating, continued to rant, but as Daryl spoke to him calmly, explaining each action he and Joann performed, the man finally quieted enough to cooperate. By the time the EMTs transported the man to the hospital emergency room for treatment, he was able to calmly recount his accident to the physician on duty.

"When people are injured, they're in pain and usually scared," Daryl explained to a shaken Joann later. "We have to stay calm and just talk to them until they understand we're only there to help them and we will be as gentle as possible. If we get in their face and try to force them to do what we want, it's only going to make matters worse. And because people who are angry and upset are most likely to sue, we can also help prevent complaints later by staying calm and professional."

From Daryl's perspective, he needed to calm the patient before he could effectively assess his injuries.

From Joann's perspective, the "difficult" patient prevented her from thinking first of her training and staying calm.

From the patient's perspective, the profuse bleeding from his wound frightened him, and he was probably going into shock, as well.

6.1 Preventing Liability Suits

Malpractice litigation not only adds to the cost of health care, it also takes a psychological toll on both patients and health care practitioners. Both sides would probably agree that prevention is preferable to litigating a malpractice claim. Health care practitioners who use reasonable care in preventing professional liability claims are least likely to be faced with defending themselves against such claims. Figure 6-1 shows the four Cs of medical malpractice prevention.

PHYSICIAN/EMPLOYERS AND MEDICAL FACILITIES

The following guidelines for physician/employers and/or medical facilities can help you evaluate the quality of care offered by your physician/employer or medical facility and make appropriate suggestions for

FIGURE 6-1 The Four Cs of Medical Malpractice Prevention

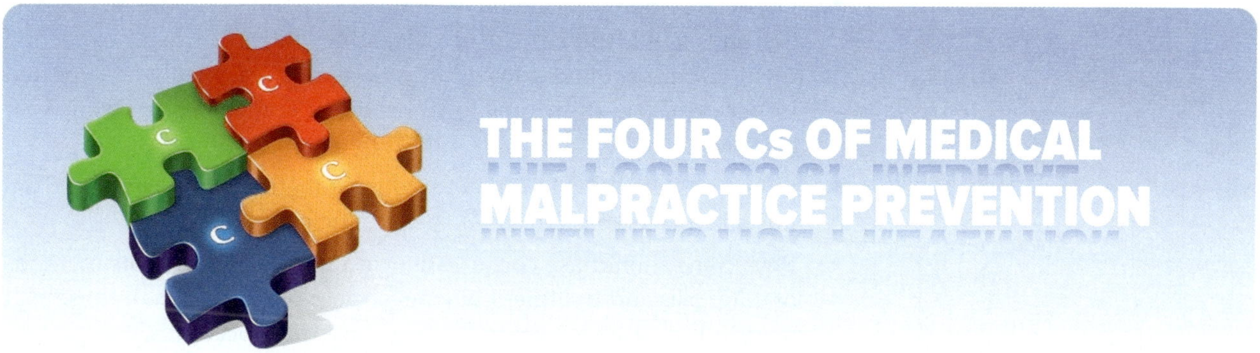

How can you protect yourself from a medical malpractice lawsuit?
By following the four Cs of medical malpractice prevention.

Caring

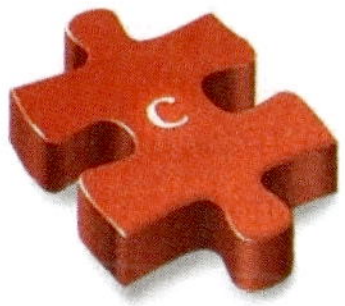

- There are two important benefits to showing your patients that you care. First is improvement in their medical condition. A secondary benefit is the decreased likelihood that your patients will feel the need to sue if treatment has unsatisfactory results, or if adverse events occur. Of course, it is important that you be sincere in your concern because others often quickly sense insincerity and may distrust you.
- Avoid destructive and unethical criticism of the work of other physicians and/or other health care practitioners. Do not discuss with a patient his or her former physician. Listen carefully to each patient's complaints and remarks about dissatisfaction with treatment, and see that the comments reach the treating physician.

Communication

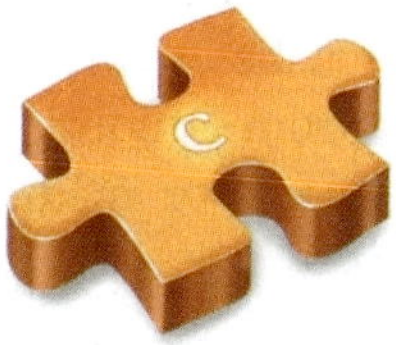

- If you communicate clearly and ask for confirmation that you have been understood, you will be more likely to earn your patients' and your colleagues' trust and respect. If your duties include taking telephone messages, relate them accurately.
- Offer to make appointments when appropriate. Remember that when health care practitioners other than physicians, or in some instances physician assistants, diagnose or prescribe, they may be charged with practicing medicine without a license. When adverse events occur, use correct procedures in reporting the event, and never avoid or ignore any patients involved.

Competence

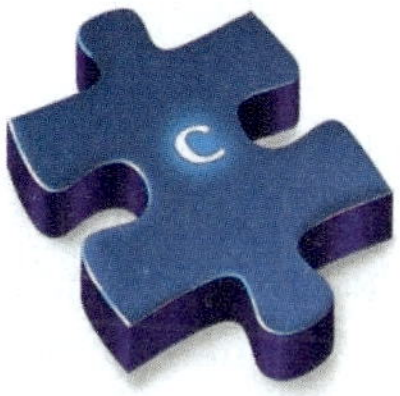

- Know your professional area well, including your limitations. Follow standards of care and appropriate procedures for medical practitioners in similar practices and in similar communities. Avoid any action that you are not fully trained or equipped to handle.
- Maintain and constantly update your knowledge and skills.
- Consult with other health care practitioners appropriately, early, and often.
- Know the requirements of good medical practice in caring for each patient.
- If you prepare or administer medications, check each drug three times: once when taking it from the supply cabinet, again when preparing the dosage, and a third time when returning the container to the shelf. All outdated medications should be discarded and promptly replaced. Prescription blanks should not be left on desktops or work areas.
- Stay informed about general medical and scientific progress by reading professional journals, attending seminars and professional association meetings, and fulfilling continuing study requirements.

Charting

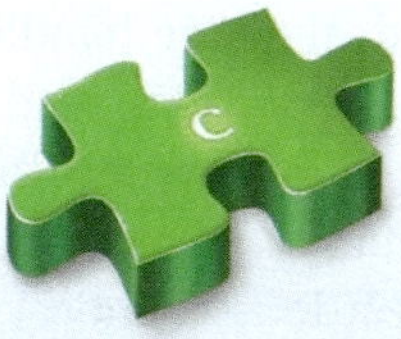

- Documentation is proof. For legal purposes, if it isn't in writing and explained completely and accurately, it wasn't done. Medical records should include X-rays, test results, progress notes, and anything else related to the patient's medical treatment.
- Document as though the patient will read his or her medical record. Never write something you would not want the patient to see.

improving patient care and reducing liability risks in the workplace environment.

- Physician/employers should carefully select and supervise all employees and should be careful in delegating duties to them, expecting them to perform only those duties they may reasonably be expected to perform, based on their qualifications, credentials, training, and experience.
- Physicians should exhaust all reasonable methods of securing a diagnosis before embarking on a therapeutic course.
- Physicians should use conservative and the least dangerous methods of diagnosis and treatment whenever possible, rather than those that involve highly toxic agents or risky surgical procedures.
- As telemedicine has become more commonplace, physicians often diagnose and prescribe medication for new patients and for established patients over the Internet. Physicians also prescribe medication for established patients over the telephone. To avoid malpractice claims, any communication with the patient, whether over the Internet or by telephone, should be properly documented in the patient's medical record. Health care practitioners who communicate with patients over the Internet should know and conform to state and federal laws regarding the practice of telemedicine.
- In ideal situations, a female medical assistant or female nurse should be present when a male physician examines a female patient, and when a female physician examines a male patient, a male medical assistant or male nurse should be present. Due to shortages of male nurses and male medical assistants, however, this may be impossible. In any case, physicians can protect themselves from unfounded patient charges by having a nurse, physician assistant, or medical assistant of either sex present during examinations.
- Physician/employers should check equipment and facilities frequently for safety, including the reception area. All employees should know safe procedures for operating equipment and should remind physician/employers when repair or replacement of equipment is necessary for continued safe operation. Employees should be alert to all hazards in the medical office that might cause injury, such as slippery floors, electric cords in unsafe places, tables with sharp edges, and so forth. The reception area at the health care facility should include a safe area for children, perhaps with such items as child-sized tables and chairs and picture books.
- When using toxic agents for diagnosis or treatment, physicians should know customary dosages or usage for such substances, any possible side effects or known toxic reactions, and the proper methods for treating reactions. Medical assistants and other medical office employees should ensure that when supplies are received, they are handled according to office policy and that all relevant literature is readily accessible to physicians. As required by the Occupational Safety and Health Administration (OSHA), employees should have access to Material Safety Data Sheets (MSDS) for each hazardous chemical in use in the medical facility. (See Chapter 10 for more information about OSHA medical workplace requirements.)

WHY DO PATIENTS SUE?

Patients sue physicians and other health care providers for a variety of reasons. A 2015 Medscape Report entitled "Top Reasons Doctors get Sued" listed seven reasons patients sue. They are:

1. Failure to diagnose.
2. Patient suffered abnormal injury.
3. Failure to treat.
4. Poor documentation of patient instructions and education.
5. Errors in medication administration.
6. Failure to follow safety procedures.
7. Improperly obtaining/lack of informed consent.

Failure to diagnose and abnormal injury accounted for 62 percent of the identified reasons. The study by Medscape surveyed nearly 4,000 primary care physicians and selected specialists to find out if and why they were sued.

COMMUNICATING WITH PATIENTS

Patients who see the medical office as a friendly place are generally less likely to sue. As a health care practitioner and/or a medical facility employee, you can help prevent medical malpractice lawsuits by:

- Developing good listening skills and nonverbal communication techniques so that patients feel the time spent with them is not rushed. For example, patients will see a health care practitioner as caring and interested if he or she sits rather than stands while interviewing

Table 6-1 Improving Communication Helps Prevent Lawsuits

Sometimes when physicians or other health care practitioners are named in lawsuits, it's not because they did something wrong. Failure to communicate, instead of medical error, is sometimes the reason behind litigation, and every medical office employee can do his or her part to help prevent lawsuits caused by failed communication.

- Polish telephone skills so you are always pleasant over the telephone.
- Don't let patients wait in line, perhaps feeling ignored, while you stare at your computer screen for several minutes before asking how you can help them.
- Check to be sure medical test results and the results of other procedures have been reported directly to the patient, rather than simply recorded on the patient's medical record.
- If you are responsible for obtaining a patient's consent to perform a procedure, don't simply ask, "Do you understand?" Instead, ask questions to determine the patient's level of understanding and allow time for the patient to ask questions to ensure that the patient is giving *informed* consent. Record the patient's questions in his or her medical record. Be sure to complete any required forms for consent and have the patient sign the form.
- It is never permissible for nonqualified office personnel to give medical advice to patients over the telephone, so always refer patients to their physicians if they telephone the office where you work asking questions you are not qualified to answer.
- Every medical office has its contingent of "difficult" patients, but use courtesy and tact when dealing with these individuals. Rudeness is never an acceptable option.

or conversing with the patient. Conversely, lack of eye contact and defensive body postures convey disinterest to a patient. In short, obey the Golden Rule when communicating with patients.

- Setting aside a certain time period during the day for returning patients' telephone calls and advising patients over the phone. Medical facility staff members responsible for answering the telephone should learn to recognize when patients' reported symptoms require the physician's immediate attention and when patients should be advised to seek emergency care.
- Reminding physicians to thoroughly explain illnesses and treatment options, including risks and possible complications, in terms the patient can understand. Patients should be encouraged to ask questions and to participate in the decision-making process. The best way to keep patients' expectations in line is through education. When dealing with accidents and bad results, a straightforward approach is desirable.
- Checking to be sure that all patients or their authorized representatives sign informed consent forms before they undergo medical and surgical procedures. Next of kin or designated representatives must also sign informed-consent forms to authorize autopsies.
- Avoiding statements that could be construed as an admission of fault on the physician's part. If a lawsuit is filed against a physician, his or her employees should say nothing to anyone except as required by the physician's attorney or the court. However, an employee may be held liable if he or she knowingly remains silent to protect a physician who has performed an illegal act.
- Using tact, good judgment, and professionalism in handling patients. Physicians should insist on a professional consultation if the patient is not doing well, if he or she is unhappy and complaining, or if the patient's family expresses dissatisfaction.
- Refraining from making overly optimistic statements about recovery or prognoses. Health care practitioners who are not physicians, physician assistants, and advanced registered nurse practitioners generally do not diagnose or prescribe, but their responsibilities may include patient education. For example, nurses and medical assistants often discuss the patient's problems and review treatment options, and this is entirely appropriate. However, such health care practitioners should not make promises on the physician's behalf, such as "The doctor will have you feeling better soon."
- Advising patients when their physicians intend to be gone for long periods of time and reminding physicians to recommend or make available qualified substitutes. The patient must not be abandoned. If a physician is retiring, moving to another location, leaving the practice of medicine, or otherwise becoming unavailable, patients should be informed, and a copy of a letter of referral, notice of a physician's intended absence from practice, or letter of dismissal should be placed in the patient's record. Notices placed in local newspapers are also appropriate if a physician retires, moves, dies, or leaves the practice of medicine. The name and telephone number of the covering physician should be available for those patients requesting care in the absence of their regular physician.

- Making every effort to reach an understanding about fees with the patient before treatment so that billing does not become a point of contention. When handling fees for the physician, employees should explain all charges to patients, detailing those that are not included in regular fees. They should also follow legal collection procedures.

DOCUMENTATION

As a legal document, a patient's medical record may be subpoenaed (via subpoena *duces tecum*) as evidence in court. When they are conscientiously compiled, medical records can prevail over a patient's recollection of events during a trial. When there is no entry in the record to the effect that something was done, there is a presumption that it was not done, and when there is an entry that something was done, the presumption is that it was done. Therefore, what is omitted from the record may be as important to the outcome of a lawsuit as what is included.

In some situations that arise in health care, such as drug testing or the examination of a rape victim, evidence may need to be collected in a certain manner to be admissible in court. When in doubt about what documentation to make, health care practitioners should contact legal authorities for advice.

Medical records should clearly show what treatment was done and when it was done. From a legal standpoint, it is important that documentation shows that nothing was neglected in the patient's care and that the care given fully met the standards demanded by law.

See Chapter 7 for a detailed discussion of what information should routinely be included in patient records.

Check Your Progress

1. Name and briefly define the four Cs of medical malpractice prevention.
2. Briefly describe how practicing effective communication skills can help prevent a medical malpractice lawsuit.
3. If a patient refuses treatment, what legal options remain for the health care practitioner in charge?
4. Name five reasons often cited for the suing of health care practitioners by patients and their families.

6.2 Types of Defenses

When, in spite of all the best efforts to avoid litigation, a medical malpractice lawsuit is filed, the physician or other health care professional must defend himself or herself against the charges.

DENIAL

Denial of wrongdoing, or the assertion of innocence, may be used as a defense in professional liability suits. If some of the alleged facts are true,

denial
A defense that claims innocence of the charges or that one or more of the four Ds of negligence are lacking.

defendants may not claim innocence. Instead, they should claim that the charge or charges do not meet all of the elements of the theory of recovery. In other words, the charge may be missing one of the four Ds of negligence.

AFFIRMATIVE DEFENSES

affirmative defenses
Defenses used by defendants in medical professional liability suits that allow the accused to present factual evidence that the patient's condition was caused by some factor other than the defendant's negligence.

Affirmative defenses that may be used by the defendant in a medical professional liability suit allow the accused to present factual evidence that the patient's condition was caused by some factor other than the defendant's negligence.

contributory negligence
An affirmative defense that alleges that the plaintiff, through a lack of care, caused or contributed to his or her own injury.

Contributory Negligence

When the defense claims **contributory negligence,** this alleges that the patient or complaining party, through a "want of ordinary care," caused or contributed to his or her own injury. The physician may deny that he or she committed a negligent act and claim the patient was totally responsible for the damage or injury. Alternatively, the physician may admit negligence but claim that the patient was also somehow at fault and so contributed to the injury.

comparative negligence
An affirmative defense claimed by the defendant alleging that the plaintiff contributed to the injury by a certain degree.

In some states, damages are apportioned according to the degree to which a plaintiff contributed to the injury. This is called **comparative negligence.** For instance, if the court decides that a patient, through his or her own negligence, contributed 20 percent toward the injury and the physician contributed 80 percent, the patient's damage award may be reduced by 20 percent.

In hearing cases alleging contributory negligence, the court will consider the patient's ability to comprehend and carry out the physician's instructions. Minors or adults who are unconscious, mentally disabled, insane, or otherwise incompetent may be judged unable to have contributed to a negligent act.

assumption of risk
A legal defense that holds that the defendant is not guilty of a negligent act because the plaintiff knew of and accepted beforehand any risks involved.

Assumption of Risk

Assumption of risk is a defense based on the contention that the patient knew of the inherent risks before treatment was performed and agreed to those risks. Informed consent (see Chapter 7) is vital to this defense because the defendant must show that the patient was fully informed of the risks prior to treatment and that the risks inherent in the treatment were the cause of the patient's injury.

For example, in one lawsuit in which the defendant used the assumption of risk defense, it was held that a physician was not liable for injuries suffered by a chronically ill woman when she fell in the examining room while attempting to undress without assistance. Because she had refused assistance, the woman had assumed the risk of injury.

In other cases, it has been held that individuals submitting to X-ray treatment assume the risk of burns from a proper exposure to X-rays but not the risk of negligence in the application of the treatment.

emergency
A type of affirmative defense in which the person who comes to the aid of a victim in an emergency is not held liable under certain circumstances.

Emergency

If services were provided during an **emergency,** this may also be used as an affirmative defense. The health care practitioner who comes to the aid of a victim in an emergency would not be held liable under common law if the defense established that:

1. A true emergency situation existed and was not caused by the defendant.
2. The appropriate standard of care was met, given the emergency situation.

Health care professionals who provide assistance in emergencies may also be protected from liability under Good Samaritan Acts, which are discussed in Chapter 7.

TECHNICAL DEFENSES

When defenses to liability suits are based on legal technicalities, instead of on factual evidence, they are called **technical defenses.** Technical defenses include those that claim the statute of limitations has run out, there is insufficient evidence to support the plaintiff's claim of negligence, and the assertion that the plaintiff has no standing to sue.

technical defenses
Defenses used in a lawsuit that are based on legal technicalities.

Release of Tortfeasor A tortfeasor is one who is guilty of committing a tort. Suppose a third party causes injury to a person as in an automobile accident and a physician treats the injured person. In most states, the party who caused the accident (the tortfeasor) is liable both for the victim's injury and for any medical negligence by the physician who treats the injured victim. This is the basis for the **release of tortfeasor** defense.

release of tortfeasor
A technical defense that prohibits a lawsuit against the person who caused an injury (the tortfeasor) if he or she was expressly released from further liability in the settlement of a suit.

If the injured party sues the tortfeasor, settles the case, and then releases the tortfeasor from further liability, the injured party cannot also sue the physician unless the victim expressly reserved that right in the release. If the victim's settlement with the tortfeasor provided compensation for all medical expenses, the release of tortfeasor is usually an absolute defense.

Laws governing release of tortfeasor contain many modifiers, which must be applied in individual cases.

Res Judicata Under the doctrine of ***res judicata***, "The thing has been decided," a claim cannot be retried between the same parties if it has already been legally resolved. For example, if a patient sues a physician for negligence and loses, the patient cannot then sue the physician for breach of contract based on evidence presented in the trial for negligence. If a patient refuses to pay a physician's fees on the grounds that the physician was negligent and the physician sues for money owed and wins, the patient cannot then sue the physician for negligence. However, if the patient fails to respond to the suit (defaults) or does not allege negligence in his or her defense, then usually he or she may sue the physician for negligence. If a physician has been sued by a nonpaying patient for negligence and does not file a counterclaim for the fee while defending the suit, the patient cannot be sued later for unpaid bills.

res judicata
"The thing has been decided." Legal principle that a claim cannot be retried between the same parties if it has already been legally resolved.

Statute of Limitations Because statutes of limitations vary with states, health care practitioners must be familiar with specific laws for their state. Statutory time limits apply to a number of legal actions, including collections, damages for child sexual abuse, retaining of medical records, wrongful death claims, medical malpractice, and many other causes of action. The **statute of limitations** for filing professional negligence suits varies with states but generally specifies 1 to 6 years, with 2 years being most common. In other words, patients may not file suit for negligence against physicians if the designated length of time has elapsed.

statute of limitations
That period of time established by state law during which a lawsuit may be filed.

COURT CASE The Unhappy Patient

In 2002, a 24-year-old patient had her first elective cosmetic procedure. After giving birth to three children and breastfeeding them, the patient was unhappy with the appearance of her post-baby body and sought to have several procedures performed to address the issues causing her displeasure. She was happy with the outcome of her first set of surgeries.

After graduating from nursing school in 2011, the patient decided to have additional elective cosmetic surgery performed to improve her appearance and to feel better about herself. Over the course of the 4 to 5 years prior to that time, although having a petite build at 5 feet in height, the patient had gained approximately 70 pounds but lost the weight, stabilizing at 114 pounds. This fluctuation in weight left her with sagging skin, loss of breast volume, and breasts that sat lower than they had after her first elective cosmetic surgery. The patient chose a different surgeon for the various procedures necessary and had surgery in June 2011.

At the patient's first post-operative visit, the surgeon reinforced his written post-operative instructions to take it easy, directing her to engage in only light activities. He also instructed the patient to return for another follow-up appointment in three weeks, which was the standard amount of time between visits, to determine if there was a decrease in swelling and to monitor any new issues with pain that might arise in the course of her post-operative recovery. The patient was instructed to follow the surgeon's verbal and written instructions with respect to her post-operative care in order to promote healing without unnecessary delay. She was also instructed to follow the schedule of post-operative appointments. She signed all written instructions.

Among the specific instructions she was given was the instruction to protect her surgical scars from sunlight for a year after surgery, since sunlight could damage her skin—even through a bathing suit. She was explicitly instructed to continuously wear a specialized support bra 24 hours a day for the first two weeks following surgery. After that period of time had passed, she was instructed to wear it at all times when she was awake. The bra served as a dressing to maintain a perfect position.

The patient was also instructed to be patient with the healing process and that the ability to heal varies on a number of factors, including genetic background, overall state of health, and lifestyle. Further, she was told that her cooperation in the healing process was extremely important and in her best interest.

After her first follow-up office visit, the patient admitted she wore the support bra for only a couple of hours each of the two days she decided to use it, removing it and making the personal choice to discontinue its use altogether because she thought it was uncomfortable. She did not communicate this information to her surgeon or his staff. She then went to Florida for a six-day vacation, going to the beach on several occasions. After her Florida vacation, she went for a week long cruise during which she again wore her two-piece bathing suit on beach excursions. She continued her membership in a tanning salon.

The patient never returned for a follow-up appointment with her surgeon. Instead, she chose to consult with her surgeon from 2002 shortly after returning from her cruise. At the patient's request, the original surgeon performed a minor revision surgery on her right breast under local anesthetic in August 2011. The surgeon indicated that it was not medically necessary.

In June 2013, the patient filed suit against the second surgeon, claiming that the scar underneath her right breast was visible when she wore her two-piece bathing suit. She asked only for her payments of almost $9,000 to the second physician be repaid so that she could afford to pay the first surgeon to attempt to fix the scar.

The second surgeon filed an answer denying negligence and denying that the medical care provided to the patient was below the appropriate standard of care. The surgeon also asserted the patient's contributory negligence as an affirmative defense. The case was tied up in a variety of motions until a two-day jury trial in mid-2015. The jury found for the surgeon. The judge vacated the jury's decision, finding for the patient-plaintiff on technical grounds. However, upon appeal, it was found that the trial court erred in overturning the jury verdict. The appellate court found in favor of the surgeon.

Source: *Stephens, M.D., and Summit Plastic Surgery Center, Appellants-Defendants, v. Jamie Fazio, Appellee-Plaintiff,* No. 02A03-1505-PL-357 Court of Appeals of Indiana, June 21, 2016.

Establishing when the statute of limitations begins also varies with state law, but the most common dates for marking the beginning of the statutory period are as follows:

- The day the alleged negligent act was committed.
- When the injury resulting from the alleged negligence was actually discovered or should have been discovered by a reasonably alert patient.
- The day the physician–patient relationship ended or the day of the last medical treatment in a series.

In some states, statutory periods may be modified for minors, for persons who are legally insane, or in certain circumstances, such as imprisonment or a situation in which foreign objects were left in the body during surgery.

Specific statutory time limits may be found in the state code, published online, and in most public and university libraries.

Check Your Progress

5. What is the difference between an affirmative defense and a technical defense?
6. Identify the type of defense described in each of the following:
   One in which the defendant claims innocence.
   One in which the accused is allowed to present factual evidence that the physician's negligence did not cause the patient's condition.
   One in which the defendant claims that the patient contributed to his or her own injury.
   One in which informed consent is a vital factor.
   One that hinges on legal technicalities, rather than factual evidence.
7. If a medical malpractice claim is dismissed due to a state's statute of limitations, does this imply that the defendant health care practitioner is exonerated? Explain your answer.

6.3 Risk Management

Because liability is a major factor in health care delivery and because health care delivery systems and practitioners seek to minimize liability whenever possible, **risk management** has become a necessary practice component. Risk management is one approach to reducing the likelihood of a malpractice lawsuit. Risk management involves identifying problem practices or behaviors and then eliminating or controlling them. Risk management activities that may help avoid litigation include providing written job descriptions for health care practice employees and providing office procedures manuals and employee handbooks that can help avoid misunderstandings and mistakes that lead to liability risks. Other common health care facility activities that may affect the likelihood or course of litigation include medical record charting,

risk management
The taking of steps to minimize danger, hazard, and liability.

patient scheduling, writing prescriptions, and communicating with patients.

quality improvement (QI) or quality assurance (QA) A program of measures taken by health care providers and practitioners to uphold the quality of patient care.

Methods used to manage risk are part of **quality improvement (QI) or quality assurance (QA):** a program of practices performed by health care providers and practitioners to uphold the quality of patient care and to reduce liability risk.

Most health care facilities and plans employ quality improvement and risk managers to oversee risk and quality issues relating to physicians and support staff. Quality improvement and risk managers may also assume responsibility for compliance with federal, state, and other health care regulations. A compliance plan is developed to help ensure that all governmental regulations are followed. Such a plan is especially beneficial for following coding and billing regulations for Medicare, Medicaid, and other government plans.

Review LO 6.1 for a variety of suggestions about how to provide patient safety and avoid liability.

Enterprise risk management (ERM) is a concept that has been used in business for many years. For the last several years, health care professional organizations have been promoting the concepts of enterprise risk management for use in health care. Risk management has traditionally been overseen by a specific department within an organization. ERM in health care links risk management and quality improvement with an organization-wide framework, rather than relying on a departmental focus. ERM looks at risk management and total value of the organization.

Although organizations differ in how they may implement ERM, risk management and quality improvement become the responsibility of all employees. Risk managers recognize that good communication is not just between provider and patient but also between departments, providers, and patients and may affect the value of the organization. According to ERM principles, good communication reduces risks and may improve outcomes.

Most health care institutions and organizations also employ individuals who are responsible for credentialing. Credentialing may be done by risk management staff or by other departments within a health care organization. Credentialing is the process of verifying a health care provider's credentials. The process may be performed by an insurance company before a provider is admitted to the network, by medical offices prior to granting hospital privileges, or by other groups that routinely employ or contract with health care providers. Credentialing usually consists of the following:

1. A provider fills out an application and attaches copies of his or her medical license, proof of malpractice insurance coverage, and other requested credentials.
2. The listed sources are asked to verify the information.
3. Medicare and Medicaid sanctions and malpractice history are checked via the National Practitioner Data Bank.
4. The findings are presented to a credentialing committee.
5. A peer review process completes the credentialing procedure.

Check Your Progress

Select the correct answer for each of the following questions.

8. Risk management has become a necessary health care practice component because
   a. Liability insurance is often unavailable.
   b. Liability is a major factor in health care delivery.
   c. Patients with bad outcomes always sue.
9. Methods used to manage risk are part of
   a. The provisions in liability insurance policies
   b. Every health care provider's practice
   c. Quality improvement or quality assurance
10. Which of the following activities help health care providers avoid litigation?
    a. Vocal disclaimers before procedures are performed
    b. Medical record charting
    c. Issuing written denials in response to accusations of wrong doing
11. Which of the following is *not* a duty of a medical practice's quality improvement and risk manager?
    a. Credentialing
    b. Checking compliance with health care regulatory agencies' requirements
    c. Scheduling patient appointments
12. Credentialing consists of
    a. Publishing health care provider job vacancies
    b. Filing health care employees' credentials with state agencies
    c. Verifying health care providers' credentials before hiring

6.4 Professional Liability Insurance

Because costs for defending a medical malpractice lawsuit can be high, **liability insurance** may be purchased to cover the costs up to the limits of the policy. For example, if a medical professional liability insurance policy covers an insured physician up to $10 million, in the event that he or she loses a malpractice suit and must pay damages, the insurance company will not pay more than that amount.

liability insurance
Contract coverage for potential damages incurred as a result of a negligent act.

The cost of liability insurance premiums for a physician is based on the physician's specialty and the dollar amount covered by the policy. Insurance for those physicians in the least risky insurance risk class (for example, family practitioners and specialists who do not perform surgery) is generally less costly than insurance for those in specialties considered riskier (for example, orthopedic surgeons and obstetricians). States vary regarding those medical specialties considered to carry the highest risk of liability and, therefore, are subject to the highest liability insurance premiums.

Some physicians drop liability insurance coverage when rates become too high. However, this can adversely affect a physician's practice because most hospitals require proof of coverage up to a predetermined minimum amount to grant hospital privileges. In addition, managed care organizations require physicians to provide proof of liability insurance coverage as a prerequisite for entering into a contractual agreement and as a component of their credentialing process.

There are two main types of medical malpractice insurance:

claims-made insurance
A type of liability insurance that covers the insured only for those claims made (not for any injury occurring) while the policy is in force.

1. **Claims-made insurance** covers the insured only for those claims made (not for any injury occurring) while the policy is in force. With this kind of insurance, the determining factor is when the claim is made, not when the injury occurs. For example, a policy in force during a previous year would cover only those claims made during that year.

occurrence insurance
A type of liability insurance that covers the insured for any claims arising from an incident that occurred or is alleged to have occurred during the time the policy is in force, regardless of when the claim is made.

2. **Occurrence insurance** (also known as *claims-incurred insurance*) covers the insured for any claims arising from an incident that occurred or is alleged to have occurred while the policy is in force, regardless of when the claim is made. For example, suppose an alleged incident of negligence by a physician occurred in September 2013, while the physician's occurrence insurance policy was in effect with XYZ Insurance Company. If a patient files a claim against the physician in January 2016, after the policy period has passed, the physician is covered under the terms of the occurrence insurance policy.

There are three types of insurance that health care practitioners can purchase to extend coverage of a canceled claims-made policy or for claims-made coverage when the insured switches to a different insurance carrier:

tail coverage
An insurance coverage option available for health care practitioners: When a claims-made policy is discontinued, it extends coverage for malpractice claims alleged to have occurred during those dates that claims-made coverage was in effect.

1. **Tail coverage.** When a claims-made policy is discontinued, tail coverage (sometimes called a reporting endorsement) is an option available to health care practitioners from their former carriers to continue coverage for those dates that claims-made coverage was in effect. Once a claims-made policy is canceled, coverage does not continue in the future for any claims that might be reported unless tail coverage or prior acts coverage is secured at the time the policy is canceled. If neither is purchased, any future claims that might arise from services performed during the policy period will no longer be covered.

prior acts insurance coverage
A supplement to a claims-made insurance policy that can be purchased from a new carrier when health care practitioners change carriers.

2. **Prior acts insurance coverage.** This is a supplement to a claims-made policy that health care practitioners can purchase from a new carrier when they change carriers. Prior acts coverage, also known as "nose" coverage, covers incidents that occurred prior to the beginning of the new insurance relationship but have not yet been brought to the insured's attention as a claim. Prior acts coverage is an alternative to a reporting period endorsement (also known as tail coverage), which is purchased from the original carrier when a change in carriers is made. Companies typically require the new insured to purchase either tail or nose coverage to protect against claims arising from prior acts.

self-insurance coverage
An insurance coverage option whereby insured subscribers contribute to a trust fund to be used in paying potential damage awards.

3. **Self-insurance coverage.** As medical malpractice insurance premiums have continued to rise, self-insurance coverage has become an option for health care practitioners in some states. It works like

this: An insurance company writes a policy with a limit of $X, and the insured parties contribute to a trust fund up to a limit of $X to be used in paying potential medical malpractice awards. The insurance company charges fees for managing the fund. One advantage to self-insurance coverage is that premiums are considerably lower than with traditional types of medical malpractice insurance. A disadvantage is that state laws regulating insurance do not always allow such plans, and even in states where such coverage is allowed, hospitals must agree to accept self-insurance plans for those physicians who apply for hospital privileges.

Physicians and other health care practitioners should notify their insurance companies immediately if advised of the possibility of a malpractice lawsuit. Insurance companies almost always provide legal representation for covered physicians, and some insurance contracts require that the insurance company's attorneys represent the insured physician.

Once a lawsuit seems imminent, the health care practitioner and/or his or her employees should not mention the suit on the telephone or in correspondence unless the insurance company's legal counsel approves such a reference.

Check Your Progress

13. If a health care practitioner covered by medical malpractice insurance receives notice of a lawsuit, he or she should first notify ______________.
14. Claims-made insurance pays for ______________.
15. Occurrence insurance pays for ______________.
16. Name two types of insurance that, in certain circumstances, extend coverage of claims-made insurance.
17. Explain how physicians might insure themselves.

Chapter Summary

<table>
<tr><th>Learning Outcome</th><th>Summary</th></tr>
<tr><td>LO 6.1 Define the four Cs of medical malpractice prevention.</td><td>What are the four Cs of medical malpractice prevention?<ul><li>Caring</li><li>Communication</li><li>Competence</li><li>Charting</li></ul>Why do patients sue?<ul><li>Failure to diagnose.</li><li>Patient suffered abnormal injury.</li><li>Failure to treat.</li><li>Poor documentation of patient instruction and education.</li><li>Errors in medication administration.</li><li>Failure to follow safety procedures.</li><li>Improperly obtaining/lack of informed consent.</li></ul>How are medical records important to the defense of a medical malpractice suit?<ul><li>They can override a patient's recall of the events.</li><li>Events not recorded are presumed not to have happened.</li><li>Events recorded are presumed to have happened.</li><li>Properly obtaining physical evidence and recording collection procedures bolster a defense.</li></ul></td></tr>
<tr><td>LO 6.2 Describe the various defenses to professional liability suits.</td><td>What types of defense may be used in a medical malpractice lawsuit?<ul><li>Denial</li><li>Affirmative<ul><li>Contributory negligence</li><li>Comparative negligence</li><li>Assumption of risk</li><li>Emergency</li></ul></li><li>Technical<ul><li>Release of tortfeasor</li><li>Res judicata</li><li>Statute of limitations</li></ul></li></ul></td></tr>
<tr><td>LO 6.3 Explain the purpose of quality improvement and risk management within a health care facility.</td><td>What purpose does risk management serve?<ul><li>Helps minimize liability</li><li>Quality improvement (QI) or quality assurance (QA)</li><li>Verifies credentials</li></ul>What is enterprise risk management in health care?<ul><li>A concept that links risk management and quality improvement within an organizational framework and makes both the responsibility of all employees</li><li>A concept that looks at risk management by extending communication among all departments and clients</li></ul></td></tr>
<tr><td>LO 6.4 Identify five different types of medical liability insurance.</td><td>What types of professional liability insurance are available to medical providers?<ul><li>Claims-made<ul><li>Tail coverage</li><li>Prior acts coverage</li></ul></li><li>Occurrence</li><li>Self-coverage</li></ul></td></tr>
</table>

Chapter 6 Review

Applying Knowledge

LO 6.1

Name the four Cs of medical malpractice prevention, and after each term, list at least one way you can comply.

1. ______________________________
2. ______________________________
3. ______________________________
4. ______________________________

Name eight guidelines for physicians and other health care practitioners to follow that may help prevent malpractice lawsuits.

5. ______________________________
6. ______________________________
7. ______________________________
8. ______________________________
9. ______________________________
10. ______________________________
11. ______________________________
12. ______________________________

LO 6.2

13. Under __________, a claim may not be retried between the same two parties if it has been legally resolved.

    a. Common law

    b. *Res ipsa loquitur*

    c. *Res judicata*

    d. Arbitration

14. The __________ is the time limit for filing a lawsuit.

    a. Affirmative defense

    b. Assumption of risk

    c. Statute of limitations

    d. Technical defense

15. Which of the following is *not* a form of affirmative defense to a professional liability suit?

    a. Contributory negligence

    b. Denial

    c. Assumption of risk

    d. Emergency

16. Under the __________ defense, a health care practitioner who comes to the aid of an accident victim at the scene would not be held liable.

   a. *Res judicata*

   b. *Res ipsa loquitur*

   c. Emergency

   d. Denial

17. When the defendant alleges that he or she did no wrong, that defense is called

   a. Negligence

   b. Contributory negligence

   c. Denial

   d. Assumption of risk

18. If the patient knew the inherent risk before treatment, the defendant may use __________ as a defense in a lawsuit.

   a. Negligence

   b. Contributory negligence

   c. Denial

   d. Assumption of risk

19. Which of the following is an affirmative defense?

   a. Release of tortfeasor

   b. Emergency

   c. *Res judicata*

   d. Statute of limitations

20. Which of the following is a technical defense?

   a. *Res judicata*

   b. Contributory negligence

   c. Comparative negligence

   d. Assumption of risk

21. When damages are apportioned according to the degree a plaintiff contributed to his or her injury, this is called

   a. Negligence

   b. Comparative negligence

   c. Denial

   d. Assumption of risk

22. The statute of limitations

   a. Is the same in each state

   b. Is a federal law

   c. Is determined by the courts

   d. Is different depending on the state

23. *Res judicata* is Latin for

   a. Buyer beware

   b. The judge is in charge.

   c. The jury is in charge.

   d. The thing has been decided.

LO 6.3

24. Risk management is a process

   a. To assess liability insurance

   b. To manage difficult patients

   c. To minimize danger, hazard, and liability

   d. None of these

LO 6.4

25. Medical malpractice insurance that covers the insured only for those claims made while the policy is in force is called

   a. Prior acts coverage

   b. Self-insurance coverage

   c. Claims-made coverage

   d. Occurrence insurance

26. Medical malpractice insurance that covers the insured for any claims arising from an incident that occurred or is alleged to have occurred during the time the policy was in force, regardless of when the claim is made, is called

   a. Prior acts coverage

   b. Self-insurance coverage

   c. Claims-made coverage

   d. Occurrence insurance

27. Which of the following is a supplemental insurance to medical liability insurance?

   a. Occurrence coverage

   b. Prior acts coverage

   c. Claims-made coverage

   d. Self-insurance coverage

Ethics Issues Defenses to Liability Suits

Use your critical thinking skills to answer the questions that follow each ethics issue.

Ethics ISSUE 1:

According to the ethical guidelines for a number of professional organizations, incompetence, corruption, or dishonest conduct on the part of health care practitioners is unethical and never acceptable. In addition to posing a real or potential threat to patients, such conduct undermines the public's confidence in the health care professions and could cause adverse events that in turn could lead to lawsuits.

Discussion Questions

Determine whether each of the following behaviors is unethical, illegal, or both, and explain how each might lead to liability.

28. A physician intentionally enters a billing code on a patient's billing sheet for an examination that was not performed. The code entered means that the patient's insurance carrier will be billed for a more expensive exam than the one that was actually performed.

29. A hospital instructs its nurses to introduce themselves by name to each new patient in this manner: "I am Susan, and I've been assigned to take care of you. I have an associate's degree in nursing [or substitute appropriate educational credentials]. I see your physician is Dr. Wellness, and I can assure you that he is an excellent doctor. Let me know if you need anything at all."

30. An anesthesiologist has never administered anesthesia to a child but conceals this fact from a surgeon who likes her and requests her for an upcoming procedure on a 6-year-old.

31. A nursing assistant slaps an elderly patient in a skilled nursing care facility for calling her a name.

32. A nurse begins a painful procedure on an elderly hospital patient and ignores the patient's requests for an explanation.

33. A phlebotomist mislabels a blood sample but later denies any responsibility for the inappropriate medical treatments that result.

Ethics ISSUE 2:

Principles of ethics and professional conduct for all health care professions emphasize that health care practitioners have a responsibility to promote and advance the patient's welfare.

After misreading an X-ray, a dentist mistakenly removes a healthy incisor from a patient's mouth, then fits the patient with a fixed bridge that will not stay in place and causes the patient great pain. The patient sees a second dentist who repairs the damage done by the first dentist and remarks about the "shoddy quality" of the first dentist's work. The patient sues the first dentist for medical malpractice, and the defendant is found not guilty. Several jurors who hear the case express the opinion that the patient bears some responsibility for his injuries simply for seeing the first dentist.

Discussion Questions

34. Was the second dentist acting ethically when she criticized the first dentist's work? Explain your answer.

35. Is the dentist who was found not guilty of medical malpractice thereby exonerated of any wrongdoing? Explain your answer.

36. Might the dentist found not guilty in this scenario be subject to sanctions from the professional organization to which the dentist belongs? Explain your answer.

37. Do you agree that the patient in this case bears some responsibility for his injuries simply for seeing the dentist in question?

Ethics ISSUE 3:

The American Medical Association's *Code of Medical Ethics* states that physicians and other health care practitioners should not provide, prescribe, or bill for services they know are unnecessary. To be fair, however, it's not difficult to understand why a reasonable doctor would want to cover all his or her bases, so to speak, because the threat of a frivolous lawsuit is always looming.

James Wilson sees his physician for intermittent chest pain. Mr. Wilson's symptoms do not include sweating, difficulty breathing, or any other indications of heart problems. After a complete examination that includes a stress test and blood work, the physician is reasonably sure Mr. Wilson does not have heart problems. To protect against liability, however, Mr. Wilson's physician orders a coronary angiogram.

Discussion Question

38. Is it ethical for a physician or any other health care practitioner to prescribe or administer a medical treatment or test just to protect against potential liability? Explain your answer.

Case Studies

Use your critical thinking skills to answer the questions that follow each case study.

LO 6.1

A patient in her midtwenties saw an ophthalmologist for a routine eye exam. Due to her young age, a glaucoma test was not performed. She later was diagnosed with glaucoma and sued the ophthalmology group, alleging negligence in failing to perform a glaucoma test.

The defense argued that the standard of care was to not administer the test to patients younger than 40 because the instance of glaucoma at younger ages was rare.

Which of the following statements do you think best describes the applicable standard of care in this case? Explain your choice.

39. The defense should prevail because the reasonable, customary, and prudent course of action followed by practitioners in the same or similar circumstances would be the same.

40. The plaintiff should prevail because all patients should be protected against glaucoma, regardless of age.

You are a phlebotomist for a community laboratory, and you report for work on an extremely busy day. You travel daily from the lab where you work to the hospital to draw blood and then back to the lab. You have finished drawing blood at the hospital and are on your way back to the lab when you get a cell phone call that the hospital needs a complete blood count and electrolytes drawn STAT for a patient who has just come into the emergency room (ER).

41. Would you turn around and go back to the ER or drop off your current blood samples and then go back to the ER? Explain your answer.

42. What does question 41 have to do with preventing medical malpractice lawsuits?

LO 6.3

A nurse on the night shift in a busy hospital sees a physician's order to administer an intravenous medication to a patient who has just been admitted through the emergency room. She does not recognize the name of the drug but notes a charge of $4,000 for the drug. Her curiosity aroused, the nurse checks the drug and discovers it should not be administered more frequently than every six weeks and any patient receiving it should be carefully monitored at 15-minute intervals. The patient tells her he received the same medication just two weeks previously.

43. What should the nurse do?

44. In checking the drug is the nurse practicing risk management? Explain your answer.

Internet Activities

LO 6.1 and LO 6.4

Complete the activities and answer the questions that follow.

45. Find the most recent Medscape Report on medical malpractice. Review the report. What are three major findings from the most recent report that are important to your chosen profession?

46. Search the Web site of the American Tort Reform Association (ATRA). Use the site to find out if your state has passed civil justice reform acts that pertain specifically to health care practitioners. If so, briefly describe the acts and how they might affect health care practitioners.

47. Do a Web search for "physician malpractice insurance" to find out how malpractice insurance premium rates vary among states. Which states seem to be in crisis regarding the cost of medical malpractice insurance? In states with lower rates, what is credited with keeping costs lower than they are in other states? What is the situation in the state where you plan to practice? Should all health care practitioners carry medical malpractice insurance? Explain your answer.

Resources

LO 6.1 and 6.2

Joel, Lucille A. *Kelly's Dimensions of Professional Nursing.* New York: McGraw-Hill, 2011.

Kubasek, Nancy, et al. *Dynamic Business Law.* New York: McGraw-Hill, 2011.

Melvin, Sean. *The Legal Environment of Business.* New York: McGraw-Hill, 2010.

Reasons physicians are sued: www.medscape.com/features/slideshow/public/malpractice-report-2015

LO 6.3

Enterprise risk management: www.ashrm.org/pubs/files/white_papers/ERM-White-Paper-8-29-14-FINAL.pdf

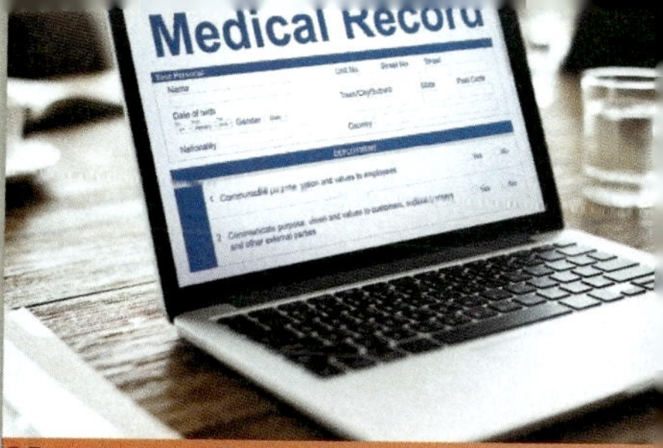

7

Medical Records, Informed Consent, and Health Information Technology

Key Terms

addendum
Confidentiality of Alcohol and Drug Abuse Patient Records
consent
doctrine of informed consent
doctrine of professional discretion
Good Samaritan acts
health information technology (HIT)
meaningful use
medical record
patient portals
social media
telemedicine

LEARNING OUTCOMES

After studying this chapter, you should be able to:

LO 7.1 Explain the purpose of medical records and the importance of correct documentation.

LO 7.2 Discuss medical records ownership, retention, storage, and destruction.

LO 7.3 Describe the purpose of obtaining a patient's consent for release of medical information.

LO 7.4 Explain the doctrine of informed consent.

LO 7.5 Briefly describe the major components of health information technology.

FROM THE PERSPECTIVE OF. . .

SALLY, MICHAEL, AND TERESA handle requests for release of patients' medical records for a Midwestern hospital serving a five-state area. They emphasize that they can release records only with signed authorization from the patient or on subpoena and that they may then release photocopies but never original medical records. When someone visits the hospital to pick up copies of a patient's records, that person is asked to show identification.

Michael lets experience be his guide and checks out any request for release of records that "doesn't feel right." For example, if a husband brings an authorization form for release of medical records that he says his wife signed, her signature should be checked against the signature on hospital admission forms. It could be that a divorce is in progress in such a situation, and the husband is seeking medical records to prove the spouse is an unfit parent.

"Never release medical records because the person making the request has intimidated you," adds Teresa. "The most officious person I've dealt with was an FBI agent who told me, 'I want this record. If you don't give it to me, I'll get it myself.' I said, 'Go for it.' Later the agent called and apologized to me."

Because the employing hospital is located in a city with an Air Force base, Sally, Michael, and Teresa often receive requests for medical records for active-duty military personnel. "We have now been told that the military can get the records they request on any active-duty person," adds Sally. "We still ask for an authorization, but it is not required because the active-duty person signs away that right when he or she signs up for the military. This applies to active-duty personnel on duty or on leave, but it does not include dependents of the person in the military."

Michael, Teresa, and Sally know that medical records contain information that can be used in ways not intended when the health care data were collected. They also know that the hospital that employs them can be legally liable for improper release of medical records. Therefore, they are extremely careful about always obtaining proper consent before releasing records.

From the perspective of individuals seeking medical records for their own purposes, not related to health care or the welfare of patients, Michael, Teresa, and Sally are unrelenting obstacles. From the perspective of the patients whose confidential medical records are conscientiously protected, Michael, Teresa, and Sally are performing their jobs well. From the perspective of their employer, Michael, Teresa and Sally are performing their jobs well and following the laws pertaining to the release of medical records.

7.1 Medical Records

medical record
A collection of data recorded when a patient seeks medical treatment.

A **medical record** is a collection of data recorded when a patient seeks medical treatment. The term *medical record*, as used in this chapter, refers to a patient's visits to one health care facility. The health record covers all of a patient's health care issues and covers all health care facilities the patient may have visited. The two terms are discussed in further detail in Chapter 8. Hospitals, surgical centers, clinics, physician offices, and other facilities providing health care services maintain patients' medical records. Medical records serve many purposes:

1. They are required by licensing authorities and provide a format for tracking, documenting, and maintaining a patient's communication data, both inside and outside a health care facility.
2. They provide documentation of a patient's continuing health care from birth to death.
3. They provide a foundation for managing a patient's health care.
4. They serve as legal documents in lawsuits.
5. They provide clinical data for education, research, statistical tracking, and assessing the quality of health care.

ENTRIES

In the past, medical records were created, maintained, and stored on paper. The "chart" was typically a physical collection of physicians' notes, X-rays, laboratory results, EEG and ECG tapes, and other detailed health care information placed inside a paper folder. Today, the common practice, and the federal government mandate, is to create, maintain, and store all medical records digitally. In addition to the data mentioned below, an electronic record today might include growth charts, flow sheets, uploaded data from glucometers, and data from implanted or wearable medical devices. Increasingly, genetic information is also part of a person's medical record, as well as data patients enter themselves through patient portals. But regardless of the method used for creating a medical record, for legal protection as well as continuity of care, the following information must be recorded in a patient's record:

- Contact and identifying information: the patient's full name, Social Security number, date of birth, and full address. If applicable, include e-mail address, home and work telephone numbers, marital status, and name and address of employer.
- Insurance information: name of policy member and relationship to patient, details such as certificate and group numbers, telephone numbers, copy of insurance card, Medicaid or Medicare numbers if applicable, and secondary insurance.
- Driver's license information, state, and number.
- Person responsible for payment and billing address.
- Emergency contact information.
- The patient's health history.
- The dates and times of the patient's arrival for appointments.
- A complete description of the patient's symptoms and reason for making an appointment.
- The examination performed by the physician.
- The physician's assessment, diagnosis, recommendations, treatment prescribed, progress notes, and instructions given to the patient, plus a notation of all new prescriptions the physician writes for the patient and of refills the physician authorizes.
- X-rays and all other test results.

- A notation for each time the patient telephoned the medical facility or was telephoned by the facility, listing date, reason for the call, and resolution.
- A notation of copies made of the medical record, including date copied and the person to whom the copy was sent.
- Documentation of informed consent, when necessary.
- Name of the guardian or legal representative to be contacted if the patient is unable to give informed consent.
- Other documentation, such as complete written descriptions; photographs; samples of body fluids, foreign objects, and clothing in cases involving criminal investigations; and so on. All items should be carefully labeled and preserved.
- Condition of the patient at the time of termination of treatment, when applicable, and reasons for termination, including documentation if the physician–patient contract was terminated before completion of treatment.
- Referrals and notations about follow-up calls to verify that an appointment was scheduled and kept.
- Missed appointments. Records should indicate "no show" or "canceled, no reschedule," as appropriate.
- Dismissals. To avoid charges of abandonment, the physician must formally withdraw from a case or formally dismiss the patient. Copies of letters of withdrawal or dismissal should be filed in the patient's record.
- Documentation of treatment refusals. Medical records should show a patient's decision to decline treatment, evaluation, or testing. "Informed refusal" should be obtained in writing with respect to any treatment or procedure that could have either diagnostic or therapeutic consequences.

Five Cs can be used to describe the necessary attributes of entries to patients' medical records. These entries must be:

1. Concise
2. Complete (and objective)
3. Clear (and legibly written)
4. Correct
5. Chronologically ordered

Medical records should never include inappropriate personal judgments or observations, or attempts at humor.

PHOTOGRAPHS, VIDEOTAPING, AND OTHER METHODS OF PATIENT IMAGING

In today's health care environment, it has become increasingly common to record patients' images through the use of photography, videotaping, digital imaging, and other visual recordings. For example, surgeons may photograph, videotape, or otherwise record procedures used during an operation for purposes of education or review. Cosmetic surgeons and physicians who treat accident victims may want to document visually the patient's condition before and after the incident. Such images then become part of the patient's medical record, subject to the same requirement for written release as the rest of the record.

Photographing or otherwise recording a patient's image without proper consent may be interpreted in a court of law as invasion of privacy. Invasion of privacy charges are most often upheld in court if the patient's image was used for commercial purposes, but such claims have also been upheld under public disclosure of embarrassing private facts. For example, "before" and "after" photographs published by a cosmetic surgeon may cause embarrassment to the patient if he or she did not give consent for the photographs to be published.

If a health care facility routinely photographs patients to document care, a special consent form should be signed stating that:

- The patient understands that photographs, videotapes, and digital or other images may be taken to document care.
- The patient understands that ownership rights to the images will be retained by the health care facility but that he or she will be allowed to view them or to obtain copies.
- The images will be securely stored and kept for the time period prescribed by law or outlined in the health care facility's policy.
- Images of the patient will not be released and/or used outside the health care facility without written authorization from the patient or his or her legal representative.

If the images will be used for teaching or publicity, a separate consent form should be used.

CORRECTIONS

Errors made when making an entry in a medical record or errors discovered later can be corrected, but corrections must be made in a specific manner so that if the medical records are ever used in a medical malpractice lawsuit, it will not appear that they were falsified. Because health care practitioners and facilities are steadily moving away from the creation or use of paper medical records, chances are health care practitioners in today's workplace will never have to know how to correct errors in paper records. But if the need arises, the prescribed legal protocol for correcting a paper medical record is as follows:

- Draw a line through the error so that it is still legible. Do not black out the information or use correction fluid to cover it up.
- Write or type in the correct information above or below the original line or in the margin. If necessary, you may attach another sheet of paper or another document with the correction on it. In this case, note in the record "See attached document A" to indicate where the corrected information can be found.
- Note near the correction why it was made (for example, "error, wrong date," or "error, interrupted by a phone call"). You can place this note in the margin or, again, add an attachment. Do not make a change in the record without noting the reason for it.
- Enter the date and time, and initial the correction.
- If possible, ask another staff member or the physician to witness and initial the correction to the record when you make it.

As detailed in the Health Information Technology (HIT) section of this chapter, the 1996 Health Insurance Portability and Accountability Act (HIPAA) required health care providers and facilities to convert from paper to electronic medical records. The act also provided for federal financial grants for health care providers and facilities to upgrade hardware and software for use in creating and maintaining electronic medical records. The federal Office of the National Coordinator for Health Information Technology (ONC) operates the ONC Health IT Certification Program. Vendors who provide electronic health records systems must meet their standards in order to be a certified program. The certified software chosen for this purpose determines general methods for correcting errors, but all correction methods used for electronic medical records must meet the more exacting requirements for correcting medical records in order to comply with federal and state law.

Most important, regardless of the software used, the system must provide for more than a simple strike-through or different-colored type to indicate changed information in a medical record. The original record must not be obscured because it could contain information vital to a patient's care. For example, say a physician is considering prescribing a certain medication for a woman of childbearing age. The medication can cause birth defects in a fetus, so the physician orders a pregnancy test. The results of the pregnancy test are positive but are mistakenly entered as negative. By the time the physician receives corrected laboratory results, the patient may have already begun taking the prescribed medication. And unless a method is in place for preserving the original medical record, the physician may not know, when he or she receives the corrected lab report, that the first report was in error.

Adding an addendum to correct an error or add to the original information is the correct method of revision, so that both the information in the original record and the information in the corrected version are available. An **addendum** is a significant change or addition to the electronic medical record.

addendum
A significant change or addition to the electronic health record (EHR).

Health care providers should have in place a policy for creating addendums to patient medical records, but typically, an addendum to a patient's electronic medical record will include the following:

a. Patient name
b. Date of service
c. Account number
d. Medical record number
e. Original report to which the addendum is to be attached
f. Date and time of the addendum and the electronic signature of the person creating the addendum

Examples of documentation errors that are corrected by addendum include wrong dates, wrong locations, duplicate documents, incomplete documents, and other errors. The amended version must be reviewed and signed by the provider.

Check Your Progress

1. Define *medical record.*
2. List five purposes served by a patient's medical record.
3. If a reconstructive surgeon wants to publish "before" and "after" photographs of patients in a brochure left in the waiting room for distribution to prospective patients, what must she do?

7.2 Medical Records Ownership, Retention, Storage, and Destruction

OWNERSHIP

It has long been the general consensus among health care providers and their legal advisors that the health care provider or facility that creates a patient's medical record owns the record. The patient, while not entitled to ownership of the original physical document with its many parts, was said to "own" the information contained in the record.

The ownership issue has become more complicated since advances in technology have led to federal legislation that mandates the conversion from paper to electronic medical records. Although ordering the digital conversion, HIPAA and other health-related federal laws do not specify who owns medical records, and state laws concerning ownership, when they exist, vary widely. As of mid-2016, only New Hampshire had a law that said patients own their own medical records. In 21 states, the law said health care providers and/or facilities own them. The rest of the states had no legislation addressing the matter, according to an analysis of state laws by Health Information & The Law, a project of the George Washington University's Hirsh Health Law and Policy Program and the Robert Wood Johnson Foundation.

Certainly, in the absence of specific state ownership laws, common sense dictates that *physical* ownership of patient medical records falls to the health care practitioners and facilities that create them because patients generally do not have the storage capacity or security measures in place to store paper or electronic records as legally required. It is certainly true, too, that patients have some control over the *information* contained in their medical records because they are free to request and obtain copies of their own medical records, request an amendment to those records, and request in writing that such records be released to third parties. Patients who disclose sensitive information about their health history and personal information such as their Social Security numbers may continue to think of that information as theirs, even if they give it to a provider for the purpose of receiving health care services. But according to the law, once a patient discloses information that becomes part of a health care provider's medical record, that information is now owned by the provider—essentially because the information has then become part of the health care provider's business records.

On signing the appropriate release, patients may usually obtain copies of the information contained in their medical records, and because that information may be extensive, it is becoming common practice for the health care practitioners and/or facilities to levy copying charges. However, under the **doctrine of professional discretion,** courts have held that in some cases, patients treated for mental or emotional conditions may be harmed by seeing their own records.

doctrine of professional discretion A principle under which a physician can exercise judgment as to whether to show patients who are being treated for mental or emotional conditions their records. Disclosure depends on whether, in the physician's judgment, such patients would be harmed by viewing the records.

Under HIPAA, patients who ask to see or copy their medical records must be accommodated, with a few exceptions. If patients need clarification, records may be reviewed in the presence of a trusted health care professional, but this cannot be made a requirement for allowing patients to see their records.

When an employer requires a job-related physical, scheduled and paid for by the employer, ownership of the medical records generated is considered the property of the health care practitioner or facility who created them, but the employer is entitled to a copy of that part of the record that is pertinent to the job-related exam. For example, an employer looking for parcel delivery employees may want to know if prospective employees can lift as much as 40 pounds; airlines need to know if prospective pilots have 20-20 vision or wear lenses that correct their vision to 20-20; stores hiring cashiers want to know if prospective employees can stand for extensive periods of time; and so on. It is not permissible, however, for employers to store employees' medical records in general personnel files; such records must be kept secure from unauthorized viewing or release.

RETENTION AND STORAGE

As a protection in the event of litigation, records should be kept until the minimal applicable statute of limitations period has elapsed, which varies with states but generally ranges from 2 to 7 years for adults. The statute of limitations period for keeping minors' medical records is different from that of adult records, with some states specifying a specific time period for keeping records (3 to 5 years is common) after the patient reaches the "age of majority" (21 in most states but may be 18 or 19).

In addition,

1. Retention of X-rays, ECG and EEG tracings, and other records may be subject to different statute of limitation periods than the rest of the record.
2. Some state medical records retention laws also specify a minimal time period for keeping a deceased patient's records, such as 3 years, 6 years, or 10 years after death.
3. Some state laws specify that when a medical record is due to be destroyed, a record summary must be maintained.
4. A state may have no statutory or regulatory specifications for the retention of medical records, but health care practitioners and facilities within those states may opt to follow the recommendation of state medical boards and medical associations.

To summarize, in the absence of specific state requirements, providers should keep health information for at least the period specified by the state's statute of limitations or for a sufficient length of time for compliance with laws and regulations. If the patient is a minor, the provider should retain health information until the patient reaches the age of majority (as defined by state law) plus the period of the statute of limitations. Legal advisors have said that a longer retention period is prudent because the statute may not begin until the potential plaintiff learns of the causal relationship between an injury and the care received. Plus, under the False Claims Act, discussed in Chapter 8, claims may be brought up to 7 years after the incident, and, on occasion, that time has been extended to 10 years.

Medical record retention requirements vary so widely that it is helpful if health care providers and facilities create a record retention schedule. Personnel responsible for setting up such schedules should compare state retention requirements and statutes of limitation and should consult with legal counsel. In addition to state law and in-house or other legal counsel, other resources for medical record retention guidelines include the following:

- Accreditation agency standards. Agencies such as the Commission on Accreditation of Rehabilitation Facilities, Medicare Conditions of Participation, and the Joint Commission have incorporated record retention schedules into their accreditation survey processes.
- American Health Information Management Association (AHIMA). The AHIMA says that, at a minimum, medical records retention schedules should include specific guidelines for what information is kept, retention time, and the storage medium on which records will be maintained (paper, microfilm, laser or other disc, magnetic tape). Retention time should also ensure patient health information is available to meet the needs of continued patient care, legal requirements, research, education, and other legitimate uses for the information. Clear destruction policies and procedures should be included, specifying appropriate methods of destruction for each medium on which information is maintained.
- Organizations with special patient populations, such as minors, and behavioral health or research patients may be governed by more specific regulations and may need to list special considerations for retention. For example, the Food and Drug Administration has required research records for cancer patients to be maintained for 30 years.

DESTRUCTION

Destruction of patient health information by a health care facility or provider must be carried out in accordance with federal and state law, and experts recommend that the process follow a written, approved retention schedule and destruction policy. Records involved in any open investigation, audit, or litigation must not be destroyed until the litigation case or open investigation has been closed.

As with record retention, there is no single standard destruction requirement. Some states require that organizations create an abstract of the destroyed patient information, notify patients when destroying patient information, or specify the method of destruction used to render the information unreadable. In the absence of any state law to the contrary, organizations must ensure paper and electronic records are destroyed with a method that provides for no possibility of reconstruction of information.

Examples of common destruction methods are as follows:

- Paper records: burning, shredding, pulping, and pulverizing
- Microfilm or microfiche: recycling and pulverizing
- Laser discs: pulverizing
- Computerized data: demagnetizing
- DVD: shredding or cutting
- Magnetic tapes: demagnetizing

The American Health Information Management Association (AHIMA) recommends that facilities destroying health records permanently maintain documentation of the destruction.

The following government Web site lists medical records minimal statute of limitation retention laws for physicians and hospitals in those states where statutes exist, as well as requirements in those states that have no laws but follow medical board/medical association guidelines: www.healthit.gov/sites/default/files/appa7-1.pdf.

Check Your Progress

4. How long should a deceased patient's medical records be retained?
5. Define *doctrine of professional discretion.*
6. If medical records are lost prior to the filing of a medical malpractice lawsuit, what might result?
7. Experts recommend that the process of destruction of medical records follow a written ________ and __________.
8. The cardinal rule for the method used to destroy medical records can be summarized as: The information must not be ______________.
9. Who owns the medical record?
10. Are you entitled to a copy of your medical record on request?

Creation and control of medical records has become a debated topic because the medical record has changed dramatically and continues to evolve, and because the security of electronically stored records must be inviolable—a condition that depends on the security measures provided by storage managers.

The "chart" used to travel within one health care facility—that is, from storage to exam room, to X-ray or lab, to the sonogram room—carried by a physician, nurse, or other health care practitioner who was charged with keeping the record secure. Now the medical record resides on a computer and is physically transported within a health care facility via a digital device. Stored on computers, the medical record is also transported over wireless networks or the Internet between health care facilities and other entities. Unfortunately, computer databases can be hacked, making complete security for the information in medical records difficult to maintain.

Because medical records contain so much personal and private information, federal and state laws have decreed that access must be restricted. In fact, violating the confidentiality of medical records is an actionable offense that can result in job loss, professional sanctions, civil suits resulting in hefty fines, and even criminal penalties.

The "rules" for health care practitioners in a position to grant access to medical records are detailed in the "Confidentiality" section.

7.3 Confidentiality

Because health care practitioners have a duty to protect the privacy of the patient, medical records should not be released to a third party without written permission signed by the patient or the patient's legal representative. Only the information requested should be released.

Requests for release of records may ask for records concerning a specific date or time span. Records may also be requested for a specific diagnosis, symptom, or body system, or for results of certain diagnostic tests. Medical records personnel should not send unsolicited records. They should carefully review the signed release form to ensure that the correct records are sent.

When medical records are requested for use in a lawsuit, a signed consent for the release of the records must be obtained from the patient, unless a court subpoenas the records. In this case, the patient should be notified in writing that the records have been subpoenaed and released.

ROUTINE RELEASE OF INFORMATION

Medical information about a patient is often released for the following purposes:

Insurance Claims. The medical office supplies specific requested information but does not usually send the patient's entire medical record. An authorization to release information signed by the patient is required before records may be released, but most health care providers incorporate the release into the patient registration form so that information can be provided in a timely manner.

Transfer to Another Physician. The physician may photocopy and send all records or may send a summary. The patient must sign an authorization to release records.

Use in a Court of Law. When a subpoena *duces tecum* is issued for certain records (the subpoena commands a witness to appear in court and to bring certain medical records), the patient's written consent to release the records is waived.

As illustrated in the chapter's opening scenario, individuals responsible for releasing medical information must follow procedure to protect against unauthorized release, even in situations in which medical records are routinely requested.

The court case "Breach of Confidentiality Declared—Damages Upheld" determined that damages were properly awarded to the plaintiff in a suit against a nurse who released confidential medical information without authorization.

While Michael, Sally, and Teresa, the medical records employees in the "From the Perspective of. . ." chapter opener, are explicitly aware of the dangers of releasing confidential medical information, all health care practitioners, like the nurse in the court case "Breach of Confidentiality Declared—Damages Upheld," also need to be constantly aware of protecting confidentiality of patients' medical records.

Health care practitioners receive subpoenas for patient medical records for a variety of reasons, including accidents involving patients, workers' compensation claims, and other nonmedical liability reasons. When this

COURT CASE

Breach of Confidentiality Declared—Damages Upheld

A 20-year-old unmarried woman who lived with her parents decided to terminate her pregnancy at the Long Island Surgi-Center. Because her parents strongly disapproved of premarital sex and were implacably opposed to abortion, she did not tell them of her decision. When she arranged for the procedure, the woman provided her cell phone number but told the clinic never to call her at home. Nevertheless, a day after the abortion, one of the clinic's nurses telephoned the young woman at home and spoke with a person she knew to be the woman's mother. Because blood test results had been received at the center that morning but had not been entered in the patient's medical record, the nurse called the patient's home to determine (1) information about the patient's blood type and (2) if the patient was experiencing vaginal bleeding. The nurse did not explicitly tell the patient's mother that her daughter had undergone an abortion, but the mother deduced the truth from the nurse's questions. The patient's relationship with her parents was irreparably damaged, and she sued the clinic, charging breaches of confidentiality, privacy, and fiduciary duty and seeking compensatory and punitive damages. The center conceded liability, and the matter proceeded to trial on the question of damages. The jury awarded the plaintiff $65,000 for past and future emotional distress and $300,000 in punitive damages. The Surgi-Center appealed the damages awarded, but the appeals court upheld the awards.

Source: *Randi A. J. v. Long Is. Surgi-Ctr.*, 2007 NY Slip Op 06953, 46 A.D. 3d 74.

occurs, the medical office sends a photocopy of the patient's medical records to the attorney who issued the subpoena.

When a physician is sued for medical malpractice, however, responsibility to comply with a subpoena to produce specified medical records in court may fall to the medical office employee in charge of medical records. In that case, the person in charge of medical records should follow these guidelines:

- Check the subpoena to be sure the name and phone number of the issuing attorney and the court docket number of the case are listed.
- If a copy of the subpoena is received, verify with the issuing attorney that it is the same as the original in every way.
- Verify that the patient named was a patient of the physician named.
- Verify the trial date and time as listed on the subpoena.
- Notify the physician that a subpoena was received, and then notify the physician's insurance company or attorney, if so directed.
- Check all subpoenaed records to be sure they are complete, but never alter them in any way.
- Document the number of pages in the record, and itemize its contents. Make a photocopy of the original to be submitted, if permitted by state law and the court.
- Offer sworn testimony regarding the record, if so instructed by the court.

Some state laws specifically address the release of confidential medical information, especially as it pertains to treatment for mental or emotional health problems, HIV testing, and substance abuse. In addition, the federal statute **Confidentiality of Alcohol and Drug Abuse Patient Records** protects patients with histories of substance abuse regarding the release of information about treatment. Under no circumstances should information of this type be released without specific, written permission from the patient to do so. The patient also has the right to rescind (cancel) consent to release information, in which case the information should not be released.

Confidentiality of Alcohol and Drug Abuse Patient Records
A federal statute that protects patients with histories of substance abuse regarding the release of information about treatment.

The following rules for authorizations for the release of medical records can serve as a general guide for medical assistants, health information technicians, and other health care practitioners:

- Authorizations should be in writing and should include the date on which consent expires.
- Authorizations should include the patient's name, address, and date of birth.
- The patient should sign authorizations, unless he or she is not a legal, competent adult. In that case, parents or guardians should sign authorizations.
- When authorizations lead to the release of patient information, only the information specifically requested should be released.
- Requests for information coming into the medical office from insurance companies, physicians, or other sources should be witnessed and dated and include the complete name, address, and signature of the party requesting the information, as well as that of the party asked to release the information.
- Requests for information should also include a specific description of the information that is needed, and the purpose for which the data will be used.

Check Your Progress

11. Name three reasons a medical facility might be requested to release a patient's medical records.
12. In which of the three situations named in question 11 might a patient's written consent to release records be waived?
13. What is needed before the medical facility can send a patient's medical record to the insurer?
14. If an insurance company submits a request for medical records pertaining to an enrolled patient's outpatient foot surgery and you are responsible for sending the records, should you send the patient's entire file to be on the safe side? Why or why not?
15. As the person who reviews requests for patients' medical records, do you need to know the purpose for which the data will be used? Explain your answer.

7.4 Informed Consent

consent
Permission from a person, either expressed or implied, for something to be done by another.

By giving **consent,** the patient gives permission, either expressed (orally or in writing) or implied, for the physician to examine him or her, to perform tests that aid in diagnosis, and/or to treat for a medical condition. When the patient makes an appointment for an examination, that patient has given implied consent for the physician to perform the exam. Likewise, when the patient cooperates with various diagnostic testing procedures, implied consent for the tests has been given.

INFORMED CONSENT

For surgery and for some other procedures, such as a test for HIV, implied consent is not enough. In these cases, it is important to ask the patient to sign a consent form, thereby documenting informed consent (see Figure 7-1).

FIGURE 7-1
A Sample Consent Form

INFORMED CONSENT for SURGERY and PROCEDURES

1. I hereby authorize staff physicians and resident staff at ______________________ to perform upon
(Name of Hospital or Facility)
______________________, such treatment, procedures and/or operations necessary to treat or diagnose the
(Name of patient)
condition(s) which appear indicated.

2. The operation(s) or procedure(s) necessary to treat and/or diagnose my condition and the risks, benefits/alternatives and options associated with them have been explained to me by ______________________, and I understand the operation(s) or
(Name of Physician or provider)
procedure(s) to be: ______________________

3. Different Provider: ☐ Not Applicable
I understand and approve that a different provider other than the physician named above may actually perform the procedure.

4. Operative Side: ☐ Not Applicable ☐ Left ☐ Right

5. Sedation & Local Anesthetics: I authorize the administration of sedation and the use of local anesthetics, drugs and medicines as may be deemed appropriate. If they will be used, the risks and benefits/alternatives of sedation have been explained to me by the procedural physician.

6. Blood and Blood Products: ☐ Not Applicable
I understand certain surgeries, procedures, or illnesses may result in loss of blood. I authorize the administration of blood and/or blood components during the procedure as well as during the course of my hospital stay. If blood will be used, the risks, benefits/alternatives have been explained to me by the physician.
Patient Initials: ______________________

7. No Blood Products: ☐ Not Applicable
I request that No blood derivative be administered to me. I hereby release the hospital, its personnel, the attending physician and its agents from any responsibility whatsoever for unfavorable reactions or any untoward results due to my refusal to permit the use of blood or its derivatives. The possible risks and consequences of such refusal on my part have been fully explained and I fully understand such risks and consequences may occur as a result of my refusal.

Signature of Patient/Responsible Person: ______________________ Relationship: ______________________

8. Unforeseen Conditions: It has been explained to me that during the course of the operation(s) or procedure(s) unforeseen conditions may be revealed that necessitate an extension of the original procedure(s) or different procedure(s) than those set forth above. I am aware that the practice of medicine is not an exact science and I acknowledge that no guarantees have been made to me concerning the result of the operation(s) or procedure(s).

9. Photography: I consent to the use of photography, closed circuit television recording and to use the photographs and other materials for study, educational and scientific purposes, in accordance with ordinary practices of the facility.

10. I consent to have my procedure/operation observed, for educational purposes, by individual(s) other than those assisting the physician during the procedure/operation.

Physician or Provider Signature | Patient's Signature (if competent) | Witness | Date | Time

Signature of Interpreter (if applicable) | Date | Time | Signature of Person Responsible Relationship | Date | Time

Witness (Telephone consent) | Date | Time | Second Physician or Provider Signature for Emergencies for incompetent patient and No family | Date | Time

Physician must initial faxed copy

The **doctrine of informed consent** is the legal basis for informed consent and is usually outlined in a state's medical practice acts. Informed consent implies that the patient understands

doctrine of informed consent
The legal basis for informed consent, usually outlined in a state's medical practice acts.

- Proposed modes of treatment
- Why the treatment is necessary
- Risks involved in the proposed treatment
- Available alternative modes of treatment
- Risks of alternative modes of treatment
- Risks involved if treatment is refused

Informed consent involves the patient's right to receive all information relative to his or her condition and then to make a decision regarding treatment based on that knowledge. Documents establishing that the patient gave informed consent prove that the patient was not coerced into treatment.

Adults of sound mind are usually able to give informed consent. Those individuals who cannot give informed consent include the following:

Minors, Persons under the Age of Majority. Exceptions include:

- Emancipated minors—those who are living away from home and responsible for their own support. A minor becomes emancipated through a court hearing in which evidence is presented that the minor should be emancipated and a judge makes a determination that the minor has met certain criteria. The minor is then declared "emancipated" and can consent to his or her health care treatment just as any adult of sound mind determines his or her health care treatment.
- Married minors
- Mature minors—those who, through the doctrine of mature minors, have been granted the right to seek birth control or care during pregnancy, treatment for reportable communicable diseases, or treatment for drug- or alcohol-related problems without first obtaining parental consent.

Persons Who Are Mentally Incompetent. Individuals judged by the court to be insane, senile, mentally challenged, or under the influence of drugs or alcohol cannot give informed consent. In these cases, a competent person may be designated by the court to act as the patient's agent.

Persons Who Speak Limited or No English. When a patient does not speak or understand English, an interpreter may be necessary to inform the patient and obtain his or her consent for treatment.

The rights of emancipated minors, married minors, and mature minors to consent to their own health care are discussed further in Chapter 11.

Other problems in obtaining informed consent may arise in situations such as when foster children need medical attention or a spouse seeks sterilization or an abortion. In each case, health care practitioners must determine who is legally able to give informed consent for treatment. When in doubt, seek legal advice.

Patient education is vital to the issue of informed consent. Stocking the medical office with brochures about various medical problems is not sufficient if the physician does not review the material with the patient. Patients who sue have successfully claimed lack of informed consent because they did not read the consent form they signed or did not read brochures handed to them. Health care personnel should be sure that patients understand all forms and all treatments and/or surgeries to be performed before signing.

Before proceeding with treatment, health care practitioners must determine whether or not patients are competent to give informed consent.

INFORMED CONSENT AND ABORTION LAW

In *Planned Parenthood v. Casey,* U.S. 833 (1992), the U.S. Supreme Court upheld a 24-hour waiting period, an informed consent requirement, a parental consent provision for minors, and a record-keeping requirement for women seeking an abortion. At the same time, the Court struck down the spousal notice requirement of a Pennsylvania statute, in addition to other specific requirements. *Casey* and *Webster v. Reproductive Health Services* before it (1989) upheld *Roe v. Wade,* the 1973 Supreme Court decision that legalized abortion in the United States (see the court case "Case Legalizes Abortion") but allowed state regulation of abortion. A number of state legislatures took the cue and passed new abortion restrictions.

Among a long list of state-imposed abortion restrictions are laws that specify certain changes in informed consent. For example, some states require that a woman seeking an abortion be clearly informed of all alternatives to abortions and be told of all risks associated with such surgeries before she can give informed consent to the abortion. In addition, before a woman can consent to an abortion in many states, she must wait a certain length of time (usually 24 hours) before actually signing a consent form.

A 1992 court case "Case Allows State Regulations" followed the landmark case of *Roe v. Wade.* This case allowed a state to regulate abortion.

Technically, abortion is legal in all 50 states, but state legislatures have added many restrictions.

Because abortion law is constantly changing, health care practitioners must stay informed about current abortion laws in their respective states. A good Web site for finding abortion laws in your state is http://statelaws.findlaw.com/family-laws/abortion.html.

HIV AND INFORMED CONSENT

State public health law varies for human immunodeficiency virus (HIV) testing, but, generally, health care practitioners must consider the following factors.

Can a minor (aged less than 18 in some states, 21 in others) consent to his or her own HIV test? Informed consent laws for minors vary, but this determination may sometimes be made without regard to age, depending on the minor's situation:

- Infants and young children do not have the capacity to consent because they do not yet have the ability to make informed decisions. The person legally designated to make health care decisions for the child has the right to decide whether the child should be tested for HIV.

LANDMARK COURT CASE

Case Legalizes Abortion

In 1970, a single woman in Texas became pregnant. She had difficulty finding work because of her pregnancy and feared the stigma of an illegitimate birth. Under the fictitious name "Jane Roe," the woman sued Henry Wade, the district attorney in Dallas County, Texas, claiming that she had limited rights to an abortion and sought an injunction against the Texas statute prohibiting abortion except to save a woman's life.

It took 3 years for the case to reach the U.S. Supreme Court, which struck down the Texas statute. The ruling came too late for Jane Roe to have the abortion she originally sought, of course, but it affected the rights of all women who would seek abortions from that time on. The Court held that the constitutional right to privacy includes a woman's decision to terminate a pregnancy during the first trimester (3 months) but that states could impose restrictions and regulate abortions after that.

Source: *Roe v. Wade,* 410 U.S. 113, 144 "n 39" (1973).

COURT CASE

Case Allows State Regulation

The Pennsylvania legislature amended its abortion control law in 1988 and 1989. Among the new provisions, the law required informed consent and a 24-hour waiting period prior to the procedure. A minor seeking an abortion required the consent of one parent (the law allowed for a judicial bypass procedure). A married woman seeking an abortion had to indicate that she notified her husband of her intention to abort the fetus. These provisions were challenged by several abortion clinics and physicians. A federal appeals court upheld all the provisions except the husband notification requirement.

The question in this case was, can a state require women who want an abortion to obtain informed consent, wait 24 hours, and, if minors, obtain parental consent without violating their right to abortions as guaranteed by *Roe v. Wade?* In a 5-to-4 decision, the Supreme Court again reaffirmed *Roe,* but it upheld most of the Pennsylvania provisions. For the first time, the justices imposed a new standard to determine the validity of laws restricting abortions. The new standard asks whether a state abortion regulation has the purpose or effect of imposing an "undue burden," which is defined as a "substantial obstacle in the path of a woman seeking an abortion before the fetus attains viability." Under this standard, the only provision to fail the undue burden test was the husband notification requirement.

Source: *Planned Parenthood v. Casey,* 505 U.S. 833 (1992).

- Married minors, emancipated minors, and minor parents may have the right to give consent for HIV testing, depending on state law.

Can an HIV-infected minor consent to his or her treatment? Generally, parental or guardian consent is required for a physician to treat a minor for HIV/AIDS, including treatment in school-based clinics. Married, emancipated, and mature minors can usually consent to their own care.

WHEN CONSENT IS UNNECESSARY

In emergency situations, when the patient is in immediate danger, the physician is not expected to obtain consent before proceeding with treatment.

All 50 states have passed **Good Samaritan acts.** These acts are intended to protect physicians and, in some states, other health care practitioners

Good Samaritan acts
State laws protecting physicians and sometimes other health care practitioners and laypersons from charges of negligence or abandonment if they stop to help the victim of an accident or other emergency.

and laypersons from charges of negligence or abandonment if they stop to help the victim of an accident or other emergency, provided they:

- Give such care in good faith.
- Act within the scope of their training and knowledge.
- Use due care under the circumstances.
- Do not bill for their services. (If a physician treats a patient as a "Good Samaritan" and later bills the patient for services, he or she may be held as having established a physician–patient relationship and may not have the immunity from civil damages that a Good Samaritan law would otherwise provide.)

While some states offer immunity to Good Samaritans, sometimes the act of rescuing an accident victim can result in a legal claim of negligent care if the injuries or illness were made worse by the volunteer's actions. Statutes typically don't exempt a Good Samaritan who acts in a willful and wanton or reckless manner in providing emergency care, advice, or assistance. Furthermore, Good Samaritan laws usually don't apply to a person rendering emergency care, advice, or assistance during the course of regular employment, such as services rendered by a health care provider to a patient in a health care facility.

Good Samaritan in legal terms refers to someone who renders aid in an emergency to an injured person on a voluntary basis. Usually, if a volunteer comes to the aid of an injured or ill person who is a stranger, the person giving the aid owes the stranger a duty of being reasonably careful. A person is not obligated by law to do first aid in most states, unless it's part of their job description. However, some states will consider it an act of negligence if a person doesn't at least call for help. Generally, where an unconscious victim cannot respond, a Good Samaritan can help on the grounds of implied consent. However, if the victim is conscious and can respond, a person should first ask permission to help.

If a person helps a victim in an emergency and is later sued, whether or not the defendant can use a state Good Samaritan law for his or her defense may depend on the court's definition of the state's law.

Check Your Progress

16. Who may give informed consent?
17. Who may not give informed consent?
18. Must consent to perform routine medical care, such as a physical examination, always be in writing? Explain your answer.
19. In which health care situations is implied consent not sufficient?
20. What consequences generally ensue if a legally competent adult is treated without consent and an adverse event occurs?

7.5 Health Information Technology (HIT)

According to the U.S. Department of Health and Human Services, **health information technology (HIT)** is "the application of information processing involving both computer hardware and software that deals with the storage, retrieval, sharing, and use of health care information, data, and knowledge for communication and decision making." The broad category *health information technology* also includes telemedicine and use of the Internet for health information purposes.

health information technology (HIT)
The application of information processing, involving both computer hardware and software, that deals with the storage, retrieval, sharing, and use of health care information, data, and knowledge for communication and decision making.

A central component of HIT is the patient's medical file. To that end, HIPAA required that all health care entities expecting reimbursement for services provided to Medicare and Medicaid patients would have an electronic medical record. The process is called **meaningful use.** In order to receive payment for Medicare and Medicaid, health care providers must attest, on a scheduled basis, that they are using certified electronic health record systems. Additionally, meaningful use sets specific objectives that health care providers must meet to qualify for incentive programs. More information about specific objectives can be found at the http://healthit.gov Web site. Table 7-1 identifies the overall goals of meaningful use.

meaningful use
A process by which health care providers use an electronic health record according to guidelines set by the federal government.

The HealthIT Web site also provides information about how many health care providers have adopted meaningful use. In 2015, 96 percent of all nonfederal acute-care hospitals had certified health IT; that is, they had met HIPAA's Stage 1 meaningful use standards. There continue to be some financial incentives to adopt meaningful use. As of March 2016, more than nine in 10 hospitals eligible for the incentive programs had achieved meaningful use of certified health IT. The latest data available at publication indicate that 78 percent of physicians had adopted an EHR as of 2015. The percentage of physicians e-prescribing (electronically prescribing) via an EHR accelerated from 7 percent in December 2008 to 70 percent in April 2014. (E-prescribing involves using software that allows health care practitioners licensed to prescribe to write and send prescriptions to participating pharmacies electronically. Benefits of e-prescribing include reduction of fraud and medication errors, increasing patient safety, and preventing patients from using more than one physician to obtain restricted drugs.)

Table 7-1 Meaningful Use Defined

- Meaningful use is using certified electronic health record (EHR) technology to:
  - Improve quality, safety, efficiency and reduce health disparities.
  - Engage patients and family.
  - Improve care coordination and population and public health.
  - Maintain privacy and security of patient health information.
- Ultimately, it is hoped that the meaningful use compliance will result in:
  - Improved population health outcomes
  - Increased transparency and efficiency
  - Empowered individuals
  - More robust research data on health systems

Source: https://www.healthit.gov/providers-professionals/meaningful-use-definition-objectives retrieved 8/5/2016.

Health care providers continue to participate in meaningful use as Stage 2 becomes a part of the process. The ultimate goal for Stage 2 is to require providers to offer patients access to a variety of electronic information services. It will be several years before compliance with Stage 2 is met.

When Hurricane Katrina hit the Louisiana and Mississippi coasts on August 29, 2005, the resulting destruction included the loss of countless paper medical records. As a result, many of the survivors couldn't remember the names of lost prescriptions or when they had last been immunized against tetanus and other diseases. In addition, storm victims who sought care from physicians had no medical records health care providers could use as a basis for treatment, and reconstruction, if even possible, would take valuable time.

By contrast, when Hurricane Sandy struck the East Coast on October 29, 2012, many health care providers had already converted paper files to digital files as part of HIPAA-mandated disaster planning. In fact, for most of the providers who suffered through Sandy, the process of compliance began long before the storm. Those providers that had disaster plans in place and had practiced them to be sure they worked were in the best position to ride out the storm without loss of critical data and services. And those providers who had duplicated all necessary electronic data at off-site data centers were also able to function during the storm or to restore function more quickly after the storm hit. For example, AtlantiCare, a health care system in New Jersey with a large regional medical center and 70 other locations throughout the state, made it through Sandy with few disruptions, thanks to advance disaster planning.

TELEMEDICINE AND SOCIAL MEDIA

telemedicine
Remote consultation by patients with physicians or other health professionals via telephone, closed-circuit television, or the Internet.

According to the American Telemedicine Association, **telemedicine** is formally defined as "the use of medical information exchanged from one site to another via electronic communications to improve a patient's clinical health status. Telemedicine includes a growing variety of applications and services using two-way video, email, smartphones, wireless tools and other forms of telecommunications technology."

When telemedicine was first used, it generally involved transmission of X-rays, sonograms, or other medical data between two distant points. In some cases, usually through closed-circuit television, a physician could examine a patient in a distant location, thus allowing patients in rural areas more complete access to medical care. As noted in the definition in the previous paragraph, telemedicine has a variety of applications beyond closed circuit television.

Telemedicine provides the following services:

- *Primary care and specialist referral services.* Primary care physicians can ask specialists to review a patient's medical history, laboratory and X-ray results, medications, and other data for help in making a diagnosis or in other aspects of the patient's care.
- *Remote patient monitoring.* Through remote transmission, medical data for homebound patients can be sent to home health agencies or remote diagnostic testing facilities for interpretation. Data can be specific to one condition, such as blood glucose levels, or they can

cover a broader area of concern. These services often supplement home health care visits.

- *Consumer medical and health information.* Through the Internet, consumers can find specific information about medical conditions, locate support and discussion groups, learn about prescribed medications, and so on. This aspect of telemedicine includes the use of **patient portals** for patients with computers or smartphones to schedule appointments with physicians, review lab results, ask for medication refills, see educational materials, and otherwise communicate with health care providers.
- *Medical education.* Physicians and other health care professionals can enroll in online courses where relevant, attend professional seminars remotely, hear specialists speak, and otherwise participate in continuing education.

patient portal
A secure online Web site that gives patients 24-hour availability to health care providers.

A big challenge for health care providers using telemedicine is that there are still a variety of policies that inhibit the use of telemedicine. Each state has different laws. If providers are treating patients in a different state from their own, there could be complications that inhibit not only their ability to treat the patient but also their ability to get paid for services they have provided.

Social media is changing the nature of health care. The term *social media* includes social networking sites, such as Facebook, LinkedIn, and Twitter, as well as media-sharing sites, blogs, microblogs, subject-specific discussion sites, and wikis, which are Web sites that allow collaborative editing of content and structure. Social media allows individuals and communities to gather, communicate, and share information, ideas, personal messages, images, and other content.

Social media
Forms of electronic communication through which users create online communities to share information, ideas, personal messages, and other content.

Many health professionals have created educational content to be shared across various social media sites. According to a 2014 study in the *Journal of Medical Internet Research*, nearly 95 percent of hospitals had a Facebook page and just over 50 percent had a Twitter account. According to an April 2016 article in *Hospitals and Health Networks,* the use of social media can benefit health care in five distinct ways:

- For those individuals seeking emotional support or tips for coping with a particular disease, social media may be very helpful. Sites provide virtual medical communities where patients can share their problems coping with a specific disease and learn more about the effects of medications and therapies.
- These sites can also deliver new clinical research insights. Sites such as PatientsLikeMe have become an analytical platform for clinicians and researchers.
- Social media can build awareness of causes or personal health crises. In 2014, the ALS (amyotrophic lateral sclerosis) Association raised $115 million for research compared to only $23.5 million in 2013. It was done by the Ice Bucket Challenge. The challenge on social media was to raise money by pouring ice on one's head, capturing it on video, and calling out another person to do the same.
- Social media gives health care consumers a voice in broadcasting opinions on everything related to health care—from hospitals to physicians to medications. Consumers may use social media to help choose their physician or hospital.

- Providers are beginning to use social media to capture patient satisfaction and feedback. Formal surveys by mail and e-mail are not always returned, and collecting information from social media may be a way to capture patient satisfaction.

According to a 2015 survey by Pew Research, about 62 percent of smartphone users get information on health care using their smartphone. Additionally, many people use either their smartphone or a wrist tracker to track their exercise, heart beat, and calorie intake.

Telemedicine, social media, and other health information technology continues to change the way health care is delivered in the twenty-first century. Optimizing the use of data to get the best results for patients will continue to be a challenge and an opportunity.

TECHNOLOGY, CONFIDENTIALITY, AND RELIABILITY

The use of technology in health care has provided us with many opportunities to improve patient care. With that technology comes a variety of cautions.

Health care workers and students posting on Facebook and Twitter, as well as other sites, even on their own time, must always be aware of confidentiality issues. For example, a student serving in an externship in allied health posted derogatory comments about a physician for whom she worked. The physician saw the student's remarks, and the student was dismissed from the program. Other incidents of unwise social media use have resulted in job loss, difficulty in obtaining a job, the permanent derailing of a career, and even legal difficulties.

When using the Internet for health care and medical information, the user should evaluate Web sites for reliability. Users should ask questions such as these:

- Who is sponsoring the site? Sites sponsored by or linked with major medical centers and groups, government agencies, and medical professionals or major medical publications are most likely to present reliable information.
- Are several reliable Web sites offering similar information? If so, the information is most likely to be reliable.
- Does the site tout miracle cures or peculiar therapies? Users should discuss any claims made with a trusted health care practitioner before sending for materials or "cures" or otherwise following such advice.

And, while advances in technology seem largely advantageous, there are still technologies that can create problems if not used properly. The following guidelines can help ensure that confidentiality is not breached when employees use photocopiers, fax machines, computers, and printers to reproduce and send medical records.

Photocopiers

- Do not leave confidential papers anywhere on the copier where others can read the information.
- Do not discard copies in a shared trash container; shred them.
- If a paper jam occurs, be sure to remove from the machine the copy or partial copy that caused the jam.

Fax Machines

- Always verify the telephone number of the receiving location before faxing confidential material.
- Never fax confidential material to an unauthorized person.
- Do not fax confidential material if others in the room can observe the material.
- Do not leave confidential material unattended on a fax machine.
- Do not discard fax copies in a shared trash container; shred them.
- Use a fax cover sheet that states, "Confidential: To addressee only. Please return if received in error."

Computers

- Locate the monitor in an area where others cannot see the screen.
- Do not leave a monitor unattended while confidential material is displayed on the screen.
- Because it is difficult to ensure the privacy of e-mail messages, sending confidential patient information via e-mail is not recommended.
- When computers are sold or otherwise recycled, it is vital that hard drives be erased or removed and destroyed.

Printers

- Do not print confidential material on a printer shared by other departments or in an area where others can read the material.
- Do not leave a printer unattended while printing confidential material.
- Before leaving the printing area, check to be sure all computer disks containing confidential material and all printed material have been collected.
- Be certain that the print job is sent to the right printer location.
- Do not discard printouts in a shared trash container; shred them.

Advances in technology have improved our ability to record, store, transfer, and share medical data electronically. They have also magnified privacy, security, and confidentiality concerns that pertain to patient medical records. Privacy and security issues are discussed at length in Chapter 8.

Check Your Progress

21. Define *health information technology.*
22. What is meaningful use?
23. How is telemedicine being used in health care?
24. How is social media used in health care?

Chapter Summary

<table>
<tr><th>Learning Outcome</th><th>Summary</th></tr>
<tr><td>LO 7.1 Explain the purpose of medical records and the importance of correct documentation.</td><td>What purposes do medical records serve?
• They are required by licensing authorities and provide a format for tracking, documenting, and maintaining a patient's communication data, both inside and outside a health care facility.
• They provide documentation of a patient's continuing health care from birth to death.
• They provide a foundation for managing a patient's health care.
• They serve as legal documents in lawsuits.
• They provide clinical data for education, research, statistical tracking, and assessing the quality of health care.
What information is entered into a patient's medical record?
• Contact and identifying information
• Insurance information
• Driver's license information
• Person responsible for payment and billing
• Emergency contact information
• Patient's health history
• Dates and times of appointments
• Descriptions of patient's symptoms and reasons for appointments
• Examinations performed
• Physician's assessment, diagnosis, recommendations, treatment, progress notes, prescriptions, and instructions to patient
• X-rays and all test results
• Notations for telephone calls
• Notations of copies made
• Documentation of informed consent
• Names of guardians or legal representatives if patient is unable to give informed consent
• All other documentation
• Condition of patient at time of termination of treatment
What are the five Cs of entries in medical records?
• Concise
• Complete
• Clear
• Correct
• Chronologically ordered
What is the accepted manner for correcting errors in a paper medical record?
• Draw a line through the error.
• Write correct information above or below original line.
• Note why correction was made.
• Enter the date and time of the correction, and initial it.
• Ask a coworker to witness and initial the correction when it is made.
What is the accepted method of correcting an electronic medical record?
• Follow the policy for software used to create the electronic medical record.
• If an addendum is added to the record, be sure it includes:
  • Patient name
  • Date of service
  • Account number</td></tr>
</table>

- Medical record number
- Original report to which the addendum is to be attached
- Date and time of the addendum and the electronic signature of the person creating the addendum

What general categories of information should be documented for legal purposes?

- What treatment was performed and when
- Referrals
- Missed appointments
- Dismissals
- Treatment refusals
- All other patient contact

LO 7.2 Discuss medical records ownership, retention, storage, and destruction.

Who owns a person's medical record?

- State laws vary, but it is generally accepted that the provider/facility that created the record owns it.

How long should medical records be kept?

- Laws vary with states, but records should be kept for the minimal statute of limitations period, plus any specified time.
- Laws also vary with states concerning minors and specific categories.

Can medical records be destroyed?

- Yes, as determined by state law and/or professional organization recommendations

LO 7.3 Describe the purpose of obtaining a patient's consent for release of medical information.

For what purposes is medical information routinely released?

- Insurance claims
- Transfer of the patient to another physician
- Use in a court of law

LO 7.4 Explain the concept of informed consent.

What information does the patient need to give informed consent?

- Proposed modes of treatment
- Why the treatment is necessary
- Risks involved
- Available alternatives
- Risks of alternatives
- Risks involved if treatment is refused

Who cannot give informed consent?

- Minors
- Persons who are mentally incompetent
- Persons who speak limited or no English

When do Good Samaritan laws protect health care practitioners who stop to help in emergencies?

- When care is given in good faith
- When caregivers act within the scope of their training and knowledge
- When caregivers use due care under the circumstances
- When caregivers do not bill for their services

LO 7.5 Briefly describe the major components of health information technology.

What is the purpose of meaningful use?

- Improve quality, safety, efficiency, and reduce health disparities
- Engage patients and family
- Improve care coordination and population and public health
- Maintain privacy and security of patient health information
- Improved population health outcomes
- Increased transparency and efficiency
- Empower individuals

	What is telemedicine? • The use of medical information exchanged from one site to another via electronic communications to improve a patient's clinical health status What is social media? • Social media allows individuals and communities to gather, communicate, and share information, ideas, personal messages, images, and other content What machines require special care in their use to prevent technological threats to confidentiality? • Photocopiers • Fax machines • Computers • Printers

Chapter 7 Review

Applying Knowledge

LO 7.1

1. Describe the difference between a medical record and a health record.
2. List the five Cs for correctly entering information into a medical record.
3. After an entry in the medical record has been written or keyed and an error is discovered, what procedure should be followed to correct the error?
   a. Use a pencil eraser to remove the entry on a written record; then write in the correction.
   b. Use the delete or backspace key if the entry was keyed in; then key in the correction.
   c. Draw a line through the error; then call the patient's physician.
   d. None of these
4. Which of the following comments should *not* be included in a patient's medical record?
   a. "Patient complained of pain in her right index finger."
   b. "Blood drawn for CBC."
   c. "Patient requests no more JELL-O."
   d. "Patient is as big as a blimp."

LO 7.2

5. Dr. Wellness works as an employee of Anytown Medical Clinic. Who owns the records of his patients?
   a. Dr. Wellness
   b. Anytown Medical Clinic
   c. Each of Dr. Wellness's patients
   d. The state in which Dr. Wellness practices
6. Dr. Wellness also sees patients at Anytown General Hospital, where he maintains records of hospital stays, procedures, and emergency room visits. To whom do these records belong?
   a. Dr. Wellness
   b. Each of Dr. Wellness's patients

c. Anytown General Hospital

d. American Hospital Association

7. How long should medical records be kept?

   a. Minimum of 2 to 7 years, depending on state statute

   b. Forever

   c. Minimum of 10 years per federal statute

   d. Twenty years, or until the patient dies

8. A physician determines that a patient being treated for a mental condition may not see his medical records. This is known as the

   a. Doctrine of informed consent

   b. Doctrine of professional discretion

   c. Doctrine of patient discretion

   d. Doctrine of medical record consent

9. Assuming that old paper medical records may be destroyed, which of the following is not an appropriate way to destroy the records?

   a. Burn the records.

   b. Shred the records.

   c. Pulverize the records.

   d. Tear each page into quarters and put in the trash.

10. The Food and Drug Administration requires research records pertaining to cancer patients be maintained for ___ years.

   a. 5

   b. 15

   c. 20

   d. 30

LO 7.3

11. What federal statute protects patients with histories of substance abuse regarding the release of information about treatment?

   a. HIV Confidentiality Act

   b. HIPAA

   c. Confidentality of Alcoholic and Drug Abuse Patient Records

   d. Release of Substance Abuse Patient Record Regulations

12. The copier malfunctions while you are photocopying a patient's medical records and prints too many copies of several pages. What will you do with the extra copies?

   a. File them with the original copy of the patient's medical records.

   b. Staple them to the photocopies because you cannot destroy them.

   c. Shred them in a paper shredder.

   d. None of these

13. Assume you are in charge of releasing medical records to a third party. Which of the following does *not* require the patient's written consent?

    a. Release of the records to the patient's insurance company

    b. Release of the records for use in a lawsuit in response to a court's subpoena

    c. Release of the records for research purposes

    d. All of these require the patient's written consent.

14. Which of the following is *not* a threat to the confidentiality of a patient's medical record?

    a. Written records are left open on a coder's desk when she takes her coffee break.

    b. A medical transcriptionist allows a friend from another office to read over his shoulder while he transcribes a physician's dictation.

    c. A medical office employee inadvertently leaves pages from a patient's medical record in the fax machine tray.

    d. A physician shows a patient's medical record to a consulting specialist.

LO 7.4

15. Which of the following individuals may not be able to give informed consent for medical treatment?

    a. A married woman who falls in her home

    b. A child injured on a school playground

    c. A pregnant teenager

    d. A person who speaks a foreign language

16. Where is the doctrine of informed consent usually outlined?

    a. American Medical Association

    b. Hospital policies

    c. Federal Medical Practice Act

    d. State medical practice acts

17. A lab technician trained in CPR and first aid stops at the scene of an auto accident. The technician administers basic first aid to the injured motorist. The motorist later sues the lab technician for malpractice. What state law will probably be used as a defense by the lab technician?

    a. Good Samaritan Law

    b. Emergency Rules of the Road

    c. Informed Consent Law

    d. Medical Practice Act

18. Elizabeth married at 16 years of age with her parents' permission. Shortly after the wedding, she learned that her husband is HIV-positive. In order for her to be tested for HIV, she must

    a. Ask her parents to authorize the test

    b. Ask her husband to authorize the test

    c. Ask a physician to administer the test and be prepared to provide proof of her marriage

    d. File a petition with the local courts to get the test done

LO 7.5

Match each definition with the correct term by writing the letter in the space provided.

_____ 19. Law that addresses the electronic storage and transmission of health information

_____ 20. Provides stages of development for patient records in a certified electronic format

_____ 21. Allows individuals and communities to gather, communicate, and share information, ideas, personal messages, images, and other content

_____ 22. Provides opportunities for providers to treat patients at a distance using various electronic formats

_____ 23. A secure Web site that allows a patient to access their health care information on a 24/7 basis

_____ 24. The application of information processing involving both computer hardware and software that deals with the storage, retrieval, sharing, and use of health care information, data, and knowledge for communication and decision making

a. Health information technology

b. HIPAA

c. Social media

d. Meaningful use

e. Patient portal

f. Telemedicine

Ethics Issues Medical Records and Informed Consent

Use your critical thinking skills to answer the questions that follow each ethics issue.

Ethics ISSUE 1:

A basic tenet of medical law and ethics is that patients have the right of self-determination. That right, however, can be effectively exercised only if patients have enough information to make an intelligent, informed choice about medical treatment.

A nurse working in a physician's office is helping the physician explain a medical diagnosis and proposed treatment plan to a middle-aged woman who is a recent immigrant from Thailand. The woman speaks no English, and her daughter is attempting to translate the conversation. The woman has metastasized lung cancer, and her prognosis is not good. The nurse notices a pronounced hesitation in the daughter's translation of this news to her mother, and she suspects the daughter has not relayed the information correctly because the patient seems undisturbed by the news.

Discussion Questions

25. As the nurse or medical assistant helping the physician in this scenario, what would you do?

26. Assume that the nurse and the physician must obtain informed consent from the patient in the scenario. Should they rely solely on the daughter's ability to translate? Explain your answer.

Ethics ISSUE 2:

You are an LPN in a reproductive services clinic, and a pregnant patient is suffering a medical condition wherein the pregnancy threatens her life. Her physician suggests that she undergo an abortion.

Discussion Questions

27. Will your personal values allow you to assist with the procedure? Explain your answer.

28. If your answer to question 27 is no, what are your alternatives?

Ethics ISSUE 3:

You have observed an LPN with whom you work in a hospital attempting to erase an entry she has made in a patient's paper medical record. She asks you not to tell that you saw her attempting to erase the entry.

Discussion Question

29. What will you do next?

Ethics ISSUE 4:

You have faxed a patient's medical record to another physician office and discover you have used the wrong fax number.

Discussion Question

30. What will you do next?

Case Studies

Use your critical thinking skills to answer the questions that follow each case study.

LO 7.3

When Ruth applied for health insurance, she listed a colonoscopy examination as part of her medical history. The insurance company asked for more information. Ruth requested, in writing, that the clinic where she had been examined send only the colonoscopy records to her insurance company. In addition to the requested information on her colonoscopy, the clinic sent all of Ruth's medical records for the past 5 years, which included the diagnoses of fibrocystic breast disease and obesity. As a result, the insurance company issued Ruth a policy but attached riders stipulating that it would not pay for any illnesses arising from the fibrocystic breast disease or obesity.

Ruth complained to the clinic administrator, explaining that she had requested that only those records concerning her colonoscopy be forwarded to the insurance company. The administrator apologized and assured Ruth that the clinic's policy concerning release of medical records would be reviewed. He also told Ruth that should she ever incur medical expenses for those conditions excepted in her insurance policy, she should contact him.

31. Did the clinic err in sending all of Ruth's medical records to the insurance company? Why or why not?
32. In your opinion, did Ruth have a legal cause for action against the clinic? Explain.
33. What would you do, in the clinic administrator's place, to rectify the situation and make sure that similar problems did not arise in the future?

A patient asked her dermatologist for the name of an internist. She visited the recommended internist several times and then learned that, without informing her, he had sent the dermatologist two detailed reports on her condition and family medical history. Because her gastrointestinal condition had nothing to do with her dermatological complaint, she believed the internist had sent the records to show his appreciation for the referral. She told the internist that she felt her privacy had been violated.

34. Do you agree with the patient? Why or why not?

LO 7.4

A 10-year-old girl suffered from a rare malignancy in her brain and around her spinal cord. She had surgery, and most of the tumor mass was removed, but residual tumor remained in the brain and around the spinal cord. The girl's doctors informed her parents that chemotherapy and radiation were possible treatment options but could cause serious problems such as sepsis, a permanent loss of IQ and stature, and even death. The parents wished to proceed with the therapy.

While their child was undergoing aggressive chemotherapy and radiation, the parents did independent research and read about several drugs being administered for cancer in other states that were not approved by the Federal Drug Administration and were illegal in their home state but were touted by physicians using them as "miracle cures." The couple sued their child's physician for failure to disclose alternative treatments, thus depriving them of informed consent.

A court awarded summary judgment to the physician.

35. In your opinion, does the court's decision seem warranted? Why or why not?
36. Did the physician involved follow the law? Did he or she act ethically? Explain your answer.
37. Under the doctrine of informed consent, should a physician be responsible for informing patients of all treatment options, even if some of the treatments are illegal or not yet proven effective? Explain your answer.

Internet Activities

LO 7.2 and LO 7.4

Complete the activities and answer the questions that follow.

38. Visit this Web site to determine how long medical records must be kept in your state:

    www.healthinfolaw.org/comparative-analysis/who-owns-medical-records-50-state-comparison

    Did you find differences in statute of limitations periods for different patients? If so, what were the differences?
39. Search online for "health information technology occupations." What occupations are listed under HIT? List three advantages to pursuing an education in HIT. If your primary interest is in patient care, would a career in HIT interest you? Explain your answer.
40. Visit the Web site for the American Medical Informatics Association (AMIA) at www.amia.org/. Find the association's ethics philosophy under "About AMIA." Briefly describe the AMIA's stance on maintaining confidentiality of electronic records.
41. Do you use social media Web sites when you have a health problem? Which sites do you use? If the health problem is severe enough that you see a provider, do you tell the provider about what you have learned at the sites you visited?

Resources

LO 7.1

http://flbog.sip.ufl.edu/risk-rx-article/correcting-errors-in-the-electronic-medical-record/

www.usfhealthonline.com/resources/healthcare/electronic-medical-records-mandate/#.V4-xgOgrI2w

LO 7.2

www.thedoctors.com/KnowledgeCenter/PatientSafety/articles/Frequently Asked-Questions-Medical-Records-Issues

http://blogs.aafp.org/cfr/freshperspectives/entry/doctor_or_patient_who_owns

https://medicopy.net/who-we-are/blog/who-owns-my-medical-record

http://medicaleconomics.modernmedicine.com/medical-economics/news/patient-records-struggle-ownership

http://library.ahima.org/PB/RetentionDestruction#.V5_FVDsrI2w

www.healthit.gov/sites/default/files/appa7-1.pdf

Chesanow, Neil. "Who Should Own a Medical Record—The Doctor or the Patient?" *Medscape*, November 16, 2016.

LO 7.4

www.law.cornell.edu/wex/informed_consent_doctrine

LO 7.5

Griffis, H. M., A. S. Kilaru, R. M. Werner, et al. 2014. "Use of Social Media Across U.S. Hospitals: Descriptive Analysis of Adoption and Utilization." *Journal of Medical Internet Research* 16(11):e264.

http://www.americantelemed.org/about-telemedicine/what-is-telemedicine

http://www.hhnmag.com/articles/7090-five-reasons-to-like-patients-use-of-social-media

http://www.pewinternet.org/2015/04/01/us-smartphone-use-in-2015/

Electronic health record: www.healthit.gov/providers-professionals/meaningful-use-definition-objectives

HIT statistics: http://dashboard.healthit.gov/quickstats/quickstats.php and https://www.healthit.gov/sites/default/files/oncdatabriefe-prescribingincreases2014.pdf

National Center for Health Statistics (HIT adoption): www.cdc.gov/nchs/data/databriefs/db236.htm

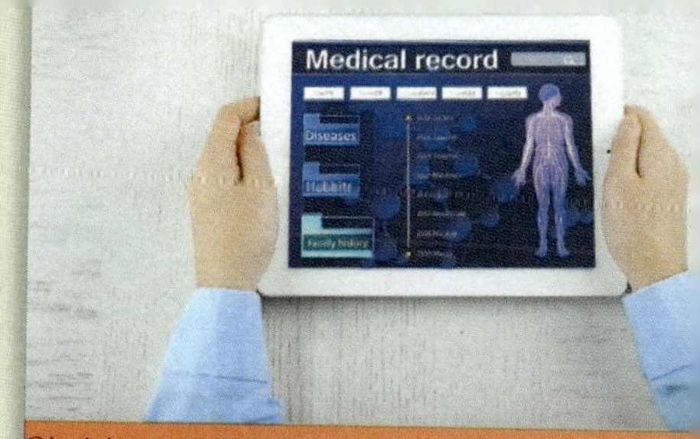

©belchonock/123 RF

8

Privacy, Security, and Fraud

LEARNING OUTCOMES

After studying this chapter, you should be able to:

LO 8.1 List the U.S. constitutional amendments and privacy laws that pertain to health care.

LO 8.2 Explain HIPAA's privacy rule.

LO 8.3 Identify those laws implemented to protect the security of health care information.

LO 8.4 Describe the federal laws that cover fraud and abuse within the health care business environment.

LO 8.5 Summarize patient rights as defined by the Patient Protection and Affordable Care Act and state statutes.

Key Terms

American Recovery and Reinvestment Act (ARRA)
breach
business associates (BA)
covered entities (CE)
Criminal Health Care Fraud Statute
de-identify
electronic health record (EHR)
electronic medical record (EMR)
Federal Anti-Kickback Law
Federal False Claims Act
Health Information Technology for Economic and Clinical Health Act (HITECH)
limited data set
Notice of Privacy Practices
permission
privacy
protected health information (PHI)
Stark Law
state preemption

FROM THE PERSPECTIVE OF. . .

ANN, AN RN IN A TEXAS HOSPITAL FOR NEARLY 25 YEARS, remembers when patients' names were posted on the doors to their rooms. She and her colleagues once freely informed telephone callers and visitors how patients were progressing. Now, Ann remarks, because of federal legislation to protect the privacy and security of health care information, times have changed. "We have to be so careful about releasing any information that when my father's dear friend was admitted to my floor in the hospital where I work, I couldn't tell him that his friend had been admitted."

From Ann's perspective, because she cares about her patients, she would like to be able to talk more freely with family members or friends who also care about her patients. But she is duty-bound to follow the law, and she knows the benefits to patients for laws that guard their privacy.

From the perspective of friends and family members who call for information about a patient, the law is harsh and hard to understand. They are often angry when they cannot learn the status of a friend or loved one.

From the perspective of some patients, the law sometimes feels overprotective and unnecessarily intrusive, but for others—such as the patient who has tried to commit suicide and failed, the one who doesn't want anyone to know he is in the hospital, or the battered spouse who doesn't want her abusive husband to find her—it's a safety net they can depend on.

8.1 The U.S. Constitution and Federal Privacy Laws

privacy
Freedom from unauthorized intrusion.

Contrary to popular belief, the term **privacy** (freedom from unauthorized intrusion) does not appear in the U.S. Constitution or the Bill of Rights. However, the U.S. Supreme Court has derived the right to privacy from the First, Third, Fourth, Fifth, Ninth, and Fourteenth Amendments to the Constitution.

LANDMARK COURT CASE
The Constitution Protects the Right to Privacy

In November 1961, the executive director and the medical director of a Planned Parenthood clinic in Connecticut were charged with violating a state statute prohibiting the dispensing of contraceptive devices to a married couple. The defendants were convicted and fined $100 each. The U.S. Supreme Court heard the case in March 1965 and issued a written opinion on June 7, 1965. Justice William O. Douglas, writing the majority opinion for the Court, held that the Connecticut statute was an unconstitutional violation of the right of privacy. Douglas noted that many rights are not expressly mentioned in the Constitution, but the Court has nevertheless found that persons possess such a right. In reviewing the many rights that Americans possess, Douglas noted the existence of "penumbras" or "zone(s) of privacy created by several fundamental constitutional guarantees."

As a result of the Supreme Court's decision in *Griswold v. Connecticut,* patients possess certain rights that affect the delivery of medical services and health care. For example, persons have the right to refuse medical treatment, and courts now recognize a person's right to die.

Source: *Griswold v. Connecticut,* 381 U.S. 479, 85 S. Ct. 1978, 14 L. Ed.2d 510 (1965).

First Amendment: Congress cannot prohibit or abridge free speech. In addition, the Establishment and Freedom of Religion clauses of this amendment prohibit the government from funding, showing preference for, or discriminating against any religion.

Third Amendment: Soldiers cannot be quartered in private homes without the consent of the owner.

Fourth Amendment: People have the right to be secure in their persons, houses, papers, and effects against unreasonable searches and seizures.

Fifth Amendment: No person must testify against himself, be tried twice for the same offense, or be deprived of life, liberty, or property without due process of law. The Miranda warning ("You have the right to remain silent . . . "), as read during criminal arrests, derives from this amendment.

Ninth Amendment: If certain rights are not explicitly mentioned in the Constitution, that does not mean they do not exist.

Fourteenth Amendment: All states must provide rights for citizens that are at least equal to those in the U.S. Constitution, and under the philosophy called federalism, states may grant citizens additional rights not specifically granted in the U.S. Constitution.

COURT CASE Fourth Amendment Right to Privacy

Every state in the nation, except Missouri, has a prescription monitoring database. The original purpose of these prescription drug monitoring program (PDMP) databases was an attempt to address the overdose deaths attributed to prescription medication, prescription drug diversion, and doctor shopping. PDMPs were intended to help law enforcement find the physicians who were overprescribing pain medications in a pattern that indicated possible fraud. Each state's laws and databases were different.

However, access to PDMPs for purposes other than limiting illicit use of opioid narcotics has created questions about Fourth Amendment rights. State laws vary in terms of what drugs are tracked and who in the law enforcement community, as well as the health care community, has access to these databases. Only 19 states require a warrant for law enforcement to access their PDMP.

Oregon created its PDMP in 2009, prioritizing patient privacy and requiring a court order for law enforcement to search the PDMP. The federal Drug Enforcement Agency (DEA) ignored that law and filed administrative subpoenas in pursuit of investigations into drug diversion. The DEA argued that it has a compelling interest that supplants privacy under the Fourth Amendment and that requiring a warrant affects its ability to conduct a timely and effective investigation.

The state of Oregon filed a lawsuit against the DEA, and the American Civil Liberties Union (ACLU) joined the case. In early 2014, a U.S. District Court granted the plaintiffs motion for summary judgment and denied the federal government's motion, with the result that the DEA must get a warrant to access the prescription records in Oregon. The DEA has appealed that decision, but as of July 2016, no decision has been reached at the federal appellate level.

In another case in July 2015, a U.S. District Court judge in Texas ruled for the DEA that an administrative subpoena may be used to search medical records. That case is also under appeal.

In July 2016, the ACLU filed a similar case in Utah.

Source: *State of Oregon v. U.S.*, DOJ Case No. 3:12-cv-02023-HA US District Court, Portland Division, February 2014; *U.S. v Zadeh* Court of Appeals, Fifth Circuit No. 15 10195, April 2016

FEDERAL PRIVACY LAWS

Concern about privacy has led to the enactment of federal and state laws governing the collection, storage, transmission, and disclosure of personal data. Privacy laws are generally based on the following considerations:

1. Information collected and stored about individuals should be limited to what is necessary to carry out the functions of the business or government agency collecting the information.
2. Once it is collected, access to personal information should be limited to those employees who must use the information in performing their jobs.
3. Personal information cannot be released outside the organization collecting it unless authorization is obtained from the subject.
4. When information is collected about a person, that person should know that the information is being collected and should have the opportunity to check the information for accuracy.

A number of federal laws concern privacy, but until the Health Insurance Portability and Accountability Act (HIPAA) of 1996, federal privacy laws have dealt with financial and credit information or the theft or illegal disclosure of electronic information. HIPAA of 1996 was the first *federal* law to deal explicitly with the privacy of medical records, and to ensure compliance, HIPAA provides for civil and criminal sanctions for violators of the law.

state preemption
If a state's privacy laws are stricter than HIPAA privacy standards, the state laws take precedence.

All states have laws governing the confidentiality of medical records, but laws vary greatly from state to state. Through **state preemption,** if a state's privacy laws are stricter than HIPAA privacy standards and/or guarantee more patients' rights, the state laws take precedence.

Table 8-1 on the next page lists eight major federal privacy laws passed since 1985.

COURT CASE

HIPAA Preempts State Law in Certain Instances

In July 2013, the U.S. Court of Appeals for the Eleventh Circuit ruled that HIPAA preempts state law in certain instances. The case centered on a Florida statute that allowed nursing homes to release medical records of a current or former resident to "spouse, guardian, surrogate, proxy or attorney in fact" of the individual. However, many Florida nursing homes refused to disclose records to surviving spouses who had not been designated as the personal representative by the probate courts. The Florida Agency for Health Care Administration (AHCA) ordered the various nursing homes to release the information, stating the surviving spouses were equal to personal representatives. OPIS Management Resources, an owner of several nursing homes in Florida, filed suit against AHCA, claiming that HIPAA standards were higher and thus the state law conflicted. The Court of Appeals held that the state statute was fatally flawed and "authorizes sweeping disclosures, making a deceased (nursing home) resident's protected health information available to a spouse or other enumerated party upon request, without any need for authorization, for any conceivable reason, and without regard to the authority of the individual making the request to act in a deceased resident's stead."

Source: *OPIS Management Resources LLC v. Secretary Florida Agency for Health Care Administration,* No. 12-12593 (11th Cir. Apr. 9, 2013).

Table 8-1 Major Federal Privacy Laws

Date Enacted	Law	Purpose
1986	Electronic Communications Privacy Act (ECPA)	Provides privacy protection for new forms of electronic communications, such as voice mail, e-mail, and cellular telephone
1994	Computer Abuse Amendments Act	Amends the 1984 act to forbid transmission of harmful computer code such as viruses
1996	Health Insurance Portability and Accountability Act (HIPAA)	Guarantees that workers who change jobs can obtain health insurance Increases efficiency and effectiveness of the U.S. health care system by electronic exchange of administrative and financial data Improves security and privacy of patient-identifying information Decreases U.S. health care system transaction costs
1999	Gramm-Leach-Bliley Act	Requires all financial institutions and insurance companies to clearly disclose their privacy policies regarding the sharing of nonpublic personal information with affiliates and third parties
2005	Patient Safety and Quality Improvement Act (PSQIA)	Helps assess and resolve patient safety and health care quality issues, encourages reporting and analysis of medical errors, and authorizes the U.S. Department of Health and Human Services (HHS) to impose civil money penalties for violations of patient safety confidentiality
2009	American Recovery and Reinvestment Act (ARRA), commonly called the Stimulus Bill	Title XIII, the Health Information Technology for Economic and Clinical Health (HITECH) Act, makes substantive changes to HIPAA, including privacy and security regulations, changes in HIPAA enforcement, provisions about health information held by entities not covered by HIPAA, and other miscellaneous changes
2010	Patient Protection and Affordable Care Act (PPACA), commonly called the Affordable Care Act or ACA	Deals mostly with the availability of health insurance coverage for all Americans but also reinforces privacy regarding protected health information
2010	Health Care and Education Reconciliation Act (HCERA)	Adds to regulations imposed on the insurance industry by PPACA

Check Your Progress

1. Does the Constitution provide specifically for the protection of privacy? Explain your answer.
2. What was the first federal law to deal explicitly with the privacy of medical records?
3. Name four considerations for protecting privacy when federal and/or state legislation is written.

Because HIPAA is the federal legal standard for privacy and security of electronic health information throughout the health care industry, health care employees must follow the law's provisions, which are contained within four standards:

Standard 1. Transactions and Code Sets. A transaction refers to the transmission of information between two parties to carry out financial or administrative activities. A code set is any set of codes used to encode data elements, such as tables of terms, medical concepts, medical diagnostic codes, or medical procedure codes.

Required code sets for use under Standard 1 include Current Procedural Terminology (CPT) and International Classification System of Diseases; Clinical Modifications 10th Edition (ICD-10-CM); and International Classification System of Diseases–Procedure Coding System 10th Edition (ICD-10-PCS).

Standard 2. Privacy Rule. Health care providers and their business associates must put in place certain policies and procedures to ensure confidentiality of written, electronic, and oral protected health information.

Standard 3. Security Rule. *Security* refers to those policies and procedures health care providers and their business associates use to protect electronically transmitted and stored PHI from unauthorized access.

Standard 4. National Identifier Standards. Provide unique identifiers (addresses) for electronic transmissions.

All four sets of HIPAA standards have been implemented, and most health care practitioners are familiar with the language and rules that make up the requirements for compliance. Anyone needing a refresher course can visit www.hipaa.com for specific information.

Of special concern in this chapter are Standard 2, the Privacy Rule and Standard 3, the Security Rule.

8.2 HIPAA's Privacy Rule

protected health information (PHI)
Information that contains one or more patient identifiers.

HIPAA's Standard 2, the Privacy Rule says that **protected health information (PHI)** must be protected against unauthorized disclosure, whether it is written, spoken, or in electronic form. PHI refers to information that contains one or more patient identifiers and can, therefore, be used to identify an individual.

The Privacy Rule has 18 items under its definition of *patient identifiers,* including name, address, and Social Security number. Even zip codes, under certain circumstances, may be considered identifiers along with e-mail addresses, medical records numbers, driver's licenses, photos, and many other items. A complete list may be found on a variety of HIPAA guidance sites. It is possible to **de-identify** health information by removing the patient identifiers listed.

de-identify
To remove from health care transactions all information that identifies patients.

More important, the Privacy Rule clearly identifies the following as protected health information:

- Past, present, or future physical or mental health condition
- Documentation of the provision of health care
- Past, present, or future payment for the provision of health care

covered entities
Health care providers who conduct administrative and financial transactions in electronic form. This includes all employees, volunteers, trainees, and all others who are under the control of the entity.

business associates
Individuals and/or organizations that provide certain functions, activities, or services on behalf of covered entities that involve access to, or the use of, disclosure of protected health information.

permission
A reason under HIPAA for disclosing patient information.

All **covered entities** (CEs) and **business associates** (BAs) are required to comply with the HIPAA Rules. Table 8-2 lists both CEs and BAs.

Health care providers and plans can use and disclose patient information (PHI), but to do so legally, they must identify a **permission**—a legal reason for each use and disclosure. To *use* PHI means that you use patients' protected health information within the facility where you work in the normal course of conducting health care business. To *disclose* PHI means that patients' protected health information is sent outside a health care facility for legitimate business or health care reasons.

Table 8-2 Who Must Comply with HIPAA Privacy Rules?

Covered Entities (CEs)	Business Associates (BAs)
Clinics, hospitals, nursing homes, and pharmacies	Health information organizations or exchanges (HIO/HIE)
Health plans	E-prescribing gateways
Health care clearinghouses	A subcontractor to a BA that creates, receives, maintains, or transmits PHI on behalf of the BA
Employees, volunteers, trainees, and all others who are under the control of the above entities	An entity that a CE contracts with to provide patients with a personal health record on behalf of the CE

Using and disclosing PHI must fall within the following six HIPAA-defined permissions:

1. Disclosures to patients. HIPAA *requires* that PHI be disclosed to any patient who asks to see his or her own medical records (unless the health care provider believes that access will do harm to the patient). This includes talking to the patient about his or her diagnosis, treatment, and medical condition, as well as allowing the patient to review his or her own medical record. Some records, however, such as psychotherapy notes, may be withheld.
2. Use or disclosure for treatment, payment, or health care operations. Health care practitioners need to use PHI within the medical office, hospital, or other health care facility for coordinating care, consulting with another practitioner about the patient's condition, prescribing medications, ordering lab tests, scheduling surgery, or for other reasons necessary to conduct health care treatment or business, such as insurance claims and billing. PHI disclosures for these purposes do not require written authorization.

   If other covered entities contact you or your employer for access to PHI, such as insurance plans, attorneys, medical survey representatives, and pharmaceutical companies, you must have the patient's written authorization to release PHI.
3. Use and disclosure with an opportunity to agree or object. According to the HHS Web site www.hhs.gov/hipaa/for-professionals/privacy/laws-regulations/index.html, informal permission may be obtained by asking the individual outright or by circumstances that clearly give the individual the opportunity to agree, comply silently or without objection, or object. Where the individual is incapacitated, in an emergency situation, or not available, covered entities generally may make such uses and disclosures, if in their professional judgment, the use or disclosure is determined to be in the best interest of the individual.
4. Incidental uses and disclosures of PHI are permitted without authorization from patients as follows:
   - Nursing care center staff members can talk about patients' care if they take reasonable precautions to prevent unauthorized individuals, such as visitors in the area, from overhearing.

- Health care practitioners can talk to patients on the phone or discuss patients' medical treatments with other providers on the phone if they are reasonably sure that others cannot overhear.
- Health care practitioners can discuss lab results with patients and among themselves in a joint treatment area if they take reasonable precautions to ensure that others cannot overhear.
- Health care practitioners can leave messages on answering machines or with family members, but information should be limited to the amount necessary for the purpose of the call. (For detailed messages, simply ask the patient to return the call.)
- You can ask patients to sign in, call patients by name in waiting rooms, or use a public address system to ask patients to come to a certain area. A patient sign-in sheet, however, must not ask for the reason for the visit.
- You can use an X-ray light board at a nursing station if it is not visible to unauthorized individuals in the area.
- You can place patient charts outside exam rooms if you use reasonable precautions to protect patient identity: Face the chart toward the wall or place the chart inside a cover while it is in place.

5. Public interest and benefit activities. The Privacy Rule permits use and disclosure of protected health information, without an individual's authorization or permission, for 12 national priority purposes, as listed on the HHS Web site www.hhs.gov/hipaa/for-professionals/privacy/laws-regulations/index.html:
   - If required by law
   - As part of public health activities
   - For victims of abuse, neglect, or domestic violence
   - In health oversight activities
   - For judicial and administrative proceedings
   - For law enforcement purposes
   - For decedents when cause of death is released to funeral home, coroners, or medical examiners
   - For cadaver organ, eye, or tissue donation
   - For research
   - In the event of serious threat to health or safety
   - For essential government functions
   - In claims for workers' compensation

limited data set
Protected health information from which certain patient identifiers have been removed.

6. Limited data set. A **limited data set** is protected health information from which certain specified, direct identifiers of individuals and their relatives, household members, and employers have been removed. A limited data set may be used and disclosed for research, health care operations, and public health purposes, provided the recipient enters into an agreement promising specified safeguards for the PHI within the limited data set.

The HIPAA Privacy Rule does not give patients the express right to sue. Instead, the person must file a written complaint with the secretary of HHS through its Office for Civil Rights. The HHS secretary then decides whether or not to investigate the complaint. Patients may have other legal standings to sue under state privacy laws. Table 8-3 provides more information about specific rights under the HIPAA Privacy Rule.

The HIPAA Privacy rules require all CEs to prominently post and distribute a **Notice of Privacy Practices** (NPP). This notice must include:

- How the CE may use and disclose an individual's PHI
- The patient's rights with respect to the information and how the patient may exercise those rights, with clear direction on how the patient may complain to the CE
- The CE's legal duties with respect to the information
- Whom patients can contact for further information

Notice of Privacy Practices
A list provided by all covered entities that demonstrates adherence to HIPAA's privacy practices rules.

Posted NPPs should be reviewed regularly to ensure that the information is up-to-date. Model NPPs may be found and downloaded at www.hhs.gov/hipaa/for-professionals/privacy/guidance/model-notices-privacy-practices/.

While HIPAA provides patients with privacy protection for their medical records, individual states may see the issue of privacy differently. The court case below illustrates that complete, total privacy may not be guaranteed by each state.

Table 8-3 Patients' Rights Under the HIPAA Privacy Rule

Patient Right	Comments	Documentation Required	Documentation Recommended
Access to medical records and the right to copy them	Access to records is guaranteed under HIPAA, but there are some limitations, as mentioned.	No	Yes
Request for amendment to designated record set	A patient has the right to request amendments to his or her PHI or other personal information. Unless a provider has grounds to deny the request, amendments must be made.	Yes	—
Request for an accounting of disclosures of PHI	You are required to account for certain disclosures during the past 3 years. Check with your privacy officer for a list. You have up to 60 days to provide the disclosure list.	Yes. Always keep a record of the appropriate disclosures, and make a copy of the disclosure report for the patient's file.	—
Request to be contacted at an alternate location	Patients can request to have you contact them at places other than work or home. You can deny the request if you cannot reasonably comply.	Yes. Obtain a request from the patient in writing. Note in the patient's electronic medical record and in a paper communication for staff members who do not have access to the patient's electronic medical record. Document reasons for denying the request if it is denied.	—
Request for further restrictions on who has access to PHI	A patient can request that certain persons or entities not have access to his or her medical record. You may deny the request if you cannot reasonably comply.	Yes. Ask the patient to complete an opt-out form that is then filed with electronic and paper records. Document reasons for denying the request if it is denied.	—
Right to file a complaint	Enforcement of the Privacy Rule is complaint-driven. Patients should be encouraged to work first with the provider. Retaliation is prohibited.	Yes. Refer the complaint to the privacy officer. Document the complaint in a privacy complaint log. Evaluate the complaint and determine how best to solve it.	—

COURT CASE

Health Privacy Law Does Not Cover Internal Use

A Wisconsin resident filed an invasion-of-privacy suit in state court that claimed that two staff members at the health care center violated a state law that broadly prohibits the release of patient health care records when the employees accessed and observed his health care records without his authorization or consent. But the court ruled, and the appellate court affirmed, that the law—Wisconsin Statute Section 146.82—applied only to the disclosure of medical records to third parties outside the medical system.

The appellate court rejected the plaintiff's contention that interpreting the statute to apply to only the disclosure of patient data to an outside party would give employees unlimited access to patient health care records, saying that its opinion "does not give employees *carte blanche* to access patient records for nefarious purposes without consequence."

The court stated that an employee's internal access to patient records is not the type of conduct governed by the state statute and added that internal use of protected health information is extensively regulated by the federal Health Insurance Portability and Accountability Act.

Source: *Wall v. Pahl et al.*, case number 2015AP001230, in the Court of Appeals of the State of Wisconsin, District III. August 2016

Check Your Progress

4. Define *protected health information.*
5. List at least three items that are considered patient identifiers.
6. Which law usually prevails, federal or state, if a state law provides greater privacy protection than a federal law? Explain your answer.
7. Define *covered entity* and *business associate*.
8. One can only legally release PHI under six HIPAA-defined ________.
9. What information may be found in a Notice of Privacy Practices?

8.3 Security of Health Care Information

As listed in Table 8-1, the American Recovery and Reinvestment Act (ARRA), commonly called the Stimulus Bill, made substantive changes to HIPAA, including privacy and security regulations, changes in HIPAA enforcement, provisions about health information held by entities not expressly covered by HIPAA, and other miscellaneous changes. All public and private health care providers and other eligible professionals across the country have adopted and demonstrated "meaningful use" of electronic medical records (EMR) in order to keep their existing Medicare and Medicaid reimbursement levels. ("Meaningful use" is explained in Chapter 7, under LO 7.5.)

When discussing medical records, it is important to note the difference between electronic medical records (EMR) and electronic health records (EHR) because, according to www.healthit.gov, an online source of information about information technology in the health industry, the two terms are not interchangeable. The **electronic medical record (EMR)** is the electronic form of a patient's medical history from just one practice. It lets health care providers in one facility:

electronic medical record (EMR) Contains all patient medical records for one practice.

- Track data over time.
- Identify with a glance which patients are due for screenings or check-ups.
- Check patients' progress within certain parameters, such as blood pressure, cholesterol and blood sugar readings, and vaccinations.
- Monitor and improve overall patient care within the practice.

By contrast, the **electronic health record (EHR)** is a more comprehensive electronic patient history, focusing on the total health of the patient and including a broader view of a patient's care. This more detailed record allows for:

electronic health record (EHR) A more comprehensive record than the EMR, focusing on the total health of the patient and traveling with the patient.

- A record that may travel with the patient, so that emergency department clinicians who see a patient in his home city or traveling across the country will know about any life-threatening allergies, or clinicians treating people injured in a disaster will know which medications the patient is taking.
- The opportunity for the patient to log on to his or her own record and see trends in lab results over time, which can help the patient plan for staying healthy.
- Specialists to see what tests, X-rays, and other procedures have already been done on a patient, thus avoiding unnecessary duplication when possible.
- Notes from any hospital stays that can help inform discharge instructions and follow-up care for the patient and can let the patient move smoothly from one care setting to another.

HIPAA'S SECURITY RULE

Before HIPAA, generally accepted security standards and general requirements for protecting health information did not exist in the health care industry. As the health care industry began to implement electronic information systems and to move away from paper records, it became necessary to establish nationwide standards for security of those electronic information systems.

While HIPAA's Standard 2 (the Privacy Rule) established national standards for the protection of certain health information, HIPAA Standard 3 is the Security Rule. The Security Rule establishes a national set of security standards for protecting certain health information that is held or transferred in electronic form. Essentially, the Security Rule operationalizes the protections set forth in the Privacy Rule. The Security Rule identifies the technical and nontechnical safeguards that CEs must have in place to secure protected health information.

Compliance with the Security Rule was required as of April 20, 2005, for most entities covered by HIPAA and by September 23, 2013, for their business associates. The authority to administer and enforce the Security Rule was transferred to the HHS Office for Civil Rights in July 2009.

While the health care workforce is more mobile and efficient, partly due to electronic clinical applications, potential security risks have increased. In addition to the clinical applications such as physician order entry and electronic transmittal of prescriptions, health insurers are providing access to claims and care management, as well as member self-service applications. The challenge for the Security Rule is to provide rules to protect the patients' privacy while allowing CEs and BAs to adopt new technologies that provide a smooth and protected flow of information to the providers.

All CEs must maintain reasonable and appropriate administrative, technical, and physical safeguards for protecting PHI. Specifically, the Security Rule requires CEs to:

1. Ensure the confidentiality, integrity, and availability of all PHI they create, receive, maintain, or transmit;
2. Identify and protect against reasonably anticipated threats to the security or integrity of the information;
3. Protect against reasonably anticipated, impermissible uses or disclosures; and
4. Ensure compliance by their workforce.

Covered entities must implement safeguards to protect the PHI. At a minimum, CEs must evaluate the likelihood and impact of potential risks to the PHI. This is called a risk analysis. Once such risks have been identified, CEs must implement appropriate security measures to address the risks found in the risk analysis. The rationale for adopting the chosen security measures must be documented. CEs must maintain continuous, reasonable, and appropriate security protections. The designation of a security official who is responsible for developing and implementing security policies and procedures is required. All staff must be trained, and appropriate sanctions against employees who violate the policies and procedures must be in place. Periodic assessment of how well the security measures are working is required by the Security Rule. A variety of physical and technical safeguards are also required. The details on all the requirements may be found at www.hhs.gov/hipaa/for-professionals/security/laws-regulations/.

As outlined in the paragraph above, a covered entity is not HIPAA-compliant if it has not taken basic steps to prepare for disaster. Data should be stored off-site or in the cloud. An easy way to test the backup is to assume that a disaster has occurred to confirm that the data can be restored. Making sure your backup works is not just a federal requirement, it is sound business practice. Beyond data breaches, fire or a severe storm can cause major problems with providers' health records. The cost of a qualified service to protect the health records may be minimal in comparison to the downtime and/or destruction of records.

Health Information Technology for Economic and Clinical Health Act (HITECH)
A section of the American Recovery and Reinvestment Act (ARRA) that strengthened certain HIPAA privacy and security provisions.

American Recovery and Reinvestment Act (ARRA)
A 2009 act that made substantive change to HIPAA's privacy and security regulations.

BREACH NOTIFICATION RULE

The Health Information Technology for Economic and Clinical Health (HITECH) Act, part of the **American Recovery and Reinvestment Act (ARRA)** of 2009, strengthened the privacy and security protections for health information established under HIPAA.

The HITECH Act requires HIPAA-covered entities to notify affected individuals, the HHS, and in some cases, the media following the discovery of a breach of unsecured PHI. Business associates are also required to notify covered entities following the discovery of a breach.

As defined by the HHS, a **breach** is an impermissible use or disclosure under the Privacy Rule that compromises the security or privacy of PHI. An impermissible use or disclosure of protected health information is presumed to be a breach unless the covered entity or business associate, as applicable, demonstrates that there is a low probability that the protected health information has been compromised based on a risk assessment that includes an analysis of the nature and extent of the PHI, who the unauthorized person is, whether the PHI was actually viewed or acquired, and the extent to which the risk has been mitigated.

breach
Any unauthorized acquisition, access, use, or disclosure of personal health information that compromises the security or privacy of such information.

Any breach of more than 500 records requires notification of the media in addition to the patients affected by the breach. This allows the public to learn of the problem early on. Source: www.hhs.gov/hipaa/for-professionals/breach-notification/index.html.

Since 2009, the HHS Office for Civil Rights (OCR) has maintained a database of PHI breaches. Through July 2016, there were 1,619 reported breaches. The biggest breach on record as of July 2016 was one that occurred in February 2015 at Anthem, a large health insurance company. Anthem reported a breach of approximately 80 million records. The records were hacked by unknown entities. Several multimillion-dollar class action lawsuits have been filed claiming that information obtained from the breach has been used in fraudulent activities. It is unlikely that this matter will be settled in 2016. The OCR is still investigating the breach.

Fines for breaches may be assessed. The OCR investigation may take several years because once a breach is reported, the OCR does an investigation of the entities' policies and procedures. Table 8-4 on the next page shows the fines for the first half of 2016.

Based on data collected by the HHS OCR, as of February 1, 2016, protected health information breaches affected more than 113 million individuals in 2015. In 2015, hacking incidents comprised nearly 99 percent of all individuals affected by breaches, and the number of reported hacking incidents, 57, comprised more than 20 percent of all reported breaches.

Check Your Progress

10. Briefly distinguish between the electronic medical record (EMR) and the electronic health record (EHR).
11. What is a *breach* of PHI?
12. A CE or BA must report a breach of _______ or more records to the media.
13. What is a risk analysis for purposes of protecting PHI?

Table 8-4 Fines for Security Breaches in Early 2016

Date	Company—Amount of Fine	Event
February 2016	Lincare—$239,800	Employee moved from one residence to another, leaving records behind in the home that was sold
February 2016	Complete PT, Pool and Land Physical Therapy—$25,000	Posted patient testimonials on a Web site without patients' permission
March 2016	Memorial Health Care—$1.55 million	Failure to implement a BA agreement and to institute organization-wide risk analysis
March 2016	Feinstein Research—$3.9 million	Laptop with PHI stolen; failure to implement appropriate security policies
April 2016	New York Presbyterian Hospital—$2.2 million	Inappropriate disclosure of two records to the media and lack of security safeguards
April 2016	Raleigh Orthopaedic Clinic of North Carolina—$750,000	Failure to execute a BA agreement before turning over patient records
June 2016	Catholic Health Care Services—$650,000	Organization is a BA for several local nursing homes; mobile phone of an employee was stolen
July 2016	University of Mississippi Medical Center—$2.75 million	Missing laptop investigation led to a variety of violations of security rules
July 2016	Oregon Health Science University—$2.7 million	Multiple breaches for unencrypted laptops; failure to implement findings from previous investigation

8.4 Controlling Health Care Fraud and Abuse

Fraud and abuse in health care include both federally funded programs such as Medicare and Medicaid, and private insurance and self-pay patients. The opportunity for fraud and abuse is great, and detecting them is difficult. According to Daniel Levinson of the HHS Office of Inspector General (OIG), it is "impossible to accurately pinpoint the true cost of fraud in federal health care programs; fraud is a significant threat to the programs' stability and endangers access to health care services for millions of Americans."

In 2007, a Medicare Fraud Strike Force was established to combine the resources of federal, state, and local law enforcement entities to prevent and combat health care fraud, waste, and abuse. As of June 2016, the Strike Force had initiated 1,522 criminal actions, had 2,185 indictments, and recovered $1.98 billion.

In May 2009, building on the work of the Medicare Fraud Strike Force, a joint task force between the HHS and the Department of Justice (DOJ) was formed. Called the Health Care Fraud Prevention & Enforcement Action Team (HEAT), this task force is made up of not only HHS investigators in the Medicare Fraud Strike Force, but also Federal Bureau of Investigation (FBI) staff members and investigators from the Office of the Inspector General. Other departments in the DOJ may also participate in this task force, depending on the investigation.

In June 2016, the U.S. Attorney General announced a nationwide sweep led by the Medicare Fraud Strike Force. Criminal and civil charges were filed against 301 individuals, including 61 doctors, nurses, and other licensed medical professionals, for their alleged participation in health care fraud schemes involving approximately $900 million in false billings.

Other examples of fraud and abuse include:

- A Dallas physician was convicted in April 2016 of eight counts of health care fraud, as well as several other counts of conspiracy, false statements, and obstruction of justice. The jury deliberated for less than 2 days before delivering its verdict on the $375 million scheme. The physician, as well as his co-conspirators, promised Medicare patients cash, food stamps, and groceries as part of their home health care scam. While several of the co-conspirators plead guilty and have been fined $25 million each and are serving 10 years in federal prison, the physician has appealed his conviction.
- A former health care clinic consultant and Medicare biller was sentenced in April 2016 to a little more than 11 years in prison and ordered to pay a $100,000 fine for her role in a $63 million healthcare fraud scheme involving a now-defunct Miami health provider. In exchange for Medicare beneficiary referrals, the defendant directed and authorized payment for kickbacks and bribes to patient brokers and others. The defendant also testified that the health provider falsified medical records.
- In a whistle-blower's lawsuit, as allowed by the False Claims Act (see "The Federal False Claims Act" in this section), a hospital in New Jersey was ordered in June 2016 to pay $450,000 to resolve allegations that it falsely billed Medicare and Medicaid for unnecessary cardiac procedures.
- As part of a Medicare fraud scheme, the owner and operator of multiple HIV/AIDS clinics in New York City paid patients kickbacks to lie to clinic doctors to facilitate fraudulent billing. The clinics also billed Medicare for medications that were either never administered or not medically necessary. The owner was sentenced in June 2016 to 5 years in prison and ordered to pay more than $12 million in restitution.
- A well-known spine surgeon failed to disclose his conflicts of interest with a leading device maker before using the company's products in surgeries. The hospital where the surgeries were performed agreed in July 2016 to pay $8.5 million to settle the two lawsuits stemming from this case.
- A medical center in South Carolina paid $17 million in fines in July 2016 to settle allegations that it violated both the Stark Law and the False Claims Act by overpaying physicians to refer to the medical center.
- A Brooklyn New York clinic fraudulently billed Medicare and Medicaid more than $70 million for services to the homeless in the local area. The owner of the clinic had to pay $8 million in restitution and was sentenced to 5 years in prison in February 2017.

Source: www.healthcarefinancenews.com/slideshow/biggest-healthcare-frauds-2016-running-list?p=5

Fraud and abuse will continue to be a problem because they can be difficult to detect: It is not easy to separate fraudulent spending from total health care dollars spent. While fines are high, some experts predict that the fraudulent activity may increase substantially over the next 10

Table 8-5 Major Federal Health Care Fraud and Abuse Laws

Date Enacted	Law	Purpose
1863—Significantly amended in 1986 and several times since	False Claims Act	Provides for civil penalties for persons knowingly making false claims to the federal government for payment
1972	Anti-Kickback Statute	Criminal law that prohibits giving, soliciting, accepting, or arranging items of value as a reward for referrals of services paid for by the government health care system
1989—Expanded in 1995	Stark Law, or Physician Self-Referral Law	Physicians or members of their immediate families cannot refer patients to health care facilities they own if the government is to pay for the care
Unknown—Part of the U.S. Code 18 Section 1347	Criminal Health Care Fraud Statute	Makes it a criminal offense to knowingly defraud a health care benefit program

years unless significantly more resources are invested to identify the fraud and abuse.

The major federal statutes addressing health care fraud and abuse are outlined in Table 8-5 and discussed following the table.

THE FEDERAL FALSE CLAIMS ACT

Federal False Claims Act
A law that allows for individuals to bring civil actions on behalf of the U.S. government for false claims made to the federal government, under a provision of the law called *qui tam* (from Latin meaning "to bring an action for the king and for oneself").

The **Federal False Claims Act** allows individuals to bring civil actions on behalf of the U.S. government for false claims made to the federal government, under a provision of the law called *qui tam* (from Latin meaning "to bring an action for the king and for oneself"). These individuals, commonly known as whistle-blowers, are referred to as *qui tam relators* and can share in any court-awarded damages.

Suits brought under the False Claims Act are most often related to the health care and defense industries. The act prohibits:

- Making a false record or statement to get a false claim paid by the government
- Conspiring to have a false claim paid by the government
- Withholding government property with the intent to defraud or willfully conceal it from the government
- Making or delivering a receipt for government property that is false
- Buying government property from someone who is not authorized to sell it
- Making a false statement to avoid or deceive an obligation to pay money or property to the government
- Causing someone else to submit a false claim by giving false information

The Justice Department secured $3.5 billion in settlements and judgments from civil cases involving fraud under the federal False Claims Act during fiscal year 2015. From January 2009 through the end of the 2015 fiscal year, the Justice Department used the False Claims Act to recover $16.5 billion in federal health care dollars. Most of these recoveries relate to fraud against Medicare and Medicaid.

In August 2016, the Department of Justice proposed a new rule to increase the percentage share that a whistle-blower may receive in a *qui tam* case.

THE FEDERAL ANTI-KICKBACK LAW

In effect since 1972 and amended many times since then, the **Federal Anti-Kickback Law** states that anyone who knowingly and willfully receives or pays anything of value to influence the referral of federal health care program business, including Medicare and Medicaid, can be held accountable for a felony. Violations of the law, which excludes from prosecution some designated "safe harbor" arrangements, are punishable by up to 5 years in prison, fines from $25,000 to $50,000, and exclusion from participation in federal health care programs.

Federal Anti-Kickback Law
Prohibits knowingly and willfully receiving or paying anything of value to influence the referral of federal health care program business.

STARK LAW

Because physicians or their family members often own health care facilities, Congress has passed legislation against self-referral called the **Stark Law.** Under this law, first enacted in 1989 and significantly expanded in 1995, physicians or members of their immediate families who have financial relationships with health care entities may not refer patients to those entities if the federal government, under Medicare or Medicaid, is responsible for payment.

Stark Law
Prohibits physicians or their family members who own health care facilities from referring patients to those entities if the federal government, under Medicare or Medicaid, will pay for treatment.

COURT CASE: University Overbilled Medicare and Medicaid for Patients Enrolled in Clinical Trial Research

Major universities often do clinical trials and treat Medicare and Medicaid patients during those trials. The clinical trial sponsor pays for the medical care and services. In this case, Emory University was also billing Medicare and Medicaid for the same services.

A lawsuit was filed by Elizabeth Elliot under the *qui tam,* or whistle-blower, provisions of the False Claims Act, which allow private citizens to bring civil actions on behalf of the United States and share in any recovery obtained. The Office of Inspector General of Health and Human Services and the FBI investigated the claims and found that Emory had billed, and in some cases received payment from, Medicare or Medicaid for services for which the clinical trial sponsor had already paid.

The U.S. Attorney's Office for the Northern District of Georgia announced a settlement in August 2013 with Emory University. Emory agreed to pay $1.5 million to settle claims that it violated the False Claims Act by billing Medicare and Medicaid for clinical trial services that were not permitted by the Medicare and Medicaid rules.

Ms. Elliot received a share of the settlement payment that resolves the *qui tam* suit that she filed. However, the claims settled in the civil settlement are allegations only, and there has been no determination of liability.

Source: *United States of America and State of Georgia ex rel. Elizabeth Elliott v. Emory University, et al.,* Civ. No. 1:09-cv-3569-AT (N.D. Ga. Dec. 18, 2009).

Generally, three questions determine whether or not a request for reimbursement is prohibited by the Stark Law: (1) Has a physician or a member of the physician's family referred a Medicare or Medicaid patient to an entity? (2) Is the referral for a "designated health service"? (3) Is there a financial relationship between the referring physician or family member and the entity providing service? If any of these three questions is answered "yes," the referral violates the Stark Law.

For years since the Stark Law was implemented, the ban on physician conflicts of interest was applied to Medicare claims but not to Medicaid. Whistle-blowers bringing suit against alleged violators called for clarification of the law, and the U.S. Justice Department agreed that the law is applicable to Medicaid as well as Medicare claims. As a result, in 2012, the Justice Department reported an all-time high of $3 billion forfeited by drug companies and health care providers via whistle-blower Stark Law lawsuits.

A common misconception is that the Federal Anti-Kickback Law and the Stark Law are the same. Table 8-6 illustrates the differences between the two laws.

Table 8-6 Comparison of the Anti-Kickback Law and the Stark Law

	The Anti-Kickback Statute (42 USC § 1320a–7b(b))	**The Stark Law (42 USC § 1395nn)**
Prohibition	Prohibits offering, paying, soliciting, or receiving anything of value to induce or reward referrals or generate federal health care program business	• Prohibits a physician from referring Medicare patients for designated health services to an entity with which the physician (or immediate family member) has a financial relationship, unless an exception applies • Prohibits the designated health services entity from submitting claims to Medicare for those services resulting from a prohibited referral
Referrals	Referrals from anyone	Referrals from a physician
Items/Services	Any items or services	Designated health services
Intent	Intent must be proven (knowing and willful)	• No intent standard for overpayment (strict liability) • Intent required for civil monetary penalties for *knowing* violations
Penalties	Criminal: • Fines up to $25,000 per violation • Up to a 5-year prison term per violation Civil/Administrative: • False Claims Act liability • Civil monetary penalties and program exclusion • Potential $50,000 civil monetary penalty per violation • Civil assessment of up to three times amount of kickback	Civil: • Overpayment/refund obligation • False Claims Act liability • Civil monetary penalties and program exclusion for *knowing* violations • Potential $15,000 civil monetary penalty for each service • Civil assessment of up to three times the amount claimed
Exceptions	*Voluntary* safe harbors	*Mandatory* exceptions
Federal Health Care Programs	All	Medicare/Medicaid

This chart is for illustrative purposes only and is not a substitute for consulting the statutes and their regulations. https://oig.hhs.gov/compliance/provider-compliance-training/files/StarkandAKSChartHandout508.pdf

CRIMINAL HEALTH CARE FRAUD STATUTE

The **Criminal Health Care Fraud Statute** (18 U.S. Code Section 1347) prohibits knowingly and willfully executing, or attempting to execute, a scheme intending to:

- Defraud any health care benefit program.
- Obtain (by means of false pretenses, representations, or promises) any of the money or property owned by, or under the custody or control of, any health care benefit program.

Criminal Health Care Fraud Statute
A section of the U.S. Code that prohibits fraud against any health care benefit program.

Proof of actual knowledge or specific intent to violate the law is *not* required. Penalties for violating the Criminal Health Care Fraud Statute may include fines, imprisonment, or both.

Under 42 U.S.C. Section 1320a-7, the HHS Office of Inspector General is required to impose exclusions from participation in all federal health care programs on health care providers and suppliers who have been convicted of:

- Medicare fraud;
- Patient abuse or neglect;
- Felony convictions for other health care–related fraud, theft, or other financial misconduct; or
- Felony convictions for unlawful manufacture, distribution, prescription, or dispensing of controlled substances.

In summary, violations of laws against health care fraud and abuse can result in imprisonment and fines, loss of professional license, loss of health care facility staff privileges, and exclusion from participation in federal and/or state health care programs.

Check Your Progress

14. The False Claims Act contains which distinguishing provision?
15. Are the Federal Anti-Kickback Law and the Stark Law exactly the same? Explain your answer.
16. What does the Criminal Health Care Fraud Statute prohibit?
17. What federal office is responsible for enforcement of the four laws discussed in this section?
18. What types of legal convictions are most likely to exclude health care providers from participation in a federal health care program?

8.5 Patients' Bill of Rights

Legislation designed to protect the health care industry and its consumers is official, that is, violation of these laws usually carries a penalty, such as fines, loss of license, or prosecution. Other methods of protecting patients exist in the form of a Patients' Bill of Rights. Depending on the legal jurisdiction, the Bill of Rights may be only recommendations or may be statute.

As discussed in 7.4 Informed Consent, an important patient right is informed consent. This means that if you need a treatment, your health care provider must give you the information you need to make a decision. Types of informed consent are established by state law.

The HIPAA Privacy Rule, discussed in Section 8.2 of this chapter, provides patients with laws to protect the privacy of their personal health information.

The Patient Protection and Affordable Care Act of 2010 also lists features at www.hhs.gov/healthcare/rights that are intended to give health care consumers more rights, but they apply only to health insurance. Insurance companies must:

- Phase out annual and lifetime limits to coverage.
- No longer limit or deny coverage to patients under 19 with a preexisting condition.
- Cover children up to age 26 on their parents' health insurance policy.
- Phase out arbitrary withdrawals of insurance coverage.
- End lifetime limits on benefits.
- Cover preventive care at no cost.
- Justify any raise in rates.
- Remove insurance company barriers to emergency service.
- Allow clients to file a complaint.

Concerns about the quality of medical care patients receive under managed care plans prompted Congress to first consider a Patients' Bill of Rights Act in 1999. The act contained provisions applicable to managed care plans for access to care, quality assurance, patient information and securing privacy, grievances and appeals procedures, protecting the physician–patient relationship, and promoting good medical practice. Congress failed to act on the bill in 1999, and it was revived in 2001 as H.R. 2563, the Bipartisan Patient Protection Act of 2001. The bill died in Congress but was revived in 2004, although it again failed to pass.

The American Hospital Association (AHA) created a Patients' Bill of Rights as early as 1973. Attempts to make it a federal law failed. In 2003, the AHA dropped the Bill of Rights and created a brochure titled "Patient Care Partnership: Understanding Expectations, Rights and Responsibilities." While it is written from a hospital perspective, it does provide guidance concerning a patient's rights.

In the last several years, some states have passed a Patients' Bill of Rights. However, depending on the state, the Bill of Rights may pertain only to hospital care or perhaps nursing homes, mental health facilities, or other health care facilities. At least four states appear to have a generalized Patients' Bill of Rights established by law.

Currently, the approach to a Patients' Bill of Rights is somewhat scattered or specifically focused on a certain area of health care. Hospitals and other health care facilities may develop their own lists of patients' rights, but these documents are probably not legally enforceable.

Check Your Progress

(There are no correct answers to the following exercises. These questions are intended solely to stimulate thought and discussion.)

19. Do you see the necessity for a Patients' Bill of Rights for health care consumers? Explain your answer.
20. Should a Patients' Bill of Rights contain the right of the patient to sue if care is demonstrably unsatisfactory? Explain your answer.
21. How can you determine if your state has a statute for a Patients' Bill of Rights?
22. Based on your own experience as a health care consumer and the experiences of your friends and family members, what rights would you list in a Patients' Bill of Rights?

Chapter Summary

Learning Outcome	Summary
LO 8.1 List the U.S. constitutional amendments and privacy laws that pertain to health care.	Which U.S. constitutional amendments and privacy laws pertain to health care? • First, Third, Fourth, Fifth, Ninth, and Fourteenth U.S. Constitutional Amendments • Health Insurance Portability and Accountability Act (HIPAA) of 1996 • American Recovery and Reinvestment Act (ARRA) of 2009 • Health Information Technology for Economic and Clinical Health Act (HITECH) • Patient Protection and Affordable Care Act (PPACA) of 2010 • Health Care and Education Reconciliation Act (HCERA) of 2010 What considerations do federal and state privacy laws share? • Information collected and stored about individuals should be limited to what is necessary to carry out the functions of the business or government agency collecting the information. • Once collected, access to personal information should be limited to those employees who must use the information in performing their jobs. • Personal information cannot be released outside the organization collecting it unless authorization is obtained from the subject. • When information is collected about a person, that person should know that the information is being collected and should have the opportunity to check it for accuracy.

LO 8.2 Explain HIPAA's Privacy Rule.	What are HIPAA's special requirements for disclosing protected health information?
	• Protected health information (PHI) can be de-identified by removing certain patient identifiers.
	• Permissions are required for releasing PHI under six categories:
	  • Disclosures to patients
	  • Disclosures for treatment, payment, or health care operations
	  • Disclosures with opportunity to agree or object
	  • Some incidental uses and disclosures permitted without authorization
	  • Disclosures for public interest and benefit activities
	  • Limited data set disclosures
	What is a covered entity?
	• Health care providers who conduct administrative and financial transactions in electronic form. This includes all employees, volunteers, trainees, and all others who are under the control of the entity.
	What is a business associate?
	• Individuals and/or organizations that provide certain functions, activities, or services on behalf of covered entities that involve access to or the use of disclosure of PHI.
	How are patients' rights defined under HIPAA?
	• Patients have the right to:
	  • Access and copy medical records.
	  • Request amendments/corrections to medical record.
	  • Request a list of disclosures.
	  • Request to be contacted at certain locations.
	  • Put further restrictions on those who have access to PHI.
	  • File a complaint.
	• Notice of Privacy Practice
	  • Requires CEs to post privacy policies.

	What are the elements of protected health information? • Past, present, or future physical or mental health condition • Documentation of the provision of health care • Past, present, or future payment for the provision of health care What must a Notice of Privacy Practices contain? • How the CE may use and disclose an individual's PHI • The patient's rights with respect to the information and how the patient may exercise those rights, with clear direction on how the patient may complain to the CE • The CE's legal duties with respect to the information • Whom patients can contact for further information
LO 8.3 Identify those laws implemented to protect the security of health care information.	What does the Security Rule require CEs and BAs to do? • Ensure the confidentiality, integrity, and availability of all PHI they create, receive, maintain, or transmit; • Identify and protect against reasonably anticipated threats to the security or integrity of the information; • Protect against reasonably anticipated, impermissible uses or disclosures; and • Ensure compliance by their workforce. What is a breach? • An impermissible use or disclosure under the Privacy Rule that compromises the security or privacy of PHI.

LO 8.4 Describe the federal laws that cover fraud and abuse within the health care business environment.	What federal laws cover fraud and abuse within the health care business environment?
	• False Claims Act
	  • Provides for civil penalties for persons knowingly making false claims to the federal government for payment.
	  • Whistle-blowers who report false claims can share in awards under *qui tam.*
	• Federal Anti-Kickback Law
	  • Criminal law that prohibits arranging items of value as a reward for referrals of services paid for by the government health care system.
	• Stark Law
	  • Physicians or members of their immediate families cannot refer patients to health care facilities they own if the government pays for care.
	• Criminal Health Care Fraud Statute
	  • A section of the U.S. Code that makes it a criminal offense to knowingly defraud a health care benefit program.

LO 8.5 Summarize patient rights as defined by the Patient Protection and Affordable Care Act and state statutes.	How are patient rights defined under HIPAA, the Patient Protection and Affordable Care Act, and other state statutes?
	• Patient Protection and Affordable Care Act (PPACA). Insurance companies must:
	  • Phase out annual and lifetime limits to coverage.
	  • No longer limit or deny coverage to patients under 19 with a preexisting condition.
	  • Cover children up to age 26 on their parents' health insurance policy.
	  • Phase out arbitrary withdrawals of insurance coverage.
	  • End lifetime limits on benefits.
	  • Cover preventable care at no cost.
	  • Justify any raise in rates.
	  • Remove insurance company barriers to emergency service.
	  • Allow clients to file a complaint.
	• Other state statutes
	  • Patient Bill of Rights may be found in some state statutes. Some health care organizations create a Patient Bill of Rights, but those do not have the full force of law.

Chapter 8 Review

Applying Knowledge

LO 8.1

1. Which U.S. Constitutional Amendments deal with the issue of privacy?
2. List the four HIPAA standards and briefly describe their purpose.

LO 8.2

3. What is a covered entity?
4. What is a business associate?
5. What is the relationship between a CE and a BA?
6. Define the six HIPAA-defined permissions.
7. What are the key elements in a Notice of Privacy Practices?
8. What are the key elements of protected health information?
9. Check each activity listed below that is permitted by HIPAA without authorization, then list the understood provision in each permitted case.

_____ A nurse discusses a patient's medical tests with her over the telephone.

_____ Two medical assistants in a medical office discuss the medical care of a patient they both know.

_____ A medical office receptionist discusses a friend's medical treatment with her family at the dinner table.

_____ Two physicians debate the possible treatment of a patient's difficult disease.

_____ A health insurance salesman telephones a medical office to speak with a medical assistant "off the record."

10. You are a medical records supervisor in a clinic. A pharmaceutical firm asks for data on patients with a certain diagnosis for a study of the numbers of people with the disease. Can you give it the information it asks for? If so, how will you provide the information?

LO 8.3

11. Would you most likely send a patient's electronic medical record or his electronic health record to a specialist collaborating on the patient's treatment with your physician employer?
12. How might a health care provider show that their EHR was as safe as possible from a breach?
13. One of the best ways to ensure against loss or corruption of medical data is to
    a. Refuse to send any medical data electronically
    b. Back up all data regularly
    c. Send only paper records to recipients of medical data
    d. Never store medical data on a computer
14. The authority to administer the Security Rule of HIPAA rests with the
    a. FBI
    b. NSA
    c. OCR
    d. DOJ

15. A risk analysis for the Security Rule is

a. Done by the federal government

b. Is voluntarily done by the health care organization

c. Is done by the individual state

d. Is a requirement for the health care organization

16. Which of the following constitutes a data breach?

a. A medical office computer is sold without erasing the hard drive.

b. A hacker accesses a hospital's list of patients with HIV.

c. A business-use laptop is stolen from a health insurance company executive while she is traveling.

d. All of these

17. A breach of more than ______ records requires notification to the media.

a. 200

b. 300

c. 400

d. 500

LO 8.4

18. Medicare fraud is not easy to estimate. Which of the following does not contribute to the challenge of determining Medicare fraud?

a. Fraud is often undetected and therefore difficult to quantify.

b. Dollar amounts spent in a single incident of fraud are increasing.

c. Fraudulent spending is not always separated from total health care dollars spent.

d. Records are destroyed yearly.

19. The False Claims Act provides for:

a. Paying any legitimate Medicare or Medicaid bill

b. Making it a criminal offense to defraud any health care benefit program

c. People bringing claims to share in any court-awarded damages

d. Jail sentences for all violators

20. A physician pays a long-term care administrator to refer all new Medicare and Medicaid patients to his medical practice. He is most likely to be accused of violating which federal law?

a. HIPAA

b. Gramm-Rudman Law

c. Federal Anti-Kickback Law

d. None of these

21. An entity may have violated the Stark Law if "yes" is answered to which of the following questions?

a. Has a physician or a member of her family referred a Medicare or Medicaid patient to an entity?

b. Is the referral for a "designated health service"?

c. Is there a financial relationship between the referring physician or family member and the entity providing service?

d. All of these

22. Which of the following statements is true?
    a. The False Claims Act covers only hospitals.
    b. The Federal Anti-Kickback Law and the Stark Law are the same.
    c. The Criminal Health Care Fraud Statute has been repealed.
    d. The Federal Anti-Kickback Law and the Stark Law are not the same.
23. Which of the following might a health care practitioner suffer if convicted of the False Claims Act, the Federal Anti-Kickback Law, the Stark Law, or the Criminal Health Care Fraud Statute?
    a. A fine
    b. A prison sentence
    c. Loss of medical license
    d. All of these

LO 8.5

24. Check all statements below that are true of a Patients' Bill of Rights:

_____ Congress passed a general Patients' Bill of Rights in 2010, and it is now law.

_____ Under HIPAA's Patients' Bill of Rights, patients may sue.

_____ The Patients' Bill of Rights for the Patient Protection and Affordable Care Act applies to insurance companies.

_____ Some health care providers publish their own Patients' Bill of Rights.

_____ A Patients' Bill of Rights is enforceable under the Criminal Health Care Fraud Statute.

Ethics Issues Privacy, Security, and Fraud

Use your critical thinking skills to answer the questions that follow each ethics issue.

Ethics ISSUE 1:

HIPAA has made it illegal, under threat of penalty, for health care practitioners to disclose confidential health information about patients to unauthorized sources.

Discussion Questions

25. Sharon, a second-year nursing student, is completing a surgical rotation in a community hospital. At the breakfast table, Sharon's husband asks her to find out what is wrong with one of his employees, who has been hospitalized for several days. He is interested in knowing when the man may be able to return to work. Is it ethical for Sharon to give her husband this information? Explain your answer.
26. What should health care practitioners do when family members or friends ask them for information about others that they have discovered in the course of their employment?

Ethics ISSUE 2:

Some sources distinguish between *privacy* in health care and *confidentiality*. According to the experts, *privacy* refers to the right of an individual to be let alone and to the fact that patients must authorize release of information. *Confidentiality* refers to limiting disclosure to authorized persons and ensuring protection of records documenting communication between providers and patients.

Discussion Questions

27. Why are privacy and confidentiality so important to patients and to health care practitioners?

28. A patient asks for a list of disclosures his physician has made of his health information within the past 6 years, and he is politely asked to submit his request in writing.

    A patient requests in writing that his health records be faxed to another physician. The person responsible for faxing the record sends the information to the wrong fax number.

    The health care practitioners in these two situations have followed the letter of HIPAA law. Have they also acted ethically? Explain why or why not.

Ethics ISSUE 3:

The Criminal Health Care Fraud Statute (18 U.S. Code Section 1347) prohibits knowingly and willfully executing, or attempting to execute, a scheme intending to defraud any health care benefit program or obtain (by means of false pretenses, representations, or promises) any of the money or property owned by, or under the custody or control of, any health care benefit program.

Discussion Questions

29. Of the following practices, which constitutes fraud?
    - Billing for services not provided.
    - Billing for services not covered under a patient's health insurance.
    - Unbundling; that is, billing separately for each stage of a procedure.
    - A licensed health care practitioner allows an unlicensed person to bill an insurer under his name.
    - A medical facility waives deductibles and copayments.

30. Are all of these practices illegal? Are all of these practices unethical?

Case Studies

Use your critical thinking skills to answer the questions that follow each case study.

LO 8.1

31. John works as an LPN at a Hollywood, California, hospital. While distributing meds to the patients on his floor, he noticed that the recently admitted patient in Room 402, named Jason Wilson, was really a well-known actor in a popular television series. John called his wife to tell her about the celebrity patient on his floor. Was John's statement to his wife a HIPAA violation?

    Can the actor sue for punitive damages?

LO 8.4

32. Patients with Alzheimer's disease sat, twice every week, unsupervised inside a small room of a memory care facility watching the movie *Forrest Gump*. Each time the patients sat in front of the television watching the movie, the facility submitted insurance claims for providing "group therapy."

    Is this practice legal and appropriate, or is it an example of health care fraud?

33. A physician assistant convinced her patients that hypnotherapy could make them more receptive to medical treatment. Fortunately, she told them, she could conduct the hypnosis sessions in the office she used for consultations. The predominant insurance company for many of the physician assistant's patients did not pay for "hypnotherapy," nor was the physician assistant qualified to provide it, so she billed the sessions as office visits, at $100 to $125 per visit.

    Was the physician assistant committing health care fraud? Explain your answer.

Internet Activities

LO 8.1, 8.2, 8.3, 8.4, and 8.5

Complete the activities and answer the questions that follow.

34. Visit www.proprofs.com/quiz-school/story.php?title=hipaa-compliance-quiz and take the privacy quiz. Answers are provided immediately after the questions. Which, if any, of the answers most surprised you and why?
35. Visit www.blueshieldca.com/bsca/about-blue-shield/fraud-prevention/quiz.sp and take the health care fraud quiz. Read the correct answer for any questions you missed.
36. Visit http://oig.hhs.gov/fraud/medicaid-fraud-control-units-mfcu/index.asp. What are the duties of the Medicaid Fraud Control Units? How would a health care practitioner report Medicaid fraud?
37. Review the court case "Fourth Amendment Right to Privacy" found in Section 8.1. See if you can find an update on the pending cases. Did the appellate courts rule on the Oregon or the Texas case? Has the Utah case been tried?
38. Does your state have a Patients' Bill of Rights in its statute? What does it say? If your state does not have a statutory Patients' Bill of Rights, find a state that does and determine what rights are protected. Hint: One of the states that does have a statutory Bill of Rights is in the southern United States, and its most southern point is 90 miles from Cuba.

Resources

LO 8.2

Privacy laws: www.hhs.gov/hipaa/for-professionals/privacy/laws-regulations/index.html

LO 8.3

HIPAA penalties: www.hhs.gov/hipaa/for-professionals/compliance-enforcement/agreements/index.html

HIPAA security: www.fiercehealthcare.com/payer/one-year-later-controversy-still-surrounds-anthem-data-breach

www.4medapproved.com/hitsecurity/disaster-recovery-hipaa-requirement/

LO 8.4

https://oig.hhs.gov/fraud/strike-force/

www.justice.gov/opa/pr/justice-department-recovers-38-billion-false-claims-act-cases-fiscal-year-2013

www.healthcarefinancenews.com/slideshow/biggest-healthcare-frauds-2016-running-list?p=5

www.healthcarefinancenews.com/slideshow/biggest-healthcare-frauds-2017-running-list

www.cms.gov/Outreach-and-Education/Medicare-Learning-Network-MLN/MLNProducts/downloads/Fraud_and_Abuse.pdf

PART THREE

Professional, Transitional, and Societal Health Care Issues

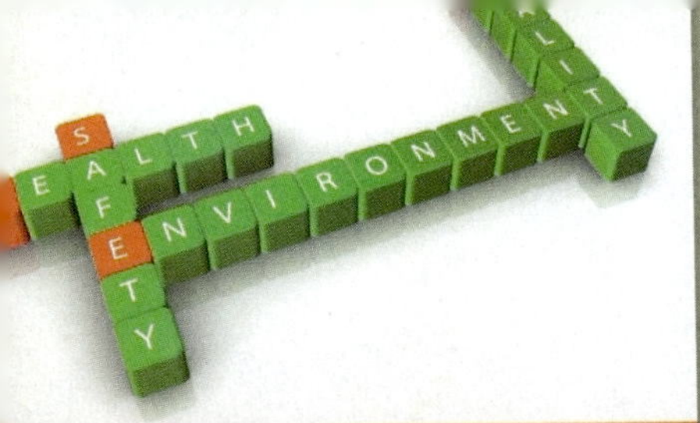

9

Public Health Responsibilities of Physicians and Other Health Care Practitioners

Key Terms

administer
Amendments to the Older Americans Act
autopsy
Child Abuse Prevention and Treatment Act
Controlled Substances Act
coroner
dispense
Drug Enforcement Administration (DEA)
federalism
Food and Drug Administration (FDA)
forensics
medical examiner
National Childhood Vaccine Injury Act
National Vaccine Injury Compensation Program (VICP)
prescribe
quarantine
Smallpox Emergency Personnel Protection Act (SEPPA)
Unborn Victims of Violence Act
vital statistics

LEARNING OUTCOMES

After studying this chapter, you should be able to:

LO 9.1 Define and determine the purpose of collecting vital statistics and identify reporting procedures.

LO 9.2 Summarize the purpose and impact of public health statutes.

LO 9.3 Cite examples of reportable diseases and injuries, and explain how they are reported.

LO 9.4 Discuss federal drug regulations, including the Controlled Substances Act.

FROM THE PERSPECTIVE OF. . .

JASON, RN, BSN, is a public health nurse working for sections of three counties in the rural Northwest. "My duties range from home visits for parenting education, to foster child care, to the mainstays of public health—communicable disease investigation and reporting—and everything in between. In fact, once during a home visit, I even delivered a baby—it was a boy," Jason says. "I enjoy the autonomy I have in my job, and I've established good rapport with the families I see regularly."

The ability to establish rapport is important, Jason explains, when he contacts individuals who have been diagnosed with a reportable disease, such as a sexually transmitted disease, also referred to as a sexually transmitted infection (STI), and their contacts. "We have a fairly high percentage of STIs in my area, and I'm often persuading people to give me the names of those with whom they have been intimate, so I can let those individuals know that they should see a doctor."

The information is kept confidential, of course, Jason continues, "but it's still a hard subject to approach. Most people are cooperative, but there are a few who don't want to talk to me. That's when my job really becomes difficult."

From Jason's perspective, his job involves helping keep families within his practice area healthy and helping hold down the spread of a contagious infection or disease once patients are diagnosed. His investigative work as a public health nurse is mandated by state law, but the process can be difficult and can feel intrusive. Nevertheless, Jason does his best to see that the people in his area are protected.

From the perspective of Jason's patients who learn they have a reportable, contagious condition, his visit is probably stressful. Those who are concerned for loved ones or others with whom they have had contact, however, are generally willing to provide names of individuals he can contact.

From the perspective of public health authorities, nurses like Jason not only see patients in their homes, where health problems often arise, but they also keep contagious diseases from becoming epidemic, and they help get vital treatment to those who have been exposed to infectious diseases.

9.1 Vital Statistics

To assess population trends and needs, state and federal governments collect **vital statistics.** Vital events for which statistics are collected include live births, deaths, fetal deaths, marriages, divorces, induced terminations of pregnancy, and any change in civil status that occurs during an individual's lifetime. Health care practitioners help in gathering this information and in filling out forms for filing with the appropriate state and federal agencies.

vital statistics
Numbers collected for the population of live births, deaths, fetal deaths, marriages, divorces, induced terminations of pregnancy, and any change in civil status that occurs during an individual's lifetime.

The information provided through the reporting of vital statistics is useful to educational institutions, governmental agencies, research scientists, private industry, and many other organizations and individuals. For example, the recording of vital statistics allows for tracking population composition and growth, measuring educational standards, and monitoring communicable diseases and other community and environmental health problems. Health care practitioners play an important role in collecting and recording valuable health data required by law; therefore, it is important that they know the correct methods and procedures for reporting public health information.

RECORDS FOR BIRTHS AND DEATHS

Birth and death certificates are permanent legal records, and a copy of a person's birth certificate is required to obtain certain government documents, such as a passport, driver's license, voter registration card, or Social Security card. Guidelines for completing the forms are as follows:

- Type or legibly print all entries. In some states, only black ink may be used.
- Leave no entries blank. Each state has specific requirements for recording information.
- Avoid corrections and erasures.
- Where requested, provide signatures. Do not use rubber stamps or initials in place of signatures.
- File only originals with state registrars.
- Verify the spelling of names.
- Avoid abbreviations, except those recommended in instructions for specific items.
- Refer any problems to the appropriate state officials.

Births All live births must be reported to the state registrar. Figure 9-1 illustrates a sample birth certificate. In some states, separate birth and death certificates must be filed for stillbirths, whereas in others, there are special forms for stillbirths that include both birth and death information. Generally, birth and death certificates are not required for fetal deaths in which the fetus has not passed the twentieth week of gestation.

Hospitals file birth certificates for babies born to mothers who have been admitted as patients. The attending physician must verify all medical information. For nonhospital births, the person in attendance is responsible for filing the birth certificate. (Jason, the public health nurse in the chapter's opening scenario, filed the birth certificate for the birth he attended.)

Deaths After a person is pronounced dead, the attending physician must complete the medical portion of the certificate of death, which generally includes the following information:

- Disease, injury, and/or complication that caused the death and how long the decedent was treated for this condition before death occurred.
- Date and time of death.
- Place of death.
- If decedent was female, presence or absence of pregnancy.
- Whether or not an autopsy was performed. An **autopsy** is a postmortem examination to determine the cause of death or to obtain physiological evidence, as in the case of a suspicious death.

autopsy
A postmortem examination to determine the cause of death or to obtain physiological evidence, as in the case of a suspicious death.

FIGURE 9-1 A Sample Birth Certificate

LOCAL FILE NO.

U.S. STANDARD CERTIFICATE OF LIVE BIRTH

BIRTH NUMBER:

CHILD

1. CHILD'S NAME (First, Middle, Last, Suffix) | 2. TIME OF BIRTH (24 hr) | 3. SEX | 4. DATE OF BIRTH (Mo/Day/Yr)

5. FACILITY NAME (If not institution, give street and number) | 6. CITY, TOWN, OR LOCATION OF BIRTH | 7. COUNTY OF BIRTH

MOTHER

8a. MOTHER'S CURRENT LEGAL NAME (First, Middle, Last, Suffix) | 8b. DATE OF BIRTH (Mo/Day/Yr)

8c. MOTHER'S NAME PRIOR TO FIRST MARRIAGE (First, Middle, Last, Suffix) | 8d. BIRTHPLACE (State, Territory, or Foreign Country)

9a. RESIDENCE OF MOTHER-STATE | 9b. COUNTY | 9c. CITY, TOWN, OR LOCATION

9d. STREET AND NUMBER | 9e. APT. NO. | 9f. ZIP CODE | 9g. INSIDE CITY LIMITS? □ Yes □ No

FATHER

10a. FATHER'S CURRENT LEGAL NAME (First, Middle, Last, Suffix) | 10b. DATE OF BIRTH (Mo/Day/Yr) | 10c. BIRTHPLACE (State, Territory, or Foreign Country)

CERTIFIER

11. CERTIFIER'S NAME: ______________________

TITLE: □ MD □ DO □ HOSPITAL ADMIN. □ CNM/CM □ OTHER MIDWIFE

□ OTHER (Specify)______________________

12. DATE CERTIFIED ____/____/______ MM DD YYYY

13. DATE FILED BY REGISTRAR ____/____/______ MM DD YYYY

INFORMATION FOR ADMINISTRATIVE USE

MOTHER

14. MOTHER'S MAILING ADDRESS: 9 Same as residence, or: State: City, Town, or Location:

Street & Number: Apartment No.: Zip Code:

15. MOTHER MARRIED? (At birth, conception, or any time between) □ Yes □ No

IF NO, HAS PATERNITY ACKNOWLEDGEMENT BEEN SIGNED IN THE HOSPITAL? □ Yes □ No

16. SOCIAL SECURITY NUMBER REQUESTED FOR CHILD? □ Yes □ No

17. FACILITY ID. (NPI)

18. MOTHER'S SOCIAL SECURITY NUMBER:

19. FATHER'S SOCIAL SECURITY NUMBER:

INFORMATION FOR MEDICAL AND HEALTH PURPOSES ONLY

MOTHER

20. MOTHER'S EDUCATION (Check the box that best describes the highest degree or level of school completed at the time of delivery)

□ 8th grade or less
□ 9th - 12th grade, no diploma
□ High school graduate or GED completed
□ Some college credit but no degree
□ Associate degree (e.g., AA, AS)
□ Bachelor's degree (e.g., BA, AB, BS)
□ Master's degree (e.g., MA, MS, MEng, MEd, MSW, MBA)
□ Doctorate (e.g., PhD, EdD) or Professional degree (e.g., MD, DDS, DVM, LLB, JD)

21. MOTHER OF HISPANIC ORIGIN? (Check the box that best describes whether the mother is Spanish/Hispanic/Latina. Check the "No" box if mother is not Spanish/Hispanic/Latina)

□ No, not Spanish/Hispanic/Latina
□ Yes, Mexican, Mexican American, Chicana
□ Yes, Puerto Rican
□ Yes, Cuban
□ Yes, other Spanish/Hispanic/Latina

(Specify)______________________

22. MOTHER'S RACE (Check one or more races to indicate what the mother considers herself to be)

□ White
□ Black or African American
□ American Indian or Alaska Native (Name of the enrolled or principal tribe)______________
□ Asian Indian
□ Chinese
□ Filipino
□ Japanese
□ Korean
□ Vietnamese
□ Other Asian (Specify)______________
□ Native Hawaiian
□ Guamanian or Chamorro
□ Samoan
□ Other Pacific Islander (Specify)______________
□ Other (Specify)______________

FATHER

23. FATHER'S EDUCATION (Check the box that best describes the highest degree or level of school completed at the time of delivery)

□ 8th grade or less
□ 9th - 12th grade, no diploma
□ High school graduate or GED completed
□ Some college credit but no degree
□ Associate degree (e.g., AA, AS)
□ Bachelor's degree (e.g., BA, AB, BS)
□ Master's degree (e.g., MA, MS, MEng, MEd, MSW, MBA)
□ Doctorate (e.g., PhD, EdD) or Professional degree (e.g., MD, DDS, DVM, LLB, JD)

24. FATHER OF HISPANIC ORIGIN? (Check the box that best describes whether the father is Spanish/Hispanic/Latino. Check the "No" box if father is not Spanish/Hispanic/Latino)

□ No, not Spanish/Hispanic/Latino
□ Yes, Mexican, Mexican American, Chicano
□ Yes, Puerto Rican
□ Yes, Cuban
□ Yes, other Spanish/Hispanic/Latino

(Specify)______________________

25. FATHER'S RACE (Check one or more races to indicate what the father considers himself to be)

□ White
□ Black or African American
□ American Indian or Alaska Native (Name of the enrolled or principal tribe)______________
□ Asian Indian
□ Chinese
□ Filipino
□ Japanese
□ Korean
□ Vietnamese
□ Other Asian (Specify)______________
□ Native Hawaiian
□ Guamanian or Chamorro
□ Samoan
□ Other Pacific Islander (Specify)______________
□ Other (Specify)______________

Mother's Name ______________

Mother's Medical Record No. ______________

26. PLACE WHERE BIRTH OCCURRED (Check one)

□ Hospital
□ Freestanding birthing center
□ Home Birth: Planned to deliver at home? 9 Yes 9 No
□ Clinic/Doctor's office
□ Other (Specify)______________

27. ATTENDANT'S NAME, TITLE, AND NPI

NAME: ______________________ NPI:

TITLE: □ MD □ DO □ CNM/CM □ OTHER MIDWIFE

□ OTHER (Specify)______________

28. MOTHER TRANSFERRED FOR MATERNAL MEDICAL OR FETAL INDICATIONS FOR DELIVERY? □ Yes □ No

IF YES, ENTER NAME OF FACILITY MOTHER TRANSFERRED FROM:

____

REV. 11/2003

Source: U.S. Department of Health and Human Services, A Sample Birth Certificate.

In most states, it is against the law for an attending physician to sign a death certificate if the death was:

- Possibly due to criminal causes
- Not attended by a physician within a specified length of time before death
- Due to causes undetermined by the physician
- Violent or otherwise suspicious

Autopsy is discussed more thoroughly in Chapter 12 "Death and Dying."

If any of these situations exist, a coroner or medical examiner must sign the death certificate. If a death occurs under suspicious circumstances, permission from next of kin is *not* needed for an autopsy to be performed. If the death did not occur under suspicious circumstances, however, consent from next of kin or a legally responsible party must be obtained for an autopsy to be performed.

When death has occurred under normal circumstances, after authorization has been obtained from the next of kin or from a legally responsible party, the body can be removed to a funeral home. In many states, the death certificate must be signed within 24 to 72 hours. The *mortician* or *undertaker* (person trained to attend to the dead) files the death certificate with the state. (See Figure 9-2 for a sample death certificate.)

If the deceased has not been under a physician's care at the time of death, the appropriate county health officer–usually the coroner or medical examiner–is responsible for completing the death certificate. A **coroner** is a public official who investigates and holds inquests over those who die from unknown or violent causes. He or she may or may not be a physician, depending on state law.

coroner
A public official who investigates and holds inquests over those who die from unknown or violent causes; he or she may or may not be a physician, depending on state law.

The purpose of a coroner's inquest is to gather evidence that may be used by the police in the investigation of a violent or suspicious death. It is not a trial, but it is a criminal proceeding, in the nature of a preliminary investigation.

Some states employ a medical examiner instead of a coroner. A **medical examiner** is a physician, frequently a pathologist, who investigates suspicious or unexplained deaths in a community. As a physician, the medical examiner can order and perform autopsies.

medical examiner
A physician who investigates suspicious or unexplained deaths.

Forensics is a division of medicine that incorporates law and medicine and involves medical issues or medical proof at trials having to do with malpractice, crimes, and accidents. Forensic scientists investigate crime scenes and present medical proof at trials and hearings. Crime scene investigators are specifically trained to determine cause of death or injury and to help identify a criminal, a victim, and others involved in crimes. Specialists in forensic medicine study such subjects as forensic pharmacology, toxicology, blood spatter interpretation, DNA (deoxyribonucleic acid) analytical techniques, and expert testimony procedures. They work for police departments and other criminal investigative bureaus, medical examiners' offices, universities, and other facilities and government agencies.

forensics
A division of medicine that incorporates law and medicine and involves medical issues or medical proof at trials having to do with malpractice, crimes, and accidents.

FIGURE 9-2 A Sample Death Certificate

U.S. STANDARD CERTIFICATE OF DEATH

LOCAL FILE NO. STATE FILE NO.

NAME OF DECEDENT ____ For use by physician or institution

To Be Completed/ Verified By: FUNERAL DIRECTOR:

1. DECEDENT'S LEGAL NAME (Include AKA's if any) (First, Middle, Last)
2. SEX
3. SOCIAL SECURITY NUMBER

4a. AGE-Last Birthday (Years)
4b. UNDER 1 YEAR — Months | Days
4c. UNDER 1 DAY — Hours | Minutes
5. DATE OF BIRTH (Mo/Day/Yr)
6. BIRTHPLACE (City and State or Foreign Country)

7a. RESIDENCE-STATE
7b. COUNTY
7c. CITY OR TOWN

7d. STREET AND NUMBER
7e. APT. NO.
7f. ZIP CODE
7g. INSIDE CITY LIMITS? □ Yes □ No

8. EVER IN US ARMED FORCES? □ Yes □ No
9. MARITAL STATUS AT TIME OF DEATH □ Married □ Married, but separated □ Widowed □ Divorced □ Never Married □ Unknown
10. SURVIVING SPOUSE'S NAME (If wife, give name prior to first marriage)

11. FATHER'S NAME (First, Middle, Last)
12. MOTHER'S NAME PRIOR TO FIRST MARRIAGE (First, Middle, Last)

13a. INFORMANT'S NAME
13b. RELATIONSHIP TO DECEDENT
13c. MAILING ADDRESS (Street and Number, City, State, Zip Code)

14. PLACE OF DEATH (Check only one: see instructions)
IF DEATH OCCURRED IN A HOSPITAL: □ Inpatient □ Emergency Room/Outpatient □ Dead on Arrival
IF DEATH OCCURRED SOMEWHERE OTHER THAN A HOSPITAL: □ Hospice facility □ Nursing home/Long term care facility □ Decedent's home □ Other (Specify):

15. FACILITY NAME (If not institution, give street & number)
16. CITY OR TOWN , STATE, AND ZIP CODE
17. COUNTY OF DEATH

18. METHOD OF DISPOSITION: □ Burial □ Cremation □ Donation □ Entombment □ Removal from State □ Other (Specify):____
19. PLACE OF DISPOSITION (Name of cemetery, crematory, other place)

20. LOCATION-CITY, TOWN, AND STATE
21. NAME AND COMPLETE ADDRESS OF FUNERAL FACILITY

22. SIGNATURE OF FUNERAL SERVICE LICENSEE OR OTHER AGENT
23. LICENSE NUMBER (Of Licensee)

To Be Completed By: MEDICAL CERTIFIER

ITEMS 24-28 MUST BE COMPLETED BY PERSON WHO PRONOUNCES OR CERTIFIES DEATH
24. DATE PRONOUNCED DEAD (Mo/Day/Yr)
25. TIME PRONOUNCED DEAD

26. SIGNATURE OF PERSON PRONOUNCING DEATH (Only when applicable)
27. LICENSE NUMBER
28. DATE SIGNED (Mo/Day/Yr)

29. ACTUAL OR PRESUMED DATE OF DEATH (Mo/Day/Yr) (Spell Month)
30. ACTUAL OR PRESUMED TIME OF DEATH
31. WAS MEDICAL EXAMINER OR CORONER CONTACTED? □ Yes □ No

CAUSE OF DEATH (See instructions and examples)

32. **PART I.** Enter the chain of events--diseases, injuries, or complications--that directly caused the death. DO NOT enter terminal events such as cardiac arrest, respiratory arrest, or ventricular fibrillation without showing the etiology. DO NOT ABBREVIATE. Enter only one cause on a line. Add additional lines if necessary.

Approximate interval: Onset to death

IMMEDIATE CAUSE (Final disease or condition ---------> resulting in death) a.____
Due to (or as a consequence of):

Sequentially list conditions, if any, leading to the cause listed on line a. Enter the **UNDERLYING CAUSE** (disease or injury that initiated the events resulting in death) **LAST**
b.____
Due to (or as a consequence of):
c.____
Due to (or as a consequence of):
d.____

PART II. Enter other significant conditions contributing to death but not resulting in the underlying cause given in PART I

33. WAS AN AUTOPSY PERFORMED? □ Yes □ No
34. WERE AUTOPSY FINDINGS AVAILABLE TO COMPLETE THE CAUSE OF DEATH? □ Yes □ No

35. DID TOBACCO USE CONTRIBUTE TO DEATH? □ Yes □ Probably □ No □ Unknown
36. IF FEMALE: □ Not pregnant within past year □ Pregnant at time of death □ Not pregnant, but pregnant within 42 days of death □ Not pregnant, but pregnant 43 days to 1 year before death □ Unknown if pregnant within the past year
37. MANNER OF DEATH □ Natural □ Homicide □ Accident □ Pending Investigation □ Suicide □ Could not be determined

38. DATE OF INJURY (Mo/Day/Yr) (Spell Month)
39. TIME OF INJURY
40. PLACE OF INJURY (e.g., Decedent's home; construction site; restaurant; wooded area)
41. INJURY AT WORK? □ Yes □ No

42. LOCATION OF INJURY: State: City or Town:
Street & Number: Apartment No.: Zip Code:

43. DESCRIBE HOW INJURY OCCURRED:
44. IF TRANSPORTATION INJURY, SPECIFY: □ Driver/Operator □ Passenger □ Pedestrian □ Other (Specify)

45. CERTIFIER (Check only one):
□ Certifying physician-To the best of my knowledge, death occurred due to the cause(s) and manner stated.
□ Pronouncing & Certifying physician-To the best of my knowledge, death occurred at the time, date, and place, and due to the cause(s) and manner stated.
□ Medical Examiner/Coroner-On the basis of examination, and/or investigation, in my opinion, death occurred at the time, date, and place, and due to the cause(s) and manner stated.

Signature of certifier:____

46. NAME, ADDRESS, AND ZIP CODE OF PERSON COMPLETING CAUSE OF DEATH (Item 32)

47. TITLE OF CERTIFIER
48. LICENSE NUMBER
49. DATE CERTIFIED (Mo/Day/Yr)
50. **FOR REGISTRAR ONLY**- DATE FILED (Mo/Day/Yr)

51. DECEDENT'S EDUCATION-Check the box that best describes the highest degree or level of school completed at the time of death.
52. DECEDENT OF HISPANIC ORIGIN? Check the box that best describes whether the decedent is Spanish/Hispanic/Latino. Check the "No" box if decedent is not Spanish/Hispanic/Latino.
53. DECEDENT'S RACE (Check one or more races to indicate what the decedent considered himself or herself to be)

Source: U.S. Department of Health and Human Services, A Sample Death Certificate.

Check Your Progress

1. Define *vital statistics.*
2. Define *autopsy.*
3. Define *coroner.*
4. Define *medical examiner.*
5. Define *forensics.*
6. Where are birth certificates and death certificates filed?
7. Birth certificates must be filed for ____________.
   The requirement to file a birth certificate for ____________ varies by state.
8. Name three circumstances in which an attending physician may not legally complete a death certificate.

9.2 Public Health Statutes

The power of the states to initiate public health statutes is inferred from the Tenth Amendment to the U.S. Constitution, included in the Bill of Rights. The amendment states: "The powers not delegated to the United States by the Constitution, nor prohibited by it to the States, are reserved to the States, respectively, or to the people." In other words, states retain police powers and all other powers not expressively granted to the federal government—a practice referred to as **federalism**—the sharing of power among national, state, and local governments.

federalism
The sharing of power among national, state, and local governments.

In all states, public health statues help guarantee the health and well-being of citizens. As part of public health law, physicians or other health care practitioners must report births, deaths, certain communicable diseases, specific injuries, and child and drug abuse to the appropriate local, state, and federal authorities. Public health statutes vary with states concerning the reporting of fetal deaths and stillbirths, time limits for filing reports, and the manner in which information must be recorded. However, all provide for:

- Guarding against unsanitary conditions in public facilities
- Inspecting establishments where food and drink are processed and sold
- Exterminating pests and vermin that can spread disease
- Checking water quality
- Setting up measures of control for certain diseases
- Requiring physicians, school nurses, and other health care workers to file certain reports for the protection of citizens

Since enforcing public health laws is vital to the health of individuals within communities, the states have enforcement power granted through each state's constitution. For example, the state can:

- Require investigations be conducted in infectious disease outbreaks.
- Make childhood vaccinations a condition for school entry.
- Ban the distribution of free cigarette samples around schools or in areas where children congregate.
- Institute smoking bans or restrictions.

- Involuntarily detain (quarantine) individuals who have certain infectious diseases.
- Seize and/or destroy property to contain the threat of toxic substances.

Table 9-1 shows how laws affect public health issues.

Table 9-1 How Laws Impact Public Health Issues

Law	Public Health Issue	How the Law Works	How the Law Is Enforced
Vaccinations to enter school	Spread of infectious disease	Parental cooperation	Requires proof of vaccination when children register for school
Smoking bans/restrictions	Diseases caused by exposure to tobacco smoke	Requires behavioral changes	Admonishment or citations for noncompliance
Child safety seat laws	Accidental injuries/death in children	Requires behavioral changes	Citations for noncompliance
Fluoridation of public water supply	Dental caries	Requires no action on the part of individuals	Periodic checking of the public water supply

Source: Adapted from CDC's *Public Health Law 101, Lesson 1,* "Key Concepts of U.S. Law in Public Health Practice," PPt Slide 11. www2.cdc.gov/phlp/phl101/.

9.3 Reportable Diseases and Injuries

Under each state's public health statutes, physicians, other health care practitioners, and anyone who has knowledge of a case must report to county or state health agencies the occurrence of certain diseases that, if left unchecked, could threaten the health and well-being of the population.

In the United States, it is mandatory that certain communicable disease cases be reported to local and state public health offices when identified by physicians, nurses, laboratory directors, infection control practitioners, health care facilities, state institutions, schools, or other health care providers. These *reportable* diseases are determined by state law and can be found online by searching "[Your State's] Reportable Diseases." The list of reportable diseases varies with states and over time. Among the infectious diseases most commonly listed as reportable are: anthrax, botulism, brucellosis, cholera, diphtheria, infectious and serum hepatitis, HIV and AIDS, various forms of influenza, Legionnaire's disease, leprosy, Lyme disease, meningococcal disease, mumps, measles/rubella, pertussis/whooping cough, plague, poliomyelitis, rabies in both animals and humans, severe acute respiratory syndrome (SARS), smallpox, tuberculosis, and typhoid fever. Other diseases that must be reported if a higher than normal incidence occurs are various types of influenza and streptococcal and staphylococcal infections. This type of required reporting uses personal identifiers, so that public health practitioners can identify cases in which immediate disease control and prevention are needed.

Requirements for reporting, such as time lapses and whether to report by telephone, mail, or online, also vary with states; therefore, health care practitioners responsible for reporting must be familiar with the specific requirements in their state. Reporting requirements are available online by searching "[Your State's] Communicable Disease Reporting Requirements."

Local public health departments must, by law, submit incident reports to the state for the diseases on the state reportable list. All public health jurisdictions are also encouraged to voluntarily report (without direct personal identifiers) incidents of certain diseases to the U.S. Centers for Disease Control and Prevention (CDC). The national *Notifiable* Infectious Disease List is available at the CDC Web site: https://wwwn.cdc.gov/nndss/conditions/notifiable/2016/infectious-diseases/. (Click on "Get Notifiable List by Year" to obtain the most current national list.) The data collected by the CDC is shared by participating national and territorial jurisdictions and is used to monitor disease trends, identify populations or geographic areas at high risk of certain diseases, develop and assess prevention and control strategies, and formulate public health policies.

Due to the ever-increasing prevalence of global travel, cases of some of the infectious diseases not routinely seen on states' reportable disease lists are now being reported within the United States. As listed on the CDC's Notifiable Infectious Disease List, these cases include the viral hemorrhagic fever diseases Ebola, Lassa, Lujo, and Marburg, and the mosquito-borne diseases malaria, dengue, West Nile virus, chikungunya, yellow fever, filariasis, Japanese encephalitis, Saint Louis encephalitis, Western and Eastern equine encephalitis, and Zika. This means that heath care practitioners and public health departments must now be concerned with protocols for dealing with the treatment and prevention of highly contagious diseases that are relatively new to the United States. Mosquito control as a method of disease prevention has also become an important activity in those areas in the United States where the climate is favorable for the infection-carrying insects to multiply.

Certain sexually transmitted infections (STIs) must be reported whenever diagnosed. *Sexually transmitted infection* is a general term that refers to any disease transmitted through sexual contact. Many STIs are transmitted through genital contact, which may or may not include sexual intercourse. For example, practicing oral sex can transmit gonorrhea from the genitals of one partner to the mouth and throat region of the other. Reportable STIs differ with states but generally include gonorrhea, syphilis, chlamydia, lymphogranuloma venereum, chancroid, granuloma inguinale (genital warts), scabies, pubic lice, and trichomoniasis. Public health practitioners use reported cases to find and treat others who may have been infected through sexual contact with the named individual.

All 50 states, the District of Columbia, and some cities now have laws that require individuals infected with HIV or their health care providers to notify past and present sexual or needle-sharing partners.

Reporting requirements for communicable diseases are usually more stringent for patients who are employed in restaurants, cafeterias, day care centers, schools, health care facilities, and other places where contagion can be rampant.

In some states, certain noncommunicable diseases must also be reported, to allow public health officials to track causes and/or treatment or to otherwise protect the public's health and safety. These diseases include cancer (to determine environmental causes); congenital metabolic disorders in newborns, such as phenylketonuria, congenital hypothyroidism, and galactosemia (to allow for prompt treatment); epilepsy and some other diseases that cause lapse of consciousness (to determine eligibility to drive a vehicle); and pesticide poisoning.

Health laws in various states allow public health officials to **quarantine** individuals who are known to have an infectious disease such as tuberculosis. The two court cases below illustrate the challenges in keeping infectious people away from family and the public.

quarantine
Used in connection to infectious diseases and illnesses, states may separate and restrict the movement of people with infectious diseases if they are a threat to public health. A court order is required.

THE NATIONAL CHILDHOOD VACCINE INJURY ACT OF 1986

Parents usually begin programs of vaccination against certain communicable diseases for their children when they are infants. When children reach school age, most states ask for proof of vaccination for children entering the public school system for the first time. Because a small percentage of vaccinated children suffer adverse effects from the vaccine administered, parents or guardians are informed of risks associated with each vaccine and must sign consent forms allowing health care practitioners to administer the vaccine.

The **National Childhood Vaccine Injury Act** of 1986 created the **National Vaccine Injury Compensation Program (VICP).** The reason for creating the VICP system was to relieve vaccine manufacturers and providers from having to pay judgments for vaccine injuries that, in turn, could lead to a shortage of vaccines due to the disincentive of legal liability. The VICP is a no-fault system designed to compensate those individuals or families of individuals who have been injured by childhood vaccines. The program serves as an alternative to suing vaccine manufacturers and providers but does not take away an injured person's right

National Childhood Vaccine Injury Act
A federal law passed in 1986 that created a no-fault compensation program for citizens injured or killed by vaccines, as an alternative to suing vaccine manufacturers and providers."

LANDMARK COURT CASE

Case Establishes Right of State to Quarantine

A California man was diagnosed with pulmonary tuberculosis, a reportable, communicable disease. A state health officer served the man with a quarantine order, and he was admitted to a hospital. The patient deserted the hospital 1 month later, but he still had tuberculosis. The man was subsequently arrested, tried, and convicted of violating the Health and Safety Code of California. He was sentenced to 180 days in jail, but the sentence was suspended, and he was placed on a 3-year probation. The health officer again served the man with an order of isolation, and he was returned to the hospital, this time to the security section. The county public health officer then served the man with successive orders of isolation for periods of 6 months each.

The man asked for a writ of habeas corpus, claiming that the Health and Safety Code of California was unconstitutional and, therefore, the health officer had no legal authority to issue consecutive certificates of quarantine and isolation.

The court held that it is the "duty of the state to protect the public from the danger of tuberculosis"; therefore, the Health and Safety Code of California was not unconstitutional. The court also held that "The health officer may make an isolation or quarantine order whenever he shall determine in a particular case that quarantine or isolation is necessary for the protection of the public health." The petition for a writ of habeas corpus was denied.

Source: In re Halko, 246 Cal. App. 2d 553, 54 Cal. Rptr. 661 (Cal. App. Dist. 2, Nov. 18, 1966).

COURT CASE Man Involuntarily Committed to Tuberculosis Treatment Facility

In April 2014, a man sought treatment at a Texas hospital for chest pain and was diagnosed with active tuberculosis. Outpatient treatment was started for the disease, but after taking only the first 10 doses of a lengthy treatment regimen, the patient stopped reporting for treatment and could not be located. In June 2014, the man was incarcerated and given a skin test for tuberculosis, which came back negative. Because previous tests were positive for tuberculosis and negative skin tests for the disease can be incorrect, the man began treatment again in early July but refused to take his medication consistently. Once he was released from jail, the public health department was unable to find him to continue treatment.

In November 2014, the man requested a free blood test for tuberculosis from the county health department where he was living. The man's blood test came back positive, and the public health department determined that he should be restarted on treatment. Public health also gave the man a written "order to implement and carry out measures for a patient with tuberculosis" and a warning letter. It informed the man that he had a "serious communicable disease" and that he was required to continue treatment or "court proceedings may be initiated against [him]." The man began treatment, but after 7 days of treatment, public health was unable to locate him until mid-December, when he was again incarcerated.

On December 17, 2014, the public health department filed an application for temporary protective custody of the man in order to complete treatment for his disease. On December 18, 2014, the public health department presented its application for extended management over the man, stating that because he "presents a threat to the public health" and had "refused to follow several written treatment orders given to him," the trial court should order involuntary inpatient treatment for him. The case then proceeded to jury trial.

The man appeared in court by teleconference to avoid the possible infection with tuberculosis of members of the public and officers of the court. A registered nurse and county tuberculosis program manager testified that in April 2014, county public health officials had diagnosed the man with active tuberculosis based on a sputum culture and chest X-ray showing a "cavitary lesion," or damage to his lung caused by the disease. The nurse also testified regarding the man's treatment history and his failure to complete a course of treatment begun in two different counties. The nurse testified that public health authorities track a patient's treatment "to prevent drug resistance and make sure people complete the entire course of treatment because it does go on for so long." She stated that drug resistance "is a real risk when you start medicine, only take it for a little while, and stop it and then restart it." She also testified that the typical course of treatment for tuberculosis lasts between 6 and 9 months.

Two of the man's family members testified in court that they had tested positive for tuberculosis and that they believed they had contracted the disease from him. Four of seven people that the man listed as contacts testified that they had also tested positive for tuberculosis.

The court ordered the man's involuntary confinement in a state tuberculosis inpatient treatment facility so that he could be treated for at least 12 months.

The man appealed his court-ordered involuntary confinement for treatment, but the order was upheld by the appeals court.

Source: IN RE COMMITMENT OF JST, 478 SW 3d 856 – Tex: Court of Appeals 2015

Smallpox Emergency Personnel Protection Act (SEPPA)
A no-fault program to provide benefits and/or compensation to certain individuals, including health care workers and emergency responders, who are injured as a result of the administration of smallpox countermeasures, including the smallpox vaccine.

to sue vaccine manufacturers and providers. The U.S. Court of Federal Claims decides who will get compensation as the result of problems caused by vaccines. Sometimes, a person may have a reaction to a vaccine that is not listed on the table (see Table 9-2). In such a case, the person or his or her family would have to prove that a vaccine caused the condition.

The **Smallpox Emergency Personnel Protection Act (SEPPA)** of 2003 established a no-fault program to provide benefits and/or compensation

Table 9-2 Vaccines Covered by the VICP

The following vaccines are covered by the VICP
Diphtheria, tetanus, pertussis (DTP, DTaP, Tdap, DT, Td, or TT)
Haemophilus influenzae type b (Hib)
Hepatitis A (HAV)
Hepatitis B (HBV)
Human papillomavirus (HPV)
Influenza (TIV, LAIV) [given each year during the flu season]
Measles, mumps, rubella (MMR, MR, M, R)
Meningococcal (MCV4, MPSV4)
Pneumococcal conjugate (PCV)
Polio (OPV or IPV)
Rotavirus (RV)
Trivalent influenza (TIV, LAIV)
Varicella (VZV)
Any combination of the vaccines above
Additional vaccines may be added in the future.
Includes all vaccines against seasonal influenza.

Source: www.hrsa.gov/vaccinecompensation/faq.html.

to certain individuals, including health care workers and emergency responders, who are injured as a result of the administration of smallpox countermeasures, including the smallpox vaccine. The program also provides benefits to anyone injured as a result of accidental smallpox inoculation through contact.

Following is a complete list of vaccinations recommended by the American Academy of Pediatrics, the American Academy of Family Practice, and the Advisory Committee on Immunization Practices of the CDC:

- Hepatitis B (HepB or HBV): Four doses as follows: the first soon after birth; the second at 1 month of age; the third at 4 months of age; and the fourth at 6 to 18 months of age.
- Diphtheria, tetanus (lockjaw), and pertussis (whooping cough) (DTP): Five doses administered at 2, 4, and 6 months; at 15 to 18 months; and at 4 to 6 years. Tetanus/diphtheria booster at age 11. Tetanus booster at 10-year intervals thereafter.
- *Haemophilus influenzae* type b (Hib): Administered at age 4 months and again at 2 years.
- Inactivated polio: Four doses: at 2 months, at 4 months, at between 6 and 18 months, and at 4 to 6 years.
- Measles, mumps, and rubella (MMR): Two doses, one administered at 12 to 15 months and the second at 4 to 6 years.
- Varicella (chicken pox): Administered during any doctor's visit at or after 12 to 18 months of age.

- Pneumococcal conjugate vaccine (PCV7): To protect against pneumonia, blood infections, and meningitis (a serious infection of the lining of the brain or spinal cord) caused by the pneumococcus bacterium. Four doses: at 2, 4, and 6 months of age, and at 12 to 15 months. Another form of the vaccine is given to children aged 2 years and over whose immune systems are vulnerable.
- Hepatitis A: Administered to children and adolescents in selected states and regions and to certain high-risk groups.
- Influenza: Administered annually to children aged 6 to 23 months who have certain risk factors, such as asthma, heart disease, sickle cell disease, human immunodeficiency virus (HIV), and diabetes.

In 2006, the FDA licensed a vaccine for the prevention of infection with the human papillomavirus (HPV), administered via three injections over 6 months. Certain types of the virus can cause genital warts and other STIs in both sexes and cancer of the cervix in women. Because of the risk of cervical cancer, vaccination is recommended for females aged 9 to 26 years. For optimum protection, the vaccine should be given to girls before they become sexually active. In October 2012, the Advisory Committee on Immunization Practices for the CDC also recommended the vaccine for 11- and 12-year-old boys.

Federal law requires that Vaccine Information Statements (VISs), prepared by the CDC, be handed out to recipients, parents, or legal representatives. The VIS explains risks and benefits of a specific vaccine.

STATE-LEVEL VACCINATION LAW

There is no federal law in the United States requiring vaccinations for everyone, but all 50 states have legislation requiring specified vaccines for children in public and private schools, and in day care settings. Some states also require specified vaccines for college or university students. In addition, health care facilities across the country are increasingly requiring health care practitioners to be vaccinated for certain vaccine-preventable diseases—notably varicella (chicken pox), pertussis (whooping cough), pneumococcal disease, and influenza—to reduce the risk of disease outbreaks or transmission in the health care workplace. In some instances, facilities have established these requirements under mandates set forth by state statutes or regulations.

All school immunization laws grant exemptions to children for medical reasons, such as HIV infection, organ transplants, or allergies to eggs used to prepare vaccines. Many states grant religious exemptions for people whose religious beliefs prohibit immunizations. Some states allow philosophical exemptions for those who object to immunizations because of personal, moral, or other beliefs. As of late 2016, the following Web site provides a map showing states that allow religious or philosophical exemptions; the site also contains a table with clickable access to each state's child immunization requirements: www.ncsl.org/research/health/school-immunization-exemption-state-laws.aspx.

The downside of vaccination exemption for nonmedical or other reasons is that children who are not vaccinated or whose vaccinations are not up-to-date are vulnerable to contracting serious infectious diseases that can lead to lifelong impairment, and even death. In addition, unvaccinated children can then pass infectious diseases on to others, creating a public health emergency. For example:

- In 2012, there were an estimated 229 cases of mumps occurring in the United States. But just 4 years later, in 2016, the number of mumps cases spiked to 4,000, across 46 states and the District of Columbia. According to the CDC, most of the mumps patients self-reported that they had received the two recommended doses of measles-mumps-rubella (MMR) vaccine. Medical experts theorized that, because the MMR vaccine is effective for about ten years, immunizations could have been out of date.
- From January 2 to November 5, 2016, 62 people from 17 states (Alabama, Arizona, California, Colorado, Connecticut, Florida, Georgia, Hawaii, Illinois, Massachusetts, Michigan, Minnesota, New York, North Carolina, Tennessee, Texas, and Utah) were reported to have measles. The majority of people who got measles were reportedly unvaccinated.
- In 2015, whooping cough was declared epidemic in West Virginia, California, Arizona, and several other states, reportedly due mostly to unvaccinated people or failure to update vaccinations. Immunization authorities in many states have recommended holding booster clinics for vaccinating those individuals whose immunity to measles, mumps, rubella, and other contagious diseases may have lapsed.

A fear that the vaccine for measles, mumps, and rubella (MMR) may cause autism in children began circulating several years ago. However, scientific studies since then have concluded that there is no relationship between the MMR vaccine and autism. The CDC continues to maintain that there is no relationship, and the American Academy of Pediatrics continues to recommend the MMR vaccine for young children.

Under current U.S. immigration law, foreign nationals who apply for immigrant visas abroad or who seek permanent resident status in the United States are required to receive vaccinations to prevent the following diseases:

- Mumps
- Measles
- Rubella
- Polio
- Tetanus and diphtheria toxoids
- Pertussis
- *Haemophilus influenzae* type B
- Hepatitis B
- Any other vaccine-preventable diseases recommended by the Advisory Committee for Immunization Practices.

Source:www.uscis.gov/news/questions-and-answers/vaccination-requirements.

The National Childhood Vaccine Injury Act, discussed above, initiated programs to educate the public about vaccine benefits and risks. The act requires physicians and other health care providers administering vaccines to report adverse events following vaccination and to keep permanent records on vaccines administered and health problems occurring after vaccination. Vaccine administrators are required to document the following in the patient's permanent medical record:

- The date the vaccine was administered
- The vaccine manufacturer
- The vaccine lot number
- The name, address, and title of the health care provider who administered the vaccine

The Vaccine Adverse Events Reporting System (VAERS), operated by the FDA and CDC, should be notified of any adverse event by the filing of a VAERS reporting form. Health care providers must report the following events:

- Any event listed in the Vaccine Injury Table, available at the Health Resources and Services Administration Web site and from the Health Resources and Services Administration Bureau of Health Professions, 5600 Fishers Lane, Rockville, MD 20857
- Any contraindicating event listed in the manufacturer's package insert.

Check Your Progress

9. State public health laws generally provide six areas of responsibility, which are ________.
10. In your opinion, why have most states passed strict antismoking laws?
11. Check the following areas in which public health laws can apply:

    ________ Public restaurants

    ________ Public swimming pools

    ________ Public schools

    ________ Private homes where residents have communicable diseases

    ________ Private schools
12. What provision has the federal government made for people who sue over vaccinations?
13. Why are certain diseases and injuries reportable to state authorities?

REPORTABLE INJURIES

In all states, physicians and other health care providers must immediately report to law enforcement officials the medical treatment of patients whose injuries resulted from certain acts of violence, such as assault, rape, or domestic violence, so that authorities can investigate the incident. (In most states, spousal abuse is reportable only if the patient says his or her injuries are due to spousal abuse.) Reportable acts of domestic violence include child abuse, spousal abuse, and elder abuse.

Child Abuse Prevention and Treatment Act
A federal law passed in 1974 requiring physicians to report cases of child abuse.

Child Abuse To help prevent violence against children, Congress in 1974 passed the **Child Abuse Prevention and Treatment Act,** mandating the reporting of cases of child abuse. All states have enacted legislation making child abuse a crime and requiring that teachers, physicians, and other licensed health care practitioners report child abuse and neglect. The report must immediately be made to the proper authorities—either in person or by telephone—and a written report is generally required within a specified time frame, such as 72 hours. Any individual reporting suspected child abuse is granted absolute immunity from criminal and civil liability resulting from the reported incident. Depending on state law, failure to report suspected cases of child abuse may be a misdemeanor.

Spousal Abuse Unlike cases of child abuse, most state laws do not specifically require a physician to report spousal abuse, unless a spouse states that his or her injuries were the result of spousal abuse. Legal remedies available to battered spouses vary from state to state, but all states have laws protecting victims of domestic abuse. Advocacy programs can explain legal options to victims and can help them cope with the legal system. Courts may issue protective, or restraining, orders, or they may issue injunctions that direct the batterer to stop abusing the victim. In some states, police may be required to arrest batterers under certain conditions. Depending on laws within the jurisdiction and the type of offense committed, a batterer may be criminally prosecuted for assault, battery, harassment, intimidation, rape, or attempted murder.

Elder Abuse The Older Americans Act was signed into law by President Lyndon B. Johnson in 1965. The act created the Administration on Aging and outlined 10 objectives aimed at preserving the rights and dignity of older citizens. The 1987 **Amendments to the Older Americans Act** defines elder abuse, neglect, and exploitation but does not deal with enforcement. The 2000 Amendments to the Older Americans Act included a 5-year reauthorization for funding, maintains the original 10 objectives, and added the National Family Caregiver Support Program for addressing the needs of caregivers to elderly individuals. The 2006 Amendments to the Older Americans Act covered a broad range of topics, including aging and disability resource centers, elder justice, elder health, the continuation of a National Family Caregiver Support Program, nutrition, transportation, and other areas of concern for older individuals.

Amendments to the Older Americans Act
A 1987 federal act that defines elder abuse, neglect, and exploitation but does not deal with enforcement.

For current information about amendments to the Older Americans Act, consult this Web site: www.aoa.gov/AoA_programs/OAA/Index.aspx.

All 50 states and the District of Columbia have enacted legislation instituting reporting systems to identify domestic and institutional elder abuse, neglect, and exploitation. In most states, reporting suspected elder abuse is mandatory for certain professionals, including physicians. (If not mandated by state law, reporting may be voluntary.) Physical, sexual, and financial abuses of elderly people are considered crimes in all states. Some forms of emotional abuse and types of neglect may be considered crimes in some states.

In addition to laws regarding child, spousal, and elder abuse, some states have passed laws protecting vulnerable adults, such as individuals who are mentally ill or mentally challenged. Some states also have statutes dealing with the prevention of fetal abuse stemming from sniffing paint and other chemicals, taking drugs, or drinking alcohol while pregnant.

The Unborn Victims of Violence Act In April 2004, Congress passed and President George W. Bush signed into law the **Unborn Victims of Violence Act,** also called "Laci and Conner's Act," after the

Unborn Victims of Violence Act
Also called Laci and Conner's Act, a 2004 federal law that provides for the prosecution of anyone who causes injury to or the death of a fetus in utero.

December 24, 2002, murder of Laci Peterson, a pregnant woman, and her 9-month-old fetus, Conner. The act provides for the prosecution of anyone who causes injury to or the death of a fetus in utero in cases in which the federal government has jurisdiction. It also states that "the punishment for that separate offense is the same as the punishment provided under Federal law for that conduct had that injury or death occurred to the unborn child's mother." Before this federal law was passed, in most states, a person accused of injuring or killing a pregnant woman was tried for offenses against the mother but not for injuring or killing her fetus as a separate individual. State law determines whether an unborn fetus is considered a "person" in cases where a pregnant woman is assaulted or otherwise injured and, as a result, her unborn baby dies.

Identifying Abuse Health care practitioners should be alert for signs of physical abuse for purposes both of mandatory reporting and of possible intervention on behalf of the victim. It is imperative, however, that medical personnel not jump to conclusions and make unsubstantiated abuse reports.

Physical signs of abuse may include but are not limited to these:

- Unexplained fractures
- Repeated injuries, especially those in unusual places or those shaped like objects such as electrical cords, hairbrushes, belt buckles, and so forth
- Burns with unusual shapes (such as a circle that may have been caused by a cigarette or the mark of an object such as an iron)
- Friction burns apparently caused by a rope or cord
- Bite marks
- Signs of malnutrition or dehydration, such as extreme weight loss, dry skin, or red-rimmed, sunken eyes
- Torn or bloody underwear
- Pain or bruising in the genital area
- Unexplained venereal disease or other genital infections

Behavioral signs of abuse may include the following:

- Illogical or unreasonable explanations for injuries
- Frequently changing physicians and/or missing medical appointments
- Attempts to hide injuries with heavy makeup or sunglasses
- Frequent anxiety, depression, or loss of emotional control
- Changes in appetite; problems at school or on the job

Observation of individuals who accompany the patient may also identify a potential abuser. One might suspect abuse, for example, if, in the presence of additional evidence, an alleged victim of abuse is accompanied by someone who smells of alcohol, exhibits pensive or obsessive behavior, seems unusually or inappropriately emotional, or shows aggressive or otherwise suspicious body language toward the patient.

When a health care practitioner suspects abuse, care and tact must be used in eliciting information from patients. Direct but tactful open-ended questions such as "Has someone harmed you?" may encourage a patient to relate what has caused his or her injuries.

Health care practitioners should emphasize to the patient that information offered will be kept confidential, as required by physician–patient confidentiality, except in those cases in which the law mandates reporting abuse. Reporting requirements for abuse should be explained during the patient's first visit. Some sources recommend having patients sign a statement indicating that they understand the reporting requirements and agree with them.

Forcing the issue to encourage an adult to leave a batterer is not always the immediate answer. Similarly, providing hotline numbers, information on safe houses, or handouts about abuse may not be helpful if the batterer is waiting in the reception area for the patient or may later find the material and be further enraged. Instead, many medical facilities have bulletins posted in restrooms telling patients where to call for help. If tear-strips with the telephone number are provided, a victim can tear off the small, easily concealed strip for future reference.

Check Your Progress

14. You are a medical assistant in a physician office, and you suspect a female patient has been abused. What signs might you look for that could indicate abuse?
15. If you see signs of abuse, but the patient does not admit that she has been abused, how might you proceed?
16. What types of injuries are health care practitioners required to report?
17. As a health care practitioner, should you report abuse if a patient asks you not to? Explain your answer.
18. In your opinion, why does the law require medical providers to report suspected abuse?

9.4 Drug Regulations

The federal government has jurisdiction over the manufacture and distribution of drugs in the United States. The **Food and Drug Administration (FDA),** an agency within the Department of Health and Human Services, tests and approves drugs before releasing them for public use. This agency also oversees drug quality and standardization.

The FDA also has responsibility for major product recalls—a function vital to maintaining public health. In August 2016, several food and drug recalls were issued to protect the public. Included on the list for that month were Laura Lynn, Key Food, and Better Valu frozen cut corn for listeria contamination; Sagent Pharmaceuticals for iron oxide particles in oxacillin intended for injection; and Whole Foods Market for undeclared egg product in croissants and chocolate croissants. A complete list of FDA recalls is available at www.recalls.gov/food.html.

Both federal and state governments regulate the sale and use of certain drugs. At the federal level, the **Drug Enforcement Administration (DEA),** a branch of the Department of Justice, regulates the sale and use of drugs by the authority granted in the Comprehensive Drug Abuse Prevention and Control Act of 1970, commonly called the **Controlled Substances Act.**

Food and Drug Administration (FDA)
A federal agency within the Department of Health and Human Services that oversees drug quality and standardization and must approve drugs before they are released for public use.

Drug Enforcement Administration (DEA)
A branch of the U.S. Department of Justice that regulates the sale and use of drugs.

Controlled Substances Act
The federal law giving authority to the Drug Enforcement Administration to regulate the sale and use of drugs.

prescribe
To issue a medical prescription for a patient.

dispense
To deliver controlled substances in some type of bottle, box, or other container to a patient.

administer
To instill a drug into the body of a patient.

General regulations mandated by the Controlled Substances Act require physicians and other health care practitioners who purchase, **prescribe, dispense, administer** or in any way handle controlled drugs to follow these procedures:

- Register with the Drug Enforcement Administration through a division office. (A list of division offices is available online at the DEA Web site.) The physician will receive a registration number that must appear on all prescriptions for controlled substances and must be renewed periodically for a specified fee. Each DEA number is issued for a specific physician in a specific location. That location is the only one at which the physician may store controlled substances, including salespeople's samples. If a physician practices in more than one state, he or she needs a DEA number for each state. The physician must notify the appropriate state authorities and the DEA whenever he or she moves from a registered location.
- Keep records concerning the administering or dispensing of a controlled drug on file for 2 years. Such records must include the patient's full name and address, the reason for use of the drug, the date of the order, the name of the drug, the dosage form and quantity of the drug, and whether the drug was administered or dispensed.
- Note on a patient's chart when controlled substances are administered or dispensed.
- Make a written inventory of drug supplies every 2 years, and keep such records for an additional 2 years.
- Keep drugs in a locked cabinet or safe, and report any thefts immediately to the nearest DEA office and the local police.

THE CONTROLLED SUBSTANCES ACT

The Controlled Substances Act is a federal law that regulates drugs under five schedules, based on their potential for abuse and their medical usefulness. If a drug has no potential for abuse, it is not listed as controlled. Table 9-3 lists the five schedules for controlled substances.

Drugs included in Schedule II require a properly executed, manually signed prescription. No refills are permitted on these prescriptions. All other scheduled drugs (Schedules III through V) may be prescribed on written or oral orders, and refills are generally permitted with certain limitations.

As of November 2016, eight states and the District of Columbia had legalized marijuana for recreational use. Laws regarding taxing and licensing differ in each state, and the amount of marijuana permitted in a person's possession differs as well. Having a small amount of marijuana in one's possession has been decriminalized in many states.

Following the November 2016 elections, medical marijuana became legal in 30 states and the District of Columbia. Definitions of medical marijuana differ by state, as do the regulations. While it is often stated that a physician's prescription is necessary, it is actually a physician's *recommendation* that is necessary. Under federal law, physicians cannot write a prescription for marijuana. However, the federal government has not prosecuted physicians for writing recommendations.

Table 9-3 Drug Schedules for Controlled Substances

Schedule I	Have no currently accepted medical use and a high potential for abuse. Some examples of Schedule I drugs are: heroin, lysergic acid diethylamide (LSD), marijuana (cannabis), 3,4-methylenedioxymethamphetamine (ecstasy), methaqualone, and peyote.
Schedule II	Have a high potential for abuse, with use potentially leading to severe psychological or physical dependence. These drugs are also considered dangerous. Some examples of Schedule II drugs are: combination products with less than 15 milligrams of hydrocodone per dosage unit (Vicodin), cocaine, methamphetamine, methadone, hydromorphone (Dilaudid), meperidine (Demerol), oxycodone (OxyContin), fentanyl, Dexedrine, Adderall, and Ritalin.
Schedule III	Have a moderate to low potential for physical and psychological dependence. The abuse potential of Schedule III drugs is less than that of Schedule I and Schedule II drugs but more than that of Schedule IV. Some examples of Schedule III drugs are: Products containing less than 90 milligrams of codeine per dosage.
Schedule IV	Have a low potential for abuse and low risk of dependence. Some examples of Schedule IV drugs are: Xanax, Soma, Darvon, Darvocet, Valium, Ativan, Talwin, Ambien, and Tramadol.
Schedule V	Have a lower potential for abuse than Schedule IV drugs and consist of preparations containing limited quantities of certain narcotics. Schedule V drugs are generally used for antidiarrheal, antitussive, and analgesic purposes. Some examples of Schedule V drugs are: cough preparations with less than 200 milligrams of codeine or per 100 milliliters (Robitussin AC), Lomotil, Motofen, Lyrica, and Parepectolin.

Source: www.dea.gov/druginfo/ds.shtml.

In 2015, attorneys general for Nebraska and Oklahoma, two states that had not legalized marijuana sales and use, asked the U.S. Supreme Court for permission to file a lawsuit directly with the Supreme Court against Colorado's law legalizing marijuana sales and use for medical and recreational purposes, alleging that Colorado's law was causing illegal marijuana to pour into their states. The two states alleged in their complaint that the U.S. attorney general was declining to enforce federal law, causing harm to those states that had not legalized marijuana sales and use. In March 2016, by a 6-to-2 vote, the Supreme Court declined to hear the case.

A map at this Web site, www.governing.com/gov-data/state-marijuana-laws-map-medical-recreational.html, shows which states have legalized marijuana use for medical and recreational purposes.

Whenever prescriptions are written for controlled substances, a copy should be filed with the patient's record. When a physician discontinues practice, he or she must return the registration certificate and any unused order forms (preferably marked "void") to the DEA. When it is necessary to dispose of controlled drugs, the physician or employee charged with disposal should contact the nearest field office of the DEA and the responsible state agency for disposal information.

State laws governing controlled substances may be as strict as or stricter than federal laws. Physicians may be required to register with the appropriate state agency, as well as the DEA, and must follow all state and federal requirements in prescribing, dispensing, and administering controlled substances. Whenever state and federal regulations differ, the more stringent regulation must be followed. For example, if federal law requires that records be held for 2 years and state law specifies 5 years, the state law takes precedence.

Because violation of a law dealing with a state-controlled and/or federally controlled substance is a criminal offense and can result in fines, jail sentences, and loss of license to practice medicine, physicians, other health care practitioners, and medical office employees should be familiar with all state and federal narcotics laws.

The role of the medical assistant concerning compliance with DEA regulations is to remind the physician of license renewal dates, to keep accurate records for scheduled drugs, to maintain an accurate inventory and inventory records, and to ensure the security of scheduled drugs kept in the office. This is accomplished by:

- Checking to be sure that all controlled substances are kept in a locked cabinet or safe
- Reminding the physician to keep his or her "black bag" in a safe place
- Keeping all prescription blanks, especially those used for narcotics, under lock and key
- Ordering prescription blanks that are serially numbered or otherwise printed to help detect alterations and theft
- Reporting to the physician any behavior by patients that would suggest an attempt to secure addictive drugs
- Checking patients' records to verify all prescriptions that may be questioned by a pharmacist

Physicians and other members of the health care team must be familiar with the laws that govern such threats as communicable disease, physical abuse, and drug abuse because they play a vital role in helping maintain healthy—and ultimately safe—communities.

Check Your Progress

Use these three terms correctly in the three sentences that follow: *prescribe, dispense, administer.*

19. Dr. Wellness will ________________ the drug to his patient, Mrs. Doe, when he starts an intravenous injection.
20. Under the law, medical assistants may not ________________ drugs for patients but may ________________ or ________________ them under a physician's direct order.
21. When a pharmacist fills a patient's prescription, he or she then will ________________ the drug to the patient.
22. What two federal agencies control the manufacture and standardization of drugs and their sale and use?
23. If state and federal regulations differ concerning the abuse of certain drugs, which law will be applied?

Chapter Summary

Learning Outcome	Summary
LO 9.1 Define and determine the purpose of collecting vital statistics, and identify reporting procedures.	What are the vital events for which the government collects statistics? • Live births • Deaths • Fetal deaths • Marriages • Divorces • Induced terminations of pregnancy • Any change in an individual's civil status What is the correct procedure for completing a birth certificate? • Type or legibly print all entries. • Leave no entries blank. • Avoid corrections and erasures. • Where requested, provide signatures. Do not use rubber stamps or initials in place of signatures. • File only originals with state registrars. • Verify the spelling of names. • Avoid abbreviations, except those recommended in instructions for specific items. • Refer any problems to the appropriate state officials. What information does a death certificate generally include? • Disease, injury, and/or complication that caused the death and time treated before death • Date and time of death • Place of death • If decedent was female, presence or absence of pregnancy • Whether or not an autopsy was performed When are autopsies performed? • When a death is suspicious • To determine cause of death, if cause is unknown When is a physician not allowed to sign a death certificate? • When death is possibly due to criminal causes • When person is not attended by a physician within a specified length of time before death • When death is due to causes undetermined by the physician • In cases of violent or otherwise suspicious deaths
LO 9.2 Summarize the purpose and impact of public health statutes.	What provisions do all public health statutes have in common? • Guard against unsanitary conditions in public facilities. • Inspect establishments where food and drink are processed and sold. • Exterminate pests and vermin that can spread disease. • Check water quality • Set up measures of control for certain diseases. • Require physicians, school nurses, and other health care workers to file certain reports for the protection of citizens.

What are some examples of the authority states have to enforce public health laws?

- Require investigations be conducted in infectious disease outbreaks.
- Make childhood vaccinations a condition for school entry.
- Ban the distribution of free cigarette samples around schools or in areas where children congregate.
- Institute smoking bans or restrictions.
- Involuntarily detain (quarantine) individuals who have certain infectious diseases.
- Seize and/or destroy property to contain the threat of toxic substances.

LO 9.3 Cite examples of reportable diseases and injuries, and explain how they are reported.

Under public health law, what diseases and conditions are generally reported to public health departments?

- Diseases that, if left unchecked, could threaten the health and well-being of the population
  - Infectious diseases
  - Sexually transmitted diseases or infections
- Other diseases that may have mandated reporting if a higher-than-normal incidence occurs.

Which no-fault federal laws compensate for vaccine injury?

- National Childhood Vaccine Injury Act of 1986
  - Established National Vaccine Injury Compensation Program (VICP)
  - Smallpox Emergency Personnel Protection Act of 2003

What information must vaccine administrators document in a patient's medical record?

- The date the vaccine was administered
- The vaccine manufacturer
- The vaccine lot number
- The name, address, and title of the health care provider who administered the vaccine
- Any adverse event listed in the Vaccine Injury Table
- Any contraindicating event as listed in the manufacturer's package insert

What injuries are reportable to the authorities under the auspices of public health?

- Spousal abuse
- Child abuse
- Elder abuse

LO 9.4 Discuss federal drug regulations, including the Controlled Substances Act.

What two federal agencies oversee drugs in the United States?

- Food and Drug Administration (FDA)
  - Oversees drug quality and standardization and must approve drugs before they are released for public use
- Drug Enforcement Administration (DEA)
  - Branch of the U.S. Department of Justice that regulates the sale and use of drugs

What are the requirements for physicians who prescribe, dispense, and administer controlled substances?

- Register with the Drug Enforcement Administration through a division office.
- Keep records concerning the administering or dispensing of a controlled drug on file for 2 years.
- Note on a patient's chart when controlled substances are administered or dispensed.
- Make a written inventory of drug supplies every 2 years, and keep such records an additional 2 years.
- Keep drugs in a locked cabinet or safe, and report any thefts immediately to the nearest DEA office and the local police.

What are schedules under which controlled substances are listed?

- Schedule I—No currently accepted medical use and high potential for abuse
- Schedule II—High potential for abuse, with use leading to high possibility of dependence
- Schedule III—Moderate to low potential for physical and psychological dependence
- Schedule IV—Low potential for abuse and low risk of dependence
- Schedule V—Lower potential for abuse than Schedule IV drugs and consist of preparations containing limited quantities of certain narcotics

What is the status of marijuana (cannabis) in the United States?

- Still listed as a Schedule I drug.
- Thirty states and District of Columbia have laws legalizing marijuana in some form.

What is the role of the medical assistant regarding controlled substances in the medical facility?

- Checking to be sure that all controlled substances are kept in a locked cabinet or safe
- Reminding the physician to keep his or her "black bag" in a safe place
- Keeping all prescription blanks, especially those used for narcotics, under lock and key
- Ordering prescription blanks that are serially numbered or otherwise printed to help detect alterations and theft
- Reporting to the physician any behavior by patients that would suggest an attempt to secure addictive drugs
- Checking patients' records to verify all prescriptions that may be questioned by a pharmacist

Chapter 9 Review

Applying Knowledge

LO 9.1

1. Four vital statistics that the government collects are __________, __________, __________, and __________.
2. Of the above, the physician should be concerned with documenting __________ and __________.
3. Which of the following is *not* recommended for completing birth and death certificates?
   a. Make entries in ink or in a typewritten form.
   b. Use rubber stamps for all signatures.
   c. Do not skip any blanks.
   d. Check entries for correct spelling.
4. Which of the following is *not* included on a death certificate?
   a. Cause of death
   b. Name of attending physician, if any
   c. Time of death
   d. Name of decedent's next of kin
5. Physicians may *not* sign a death certificate in which of the following situations?
   a. Death is suspicious.
   b. Physician was treating the patient.
   c. Death occurred in the home.
   d. Death occurred in the hospital.

6. Which of the following best defines a coroner?
   a. A public official who must be a physician
   b. A public official who is elected by popular ballot
   c. A public official who is appointed by the governor
   d. A public official who investigates and holds inquests over those who die from unknown or violent causes
7. A coroner or medical examiner signs a death certificate if
   a. The death is possibly due to criminal causes or is otherwise suspicious.
   b. The death was not attended by a physician within a specified length of time.
   c. The death is due to causes undetermined by the physician.
   d. All of these

LO 9.2

8. State public health laws derive indirectly from
   a. A federal law called U.S. Public Health Law
   b. The Tenth Amendment to the U.S. Constitution
   c. City ordinances
   d. None of these
9. Briefly define the term *federalism.*
   a. Cooperation among federal, state, and local governments.
   b. Federal law is accepted as the law of the land.
   c. State law overrides federal law.
   d. Municipal law overrides state law.
10. Which of the following falls within the supervision of a state's public health department?
    a. Licensing of public health nurses
    b. Admitting cases of infectious disease to hospitals
    c. Mandatory vaccinating of schoolchildren
    d. Prescribing treatment for STIs

LO 9.3

11. Which of the following should be reported to the health department?
    a. Otitis media (middle ear infection)
    b. Strep throat
    c. Influenza
    d. Human immunodeficiency virus (HIV)
12. Which of the following will most likely require notification of the appropriate health agencies?
    a. Auto accident
    b. Staph infection
    c. Strep throat
    d. Phenylketonuria (PKU—a genetic disease sometimes diagnosed in infants)

13. Which no-fault federal law compensates for childhood vaccine injury?

a. Tenth Amendment to the U.S. Constitution

b. National Childhood Vaccine Injury Act of 1986

c. Smallpox Emergency Personnel Protection Act of 2003

d. None of these

14. Which of the following vaccination information is *not* documented in a patient's medical record?

a. The date the vaccine was administered

b. The vaccine manufacturer

c. The vaccine lot number

d. The date the vaccine was ordered

15. Which of the following injuries are reportable to law enforcement or to the health department?

a. A restaurant worker falls off a ladder while changing a lightbulb.

b. A woman tells her physician that her broken ribs occurred when her husband beat her.

c. A child is severely injured in an automobile accident.

d. None of these

LO 9.4

16. Which of the following is *not* the responsibility of the medical assistant working in a facility where physicians prescribe and administer controlled substances?

a. Checking to be sure that all controlled substances are kept in a locked cabinet or safe

b. Reminding the physician to keep his or her "black bag" in a safe place

c. Ordering prescription blanks that are serially numbered or otherwise printed to help detect alterations and theft

d. Checking with the patient's pharmacist to be sure prescriptions have been filled

17. Prescriptions for which of the following categories of drugs may *not* be renewed?

a. Schedule I

b. Schedule II

c. Schedule IV

d. Schedule V

18. With one exception, drugs in this category have no accepted medical use and are used for research purposes only.

a. Schedule V

b. Schedule II

c. Schedule I

d. Schedule III

19. Who must be notified if controlled substances are stolen from a medical facility?

a. All patients who currently have prescriptions for the stolen drug

b. The state medical board

c. The nearest DEA office and the local police

d. The nearest FDA office

20. A medical facility must keep records concerning the administering or dispensing of a controlled drug on file for __________.

    a. 6 years

    b. 9 years

    c. 10 years

    d. 2 years

21. Which of the following is *not* a requirement for physicians who prescribe, dispense, and administer controlled substances?

    a. Register with the Drug Enforcement Administration through a division office.

    b. Note on a patient's chart when controlled substances are administered or dispensed.

    c. Make a written inventory of drug supplies every 2 years, and keep such records an additional 2 years.

    d. Renew permits for prescribing and dispensing controlled substances every 6 months.

Match each definition with the correct term by writing the letter in the space provided.

_____ 22. Tests and approves drugs for public use.

_____ 23. Also known as the Comprehensive Drug Abuse Prevention and Control Act of 1970.

_____ 24. As a branch of the Department of Justice, regulates the sale and use of drugs.

_____ 25. Require reports of communicable diseases and certain injuries, as mandated by state laws.

_____ 26. Mandates reporting of child abuse.

_____ 27. Created a no-fault compensation program for health care practitioners and/or emergency responders injured by the smallpox vaccine.

_____ 28. The federal law that makes killing or injuring a fetus a crime separate from killing or injuring the pregnant mother in cases where the federal government has jurisdiction.

a. Unborn Victims of Violence Act

b. Drug Enforcement Administration (DEA)

c. Smallpox Emergency Personnel Protection Act of 2003 (SEPPA)

d. Food and Drug Administration (FDA)

e. Amendments to the Older Americans Act

f. Controlled Substances Act

g. Child Abuse Prevention and Treatment Act of 1974

h. Public health statutes

Ethics Issues Public Health Responsibilities of Physicians and Other Health Care Practitioners

Use your critical thinking skills to answer the questions that follow each ethics issue.

Ethics ISSUE 1:

"Herd immunity" is one of the primary considerations for mandatory vaccinations in the United States. That is, when a large segment of the population is inoculated against certain infectious diseases, individuals—both vaccinated and unvaccinated—benefit, as well as the community as a whole. A true mandate for vaccinating all schoolchildren in the United States has not been enacted since World War I. Today, every state except Mississippi and West Virginia has exceptions that allow parents to exempt their children from state vaccination requirements on the basis of religious or other personal beliefs. Recent epidemics of childhood diseases such as measles, mumps, and pertussis in the United States indicate that objections to mandatory vaccinations have increased.

Discussion Questions

29. In your opinion, does a parent's failure to vaccinate his or her child constitute a lack of social responsibility? Explain your answer.
30. Should one's concern for others supersede objections to vaccination on personal or religious grounds? Explain your answer.
31. Should your role as a health care practitioner include encouraging parents to have their children vaccinated? Explain your answer.
32. As a health care practitioner, are you ethically bound to be vaccinated for common contagious diseases?

Ethics ISSUE 2:

A young woman is diagnosed with a sexually transmitted infection and is subsequently reported to the public health department. A public health nurse visits her, but she refuses to name her sexual contacts.

Discussion Questions

33. Should the woman be compelled by law to name her sexual contacts? Why or why not? Do the best interests of the woman's sexual contacts and their contacts supersede the woman's right to privacy? Explain your answer.
34. What values are involved in Ethics Issue 2?
35. What is the first duty of health care practitioners caring for the woman in Ethics Issue 2?

Ethics ISSUE 3:

Laws that require the reporting of cases of suspected abuse of children and elderly persons often create a dilemma for health care practitioners. The parties involved, both the suspected offenders and the victims, will often plead that the matter be kept confidential and not be disclosed or reported for investigation by public authorities.

Discussion Questions

36. Assume you are a member of the health care team that has repeatedly treated a woman for injuries that appear to have been inflicted by another. How might you phrase an opening question to learn whether or not she is the victim of abuse?
37. If the woman protests that she is simply "accident prone," how might you phrase your response? Would you drop the matter at this point or continue to question the woman?
38. What could you do to protect the woman if she does not admit abuse, but you are reasonably sure that she is being abused?

Case Studies

Use your critical thinking skills to answer the questions that follow each case study.

LO 9.4

One of a physician's patients, a well-respected citizen in a small community, saw the doctor with a complaint of blood in his urine (hematuria). The physician asked the patient if he'd had any new sexual partners recently, and the patient admitted that he had. The physician explained to the patient that his urine specimen had been positive for the STI chlamydia. The physician urged the patient to discuss his medical condition with the patient's wife, who was also the physician's patient, but the man was reluctant.

39. If the patient refuses to confide in the wife, what should the physician do?
40. What are the legal issues in this case? What are the ethical issues?

Barbara, a medical assistant, noticed that her aunt, who suffered chronic pain from a neck injury, carried two bottles of Percodan in her purse. "Two doctors write prescriptions for me," Barbara's aunt confided, "but neither knows about the other. That's the only way I can get enough medication to control my pain."

41. In Barbara's place, would you report your aunt's deception to the physicians named on her prescriptions? Explain your answer.
42. What would you tell your aunt?
43. How can physicians guard against such abuses by patients?

Internet Activities

LO 9.1 and LO 9.3

Complete the activities and answer the questions that follow.

44. Visit this Web site to view the most recent National Vital Statistics Report for births in the United States: www.cdc.gov/nchs/data/nvsr/nvsr64/nvsr64_12.pdf. Was there a change in the birth rate for your state over the last reporting period? If so, what was it? Name those states that show an increase in birth rates. What conclusions, if any, can you draw from this data? Name three conclusions drawn from federal analysis of the data collected and published at this Web site.
45. Visit the CDC Web site www.cdc.gov/nchs/fastats/ for "leading causes of death [last year]." Name the top four. Name three additional types of population statistics available at this Web site.
46. Visit the Web site for the National Vaccine Injury Compensation Program (VICP) at www.hrsa.gov/vaccinecompensation/. Who is eligible to file a petition (claim)?
47. Find the Web site for your state's department of health. Which communicable diseases must be reported in your state? To whom must you report communicable diseases? What is the process involved? At this Web site, can you tell which diseases are prevalent in your state? How?

Resources

LO 9.1

National Vital Statistics System: www.cdc.gov/nchs/nvss/about_nvss.htm

LO 9.2

Public health law (slides): www.cdc.gov/phlp/docs/phl101/phl101-unit-1—16jan09-secure.pdf

Public Health Law Program (CDC): www.cdc.gov/phlp/index.html

LO 9.3

National Notifiable Diseases Surveillance System: https://wwwn.cdc.gov/nndss/conditions/notifiable/2016/infectious-diseases/

Reportable diseases: https://wwwn.cdc.gov/nndss/conditions/notifiable/2016/infectious-diseases/

National Childhood Vaccine Injury Act: www.nvic.org/injury-compensation/origihanlaw.aspx

Vaccines:

www.cdc.gov/vaccines/index.html

www.ncsl.org/research/health/school-immunization-exemption-state-laws.aspx

www.cdc.gov/vaccines/imz-managers/laws/

Measles outbreak: www.cdc.gov/measles/cases-outbreaks.html

Mumps outbreaks: https://search.cdc.gov/search?query=mumps+outbreaks&utf8=%E2%9C%93&affiliate=cdc-main

www.scientificamerican.com/article/whats-behind-the-2016-mumps-spike-in-the-u-s/

Disease epidemics, 2015: http://time.com/27308/4-diseases-making-a-comeback-thanks-to-anti-vaxxers/

www.immunize.org/

Vaccine compensation: www.hrsa.gov/vaccinecompensation/vaccineinjurytable.pdf

www.hrsa.gov/vaccinecompensation/coveredvaccines/index.html

Vaccine schedules: www.cdc.gov/vaccines/schedules/

www.cdc.gov/vaccines/parents/downloads/parent-ver-sch-0-6yrs.pdf

Older Americans Act: www.aoa.gov/AoA_programs/OAA/Index.aspx

The MMR vaccine and autism: Sensation, refutation, retraction, and fraud:

www.ncbi.nlm.nih.gov/pmc/articles/PMC3136032/

LO 9.4

DEA drug schedules: www.dea.gov/druginfo/ds.shtml

State marijuana laws: www.governing.com/gov-data/state-marijuana-laws-map-medical-recreational.html

Marijuana: www.governing.com/topics/public-justice-safety/tns-scotus-marijuana-nebraska-colorado.html

www.scotusblog.com/2014/12/two-states-sue-to-block-colorado-marijuana-markets/

http://medicalmarijuana.procon.org/view.resource.php?resourceID=000881

Supreme Court case: www.scotusblog.com/wp-content/uploads/2015/12/Original-No.-144-US-CVSG-Br.pdf

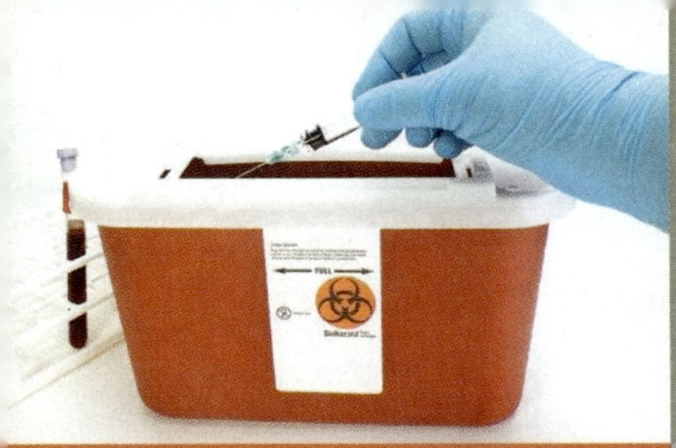

10 Workplace Legalities

Key Terms

affirmative action
background check
Chemical Hygiene Plan
Clinical Laboratory Improvement Act (CLIA)
discrimination
employment-at-will
General Duty Clause
Hazard Communication Standard (HCS)
just cause
Medical Waste Tracking Act
Occupational Exposure to Bloodborne Pathogen Standard
Occupational Safety and Health Administration (OSHA)
public policy
right-to-know laws
United Nations Globally Harmonized System of Classification and Labeling of Chemicals (GHS)
workers' compensation
wrongful discharge

LEARNING OUTCOMES

After studying this chapter, you should be able to:

LO 10.1 Identify federal laws regarding hiring and firing, discrimination, and other workplace regulations.

LO 10.2 Describe the Occupational Safety and Health Administration's (OSHA) top workplace priorities.

LO 10.3 Examine the role of health care practitioners in following OSHA, Centers for Disease Control and Prevention (CDC), and Clinical Laboratory Improvement Act (CLIA) standards for workplace safety.

LO 10.4 Summarize the purpose of workers' compensation laws and unemployment insurance.

LO 10.5 Determine the appropriate legal process for hiring employees and maintaining the required paperwork while a person is employed.

FROM THE PERSPECTIVE OF. . .

MARILYN is a supervisory medical technologist in the laboratory of a small clinic in the Midwest. Because the clinic does not employ phlebotomists to do blood draws, Marilyn performs this task, as well as all the analytical duties of a medical technologist. When asked the most frequent cause of analytical errors, she says preanalytical personnel practices, rather than equipment malfunction, are most often at fault. "For example, one day a technologist found that the instrument we use for analyzing urine dipsticks was consistently reporting positive for leukocytes on every patient. She asked me if the instrument needed to be checked, and I couldn't find anything wrong with it, so I watched her do a couple of analyses. The manual for the instrument emphasizes cleaning the work table daily after each use, and the technologist admitted that this hadn't been done. In fact, the work table hadn't been adequately cleaned for several days."

The technologist cleaned the work table before the next urine sample was tested, and no leukocytes were reported. "Apparently there was cross contamination from some previous urines with positive leukocyte readings. After that, the technologist made sure to clean the work table thoroughly and often. In the lab, we need to be especially careful about using the instruments according to manual instructions and about preventing cross contamination of specimens."

From Marilyn's perspective as a laboratory supervisor, sloppy or inattentive work habits can cause inaccurate test results, which can alter a patient's course of medical treatment and cause unnecessary stress and sometimes legal action. Therefore, she generally observes the work habits of employees she supervises before assuming equipment malfunction.

From the technologist's perspective, she realized that the urinalyses results were probably incorrect and asked her supervisor for help. She was eager to correct any errors in preanalytical technique and took steps to ensure her test results were accurate.

From the perspective of the patients who provided specimens for analysis and the physicians who ordered the tests, employees who are vigilant and eager to improve job performance are the first line of defense against errors in medical diagnosis and treatment.

10.1 Basic Employment Law

This chapter provides an overview of workplace law, but it does not cover every employment statute and situation. For more detail, consult U.S. and state codes and/or an attorney specializing in employment law.

Many federal and state laws govern the workplace. Federal laws may apply only to those businesses with a certain number of employees (such as 15, 20, or 50) who work for a minimum number of weeks during the year. State laws may apply to those areas not covered by federal law, or they may extend or overlap existing federal law.

Traditionally, employment followed the principle of **employment-at-will.** This meant that employees could be refused employment and could

employment-at-will
A concept of employment whereby either the employer or the employee can end the employment at any time, for any reason.

be disciplined or fired for any or no reason. In fact, either the employer or the employee could end the employment at any time. Now employment-at-will is affected not only by federal and state statutes, executive orders, and case law but also by contracts between a worker and an employer, collective bargaining agreements between companies and unions, and civil service rules for government workers.

HIRING AND FIRING

wrongful discharge
A concept established by precedent that says an employer risks litigation if he or she does not have just cause for firing an employee.

just cause
An employer's legal reason for firing an employee.

public policy
The common law concept of wrongful discharge when an employee has acted for the "common good."

Employees generally cannot sue their employers simply because they have been fired, but an employer cannot fire an employee for an illegal reason. When no law exists that prohibits a specific reason for firing an employee, the discharged worker may have cause for litigation under precedent for **wrongful discharge.** Generally, in such cases the employer must have documentation that shows **just cause** (a legal reason) for dismissing the employee. Promises made to the employee orally, in a written contract, or in a company handbook may be used as evidence, should a suit involving wrongful discharge be filed against his or her employer.

State courts vary in their willingness to accept the common law concept of wrongful discharge, but most recognize **public policy** or "common good" reasons for lawsuits brought by fired employees, such as refusing to commit an illegal act, whistle-blowing, performing a legal duty, or exercising a private right.

COURT CASE Employee Wins Wrongful Discharge Case

In July 2015, a clinical manager e-mailed her supervisor and a regional director of the home health agency at which she was employed to express concern regarding the agency's noncompliance with Pennsylvania state laws. The clinical manager cited specific instances in which the home health agency had accepted patients despite being unable to meet the patients' needs. Specifically, nurses who did not have training in central catheter procedures were being scheduled with patients who needed the procedure, and mental health nurses were being scheduled with patients whose needs required physical care, not mental health care. The clinical manager was concerned that these were violations of Pennsylvania law. Additionally, the clinical manager wrote that if she were to comply with the home health agency's instructions, she would be violating Pennsylvania's Standards of Nursing Conduct. The clinical manager specifically stated that her concerns would be reported in accordance with state and federal reporting requirements. Failure on the part of the supervisor and regional manager to promptly respond to the clinical manager's e-mail caused the clinical manager to convey her concerns to the corporate compliance office. She was assured by corporate compliance staff that her concerns were justified and that her supervisor would be tasked with ensuring future compliance with Pennsylvania law. The day following the response from corporate compliance, the clinical manager was terminated and offered a separation agreement with severance pay, which the clinical manager rejected.

She filed suit in December 2015 in U.S. District Court claiming that the home health agency violated Pennsylvania public policy by wrongfully discharging her in retaliation for her refusal to engage in conduct prohibited by law. In July 2016, the court determined that due to the technical language in the Pennsylvania Whistle Blowers Act, the clinical manager did not have protection under that law. However, the court did find that the clinical manager had sufficient facts to support a wrongful discharge claim. The court also ruled that the clinical manager had sufficient facts to support a claim for relief under the federal Patient Safety and Quality Improvement Act.

This case is still being litigated as of August 2016.

Source: *Tracey Eaves-Voyles v Almost Family, Inc, d/b/a as Omni Home Care*, Civ. No 1:15-CV2421, United States District Court MD Pennsylvania 7/27/16.

COURT CASE Employee Loses Wrongful Discharge Case

In early 2011, the director of care delivery (DCD) in a large skilled nursing facility was fired from her job. The DCD was hired in March 2010. The DCD experienced significant weight gain and edema (excess fluid that makes tissues appear doughy). The DCD believed that she was suffering from kidney failure. A variety of physicians saw the DCD as a patient, but no provider had a certain diagnosis of chronic kidney disease or kidney failure. She was referred to a kidney specialist who diagnosed stage one chronic kidney disease with obesity.

While seeing the different physicians, the DCD missed a significant amount of time at work. The staff reporting to the DCD complained to Human Resources about her job performance. Her supervisor, in conjunction with Human Resources, issued a third written warning on February 21, 2011, for violation of work rules, citing negative comments about her work where patients could overhear, extended lunch breaks, arriving late, leaving early or calling in, and failing to attend patient care conferences. The employee was provided with a written Performance Improvement Plan along with the clear notice that further performance issues could result in termination.

It was not until this meeting that the DCD asked about whether the provisions of the Family Medical Leave Act (FMLA) would apply in her situation as some of the work time missed was due to being ill or seeing a health care provider for her edema issues. She was advised that she was not eligible for FMLA at this point in her employment.

Several days later, she was cited by her supervisor for failure to complete work tasks. The DCD left for the day without completing the overdue work tasks. The following week, the DCD was terminated from her position.

The case was first heard in the district court and then appealed to the federal court as a violation of FMLA. The appellate court ruled that "we do not doubt that edema and fluid retention may be signs of a potentially serious condition such as congestive heart failure, liver disease, or primary kidney disease. But no such condition was ever diagnosed, and the skilled nursing facility did not interfere with the DCD's frequent medical appointments to obtain needed diagnosis and treatment."

Source: *Lucinda Dalton v ManorCare of West Des Moines IA, LLC*, United States Court of Appeals, Eighth Circuit, 2 F.3d 955 (2015) No 13-3743 April 2015.

DISCRIMINATION

Federal laws forbid **discrimination** when it comes to any aspect of employment, including hiring, firing, pay, job assignments, promotions, layoff, training, fringe benefits, and any other term or condition of employment for any of the following reasons:

discrimination
Prejudiced or prejudicial outlook, action, or treatment.

- Being of a particular race, color, religion, or national origin, or being male, female, or transgender
- Being over 40 years of age
- Having a history of a disability or having a disability that may be accommodated
- Having a particular genetic disposition
- Being pregnant
- Joining a union or engaging in political activity

Most states have passed laws that add to the federal list of prohibited discriminatory employment practices. Title VII of the Civil Rights Act makes sexual discrimination illegal, and sexual harassment is considered a form of sexual discrimination. The Equal Employment

Opportunity Commission (EEOC) identifies sexual harassment as follows:

> Unwelcome sexual advances, requests for sexual favors, and other verbal or physical conduct of a sexual nature constitute sexual harassment when (1) submission to such conduct is made either explicitly or implicitly a term or condition of an individual's employment; (2) submission to or rejection of such conduct by an individual is used as a basis for employment decisions affecting such individual; or (3) such conduct has the purpose or effect of unreasonably interfering with an individual's work performance or creating an intimidating, hostile, or offensive working environment.
>
> Source: 1980, the Equal Employment Opportunity Commission (EEOC).

Parts 1 and 2 of this definition prohibit what is known as *quid pro quo* (from Latin, meaning "something for something") sexual harassment. Part 3 prohibits conduct that interferes with an employee's work performance or creates a hostile working environment.

Court decisions have affirmed that sexual harassment of employees, male or female, is cause for legal action. Employers may be found liable even though an employee actually committed the offense. For example, if the offending employee is a supervisor, the employer is usually automatically held liable. If a nonsupervisory employee sexually harasses another worker, the employer is held liable only if he or she knew or should have known about the offense and did nothing to stop it.

LANDMARK COURT CASE

A History-Making Sexual Harassment Case

A bank employee worked for Meritor Savings Bank for more than four years. During that time, she claimed that her supervisor continued to make sexual propositions. She finally complied, fearing for her job. She also claimed that her supervisor publicly fondled her and forcibly raped her. When she was fired after an indefinite sick leave, she sued for sexual harassment.

A trial court ruled for the bank, finding no *quid pro quo* discrimination, but the employee appealed, and the appellate court found in her favor. The bank appealed, but the U.S. Supreme Court upheld the appellate court's decision in the plaintiff's favor. In a precedent-setting pronouncement, the Court said, "A plaintiff may establish a violation of Title VII by proving that discrimination based on sex has created a hostile or abusive work environment." The court remanded the case to the district court for further proceedings.

Source: Meritor Savings Bank, FSB v. Vinson, 106 S.C. 2399, 91 L.Ed.2d 49, 447 U.S. 57 (U.S. Sup. Ct., 1986).

Check Your Progress

1. Define *employment-at-will.*
2. Define *wrongful discharge.*
3. Define *just cause.*
4. Define *public policy.*
5. Who is liable if sexual harassment in the workplace occurs?
6. The demand for sexual favors in exchange for employment benefits is called ___________.

FEDERAL LABOR AND EMPLOYMENT LAWS

The following federal laws cover discrimination in hiring and firing, workers' wages and hours, worker safety, and other workplace issues.

Employment Discrimination Laws These laws address discrimination in hiring and firing:

Wagner Act of 1935. This act makes it illegal to discriminate in hiring or firing because of union membership or organizational activities.

Title VII of the Civil Rights Act of 1964. This act applies to businesses with 15 or more employees working at least 20 weeks of the year. The law prevents employers from discriminating in hiring or firing on the basis of race, color, religion, sex, or national origin. Some states have laws that also prohibit discrimination based on marital status, parenthood, mental health, mental retardation, sexual orientation, personal appearance, or political affiliation.

Title VII also specifically prevents federal judges from using **affirmative action** plans—programs intended to remedy the effects of past discrimination—just to correct an imbalance between the percentage of minority persons working for a specific employer and the percentage of qualified minority members in the workplace. Federal judges can order affirmative action plans only when they decide an employer has intentionally discriminated against a minority group.

affirmative action
Programs that use goals and quotas to provide preferential treatment for minority persons determined to have been underutilized in the past.

Title VII created the U.S. Equal Employment Opportunity Commission (EEOC). The EEOC enforces Title VII provisions, the Age Discrimination in Employment Act, the Equal Pay Act, and Section 501 of the Rehabilitation Act. EEOC field offices handle charges or complaints of employment discrimination.

Age Discrimination in Employment Act (ADEA) of 1967. This act applies to businesses with 20 or more employees working at least 20 weeks of the year. It prohibits discrimination in hiring or firing based on age for persons aged 40 or older.

Rehabilitation Act of 1973. This act applies to employers with federal contracts of $2,500 or more. It prohibits discrimination in employment practices based on physical disabilities or mental health. It also requires federal contractors to implement affirmative action plans in hiring and promoting employees with disabilities.

1976 Pregnancy Discrimination Act. This is an amendment to Title VII of the Civil Rights Act that makes it illegal to fire an employee based on pregnancy, childbirth, or related medical conditions.

Titles I and V of the Americans with Disabilities Act of 1990. This act applies to all employers with 15 or more employees working at least 20 weeks during the year. Titles I and III of the act ban discrimination against persons with disabilities in the workplace, mandate equal access for workers who are disabled to certain public facilities, and require all commercial firms to make existing facilities and grounds more accessible to persons with disabilities.

Civil Rights Act of 1991. This act provided two new important benefits for employees who prove discrimination: (1) Employees may collect punitive damages; (2) employees may collect damages for emotional distress associated with incidents of discrimination.

Genetic Information Nondiscrimination Act of 2008 (GINA). The act prohibits discrimination in health insurance and employment based on genetic information. It is discussed in more detail in Chapter 11.

Lilly Ledbetter Fair Pay Act of 2009. This law responded to the Supreme Court's decision in *Ledbetter v. Goodyear Tire and Rubber Company* (see the court case "Employee Alleges Pay Discrimination"). It revised sections of the Civil Rights Act of 1964, the Age Discrimination in Employment Act of 1967, the Americans with Disabilities Act of 1990, and the Rehabilitation Act of 1973. The revisions were concerned primarily with statutes of limitation trigger dates, extending the class of plaintiffs to any individual who is "affected by" unlawful discrimination, and recovery of back pay.

Wage and Hour Laws The following laws address wages and hours of work:

1935 Social Security Act. Funded by the Federal Insurance Contribution Act (FICA), the act now encompasses "old age" and survivors insurance (OASI), public disability insurance, unemployment insurance (through the Federal Unemployment Tax Act), and the hospital insurance program Medicare.

1938 Fair Labor Standards Act. This act prohibits child labor and the firing of employees for exercising their rights under the act's wage and hour standards. It also provides for overtime pay and a minimum wage. In May 2016, by Executive Order of the President, the wage and hour rules were updated with an effective date of December 1, 2016. The new rules guarantee overtime pay protection to workers earning less than $47,476 annually. Other thresholds were set for highly compensated employees. Future automatic updates to these thresholds will occur every three years, beginning on January 1, 2020. Some nurses may receive overtime pay, depending on how they are paid—hourly or by salary—and licensed practical nurses "and other similar health care employees" are guaranteed overtime pay. Several states challenged the Executive Order, and in mid-November 2016, a federal court issued a temporary injunction halting implementation of the Executive Order.

Equal Pay Act of 1963. As an amendment to the Fair Labor Standards Act, this act requires equal pay for men and women doing equal work.

Employee Retirement Income Security Act (ERISA) of 1974. This act regulates private pension funds and employer benefit programs. As part of its provisions, employers cannot prevent employees from collecting retirement benefits from plans covered by the act.

Workplace Safety Laws One important law addresses health and safety in the workplace:

Occupational Safety and Health Act of 1970. This act ensures the safety of workers and prohibits firing an employee for reporting workplace safety hazards or violations.

Other Terms of Employment Labor and employment laws may also address employees' family emergencies and other family situations.

Family Medical Leave Act (FMLA) of 1991. This act applies to employers with 50 or more employees. It mandates allowing employees to take unpaid leave time for maternity, for adoption, or for caring for ill family members.

LANDMARK COURT CASE

Employee Alleges Pay Discrimination

Lilly Ledbetter retired from Goodyear Tire and Rubber Company in 1998 after working for 19 years as a night supervisor in the Gadsden, Alabama, plant—a job most often performed by men. Ledbetter discovered 6 years before her retirement that for most of her career, she had earned 20 percent less than her male counterparts, and she filed a charge with the EEOC alleging pay discrimination. Title VII of the Civil Rights Act of 1964 specified that charges of unlawful employment practice must be filed within 180 days of the practice (some states allow filing within 300 days of the practice), but despite this statute of limitations requirement, a lower court declared Goodyear guilty of pay discrimination under Title VII. The case reached the U.S. Supreme Court, where Ledbetter argued that each paycheck she received was an unlawful employment practice and should reset the clock regarding the statute of limitations for filing a claim. The Supreme Court threw out the case on grounds that the statute of limitations, as mandated in Title VII, had run out. This triggered Congress to pass legislation dealing with the statute of limitations issue, and President Barack Obama signed the bill into law on January 29, 2009, eight days after his inauguration.

While Lilly Ledbetter ultimately lost her case against Goodyear, her lawsuit triggered legislation that would help other employees with similar discrimination claims against their employers.

Source: Ledbetter v. Goodyear Tire and Rubber Company, 550 U.S. 618, 127 S. Ct. 2162 (2007).

Check Your Progress

7. What federal act makes it illegal for employers to discriminate against employees or potential employees on the basis of race, color, religion, sex, or national origin?
8. Which act protects the rights of pregnant employees?
9. Social Security benefits are disbursed under the authority of which act?
10. Which federal act would apply if a job applicant were denied employment because she admitted a family history of Huntington's disease?
11. Which law affected trigger dates for the statute of limitations on alleged acts of discrimination in the workplace?
12. What is the salary level put in place in May 2016 that guarantees overtime pay protection? Did it go into effect?

10.2 OSHA's Workplace Priorities

Certain federal and state laws provide specifically for employee safety and welfare. Major areas covered include workplace safety, such as medical hazards, job-related injuries and illnesses, and unemployment or reemployment.

OCCUPATIONAL SAFETY AND HEALTH ADMINISTRATION (OSHA)

In the 1960s, job-related disabilities and injuries caused more lost workdays in U.S. companies than did strikes. As a result of increasing concern over such statistics, in 1970 Congress passed the Occupational Safety and Health Act. The act established the **Occupational Safety and Health Administration (OSHA),** charged with writing and enforcing compulsory standards for health and safety in the workplace.

Occupational Safety and Health Administration (OSHA) Established by the Occupational Safety and Health Act of 1970, the organization that is charged with writing and enforcing compulsory standards for health and safety in the workplace.

The act covers all employers and employees with few exceptions. Standards cover four areas of employment–general industry, maritime, construction, and agriculture–and include regulations for the physical workplace, machinery and equipment, materials, power sources, processing, protective clothing, first aid, and workplace administration.

All employers must know those standards that apply to their business. The Web site www.osha.gov is the primary source of information for OSHA standards.

Under the authority of the U.S. secretary of labor, OSHA inspectors may conduct workplace inspections unannounced; issue citations to employers for violations of the act; and, in some cases, levy fines. The millions of workplaces covered by the Occupational Safety and Health Act cannot be inspected at one time; therefore, priorities have been established for inspecting the worst situations first. The priority of workplace inspections is as follows:

1. Imminent danger situations receive top priority. An imminent danger is any condition in which there is reasonable certainty that a danger exists that can be expected to cause death or serious physical harm immediately or before the danger can be eliminated through normal enforcement procedures.

If an OSHA inspector finds an imminent danger situation, he or she will ask the employer to voluntarily remedy the situation so that employees are no longer exposed to the dangerous situation. If the employer fails to do this, an OSHA compliance officer may apply to the federal district court for an injunction to stop work until unsafe conditions are corrected.

2. Second priority goes to the investigation of fatalities and accidents resulting in a death or hospitalization of three or more employees. The employer must report such catastrophes to OSHA within 8 hours. OSHA investigates to determine the cause of these accidents and whether existing OSHA standards were violated.
3. Third priority goes to formal employee complaints of unsafe or unhealthful working conditions and to referrals from any source about a workplace hazard. The act gives each employee the right to request an OSHA inspection when the employee believes he or she is in imminent danger from a hazard or when he or she thinks that there is a violation of an OSHA standard that threatens physical harm. OSHA will maintain confidentiality, if requested, and will inform the employee of any action taken.
4. Fourth in priority are programmed inspections aimed at specific high-hazard industries, workplaces, occupations, health substances, or other industries identified in OSHA's current inspection procedures. OSHA selects industries for inspection on the basis of such factors as injury incidence rates, previous citation history, employee exposure to toxic substances, or random selection.
5. Last on the list of priorities for OSHA inspections are follow-up inspections. A follow-up inspection determines if the employer has corrected previously cited violations. If an employer has failed to abate a violation, the OSHA compliance officer informs the employer that he or she is subject to "Failure to Abate" alleged violations. This involves proposed additional daily penalties until the employer corrects the violation.

Fines are imposed as penalties for violations. Employers and employees may appeal under some circumstances.

Under OSHA standards, both employers and employees have certain rights and responsibilities. Employers must provide a hazard-free workplace and comply with all applicable OSHA standards. Employers must also inform all employees about OSHA safety and health requirements, keep certain records, and compile and post an annual summary of work-related injuries and illnesses. It is the employer's responsibility to ensure that employees wear safety equipment when necessary, to provide safety training, and to discipline employees for violation of safety rules. The law prohibits employers from retaliating in any way against employees who file complaints under the act.

For their part, employees must comply with all applicable OSHA standards, report hazardous conditions, follow all safety and health rules established by the employer, and use protective equipment when necessary. Many states have employee **right-to-know laws,** which allow employees access to information about toxic or hazardous substances, employer duties, employee rights, and other health and safety issues.

right-to-know laws
State laws that allow employees access to information about toxic or hazardous substances, employer duties, employee rights, and other workplace health and safety issues.

Federal OSHA authority extends to all private-sector employers with one or more employees, as well as to federal civilian employees. In addition, many states administer their own occupational safety and health programs through plans approved under section 18(b) of the federal OSHA act.

Check Your Progress

13. OSHA provides for ________________ in the workplace.
14. What state laws allow employees access to information about toxic or hazardous substances?
15. As an employee in a health care facility, what are your general responsibilities under OSHA standards?

10.3 OSHA, CDC, and CLIA Guidelines and Regulations

OSHA standards for medical settings and health care workers often are influenced by and/or closely associated with guidelines issued by the Centers for Disease Control and Prevention (CDC). Following are summaries of six OSHA standards and CDC guidelines that most often affect health care practitioners working in medical settings.

Occupational Exposure to Bloodborne Pathogen Standard An OSHA regulation designed to protect health care workers from the risk of exposure to bloodborne pathogens.

1. The Occupational Exposure to Bloodborne Pathogen Standard is an OSHA regulation passed in 1991. The standard is designed to protect workers in health care and related occupations from the risk of exposure to bloodborne *pathogens* (disease-causing organisms), such as the human immunodeficiency virus (HIV), hepatitis B virus (HBV), and hepatitis C virus (HCV). The standard requires posting of safety guidelines, exposure incident reporting, and formulation of a written exposure control plan that outlines the protective measures an employer will take to eliminate or minimize employee exposure to blood and other body fluids. The plan must be available to OSHA inspectors and to employees.

As mandated by the Needlestick Safety and Prevention Act, passed by Congress in 2000, the Occupational Exposure to Bloodborne Pathogen Standard, 29 CFR 1910.1030, was revised in 2001 to include new provisions requiring employers to maintain a sharps injury log and to involve nonmanagerial employees in selecting safer medical devices.

By authority of the Bloodborne Pathogen Standard, OSHA can levy fines for violations leading to employee exposure to bloodborne pathogens, based on guidelines issued by the CDC. The CDC provides guidelines for universal precautions that include the following:

- Do not contaminate the outside of containers when collecting specimens. All specimen containers should have secure lids.
- Wear gloves when processing patients' specimens, including blood, body fluids containing blood, and other fluids. Masks and goggles should be worn if splashing or aerosolization may occur. Change gloves and wash hands after handling each specimen.

- Use biological safety cabinets for blending and vigorous mixing whenever there is a potential for droplets.
- Do not pipette fluids by mouth. Use mechanical pipetting devices.
- Use extreme caution when handling needles. Do not bend, recap, or remove needles from disposable syringes. Place entire needle assembly in a clearly marked, puncture-resistant, leak-proof container.
- Decontaminate work surfaces with a chemical germicide after spills and daily when work is completed. (A clean work surface proved essential in the laboratory scenario at the beginning of this chapter.)
- Clearly and permanently label tissue or serum specimens to be stored as potentially hazardous.
- Never eat, drink, smoke, or apply cosmetics or lip balm in the laboratory.
- Remove protective clothing and wash hands before leaving the laboratory.

2. The Hazard Communication Standard (HCS) is an OSHA standard that is intended to increase all employers' and employees' awareness of risk, improve work practices and appropriate use of personal protective equipment, and reduce injuries and illnesses.

In March 2012, OSHA published the first major revision to the Hazard Communication Standard. The changes aligned the standard with the **United Nations Globally Harmonized System of Classification and Labeling of Chemicals (GHS).** New wording, taken from GHS, was intended to transform the right of employees to know about workplace hazards to the "right to understand" workplace hazards.

GHS established objective criteria for classifying and identifying chemical hazards. The goal was to ensure the safe use of chemicals by providing practical, reliable, consistent, and easy-to-understand information for workers and students everywhere. For example, to alleviate confusion over "toxicity" as opposed to "toxic," the following phrases are used:

- Fatal if swallowed
- Toxic if swallowed
- Harmful if swallowed
- May be harmful if swallowed.

GHS Pictograms (See Figure 10-1.) As of June 1, 2015, the HCS requires pictograms on labels to alert users to the chemical hazards to which they may be exposed. Each pictogram consists of a symbol on a white background framed within a red border and represents a distinct hazard or hazards. The pictogram on the label is determined by the chemical hazard classification.

Under GHS provisions, there are more than 80 specific hazard statements and several hundred precautionary statements for use in labeling. Following is an example of the hazard and precautionary statement for ethanol (ethyl alcohol):

> **Hazard Statement(s):** Highly Flammable Liquid and Vapor H315 and H320 Causes skin and eye irritation; H335 May cause respiratory irritation; H401 Toxic to aquatic life.
>
> **Precautionary Statements:** P210 Keep away from heat/sparks/ open flames/hot surfaces. No smoking; P261 Avoid breathing dust/ fume/gas/mist/ vapors/spray; P305 + P351 + P338 IF IN EYES: Rinse cautiously with water for several minutes. Remove contact lenses, if present and easy to do. Continue rinsing.

Hazard Communication Standard (HCS)
An OSHA standard intended to increase health care practitioners' awareness of risks, improve work practices and appropriate use of personal protective equipment, and reduce injuries and illnesses in the workplace.

United Nations Globally Harmonized System of Classification and Labeling of Chemicals (GHS)
Led to a 2012 revision of the Hazard Communication Standard in order to transform "right to know" to "right to understand," in line with GHS.

FIGURE 10-1 GHS Mandates Nine Pictograms for Chemical and Physical Hazards

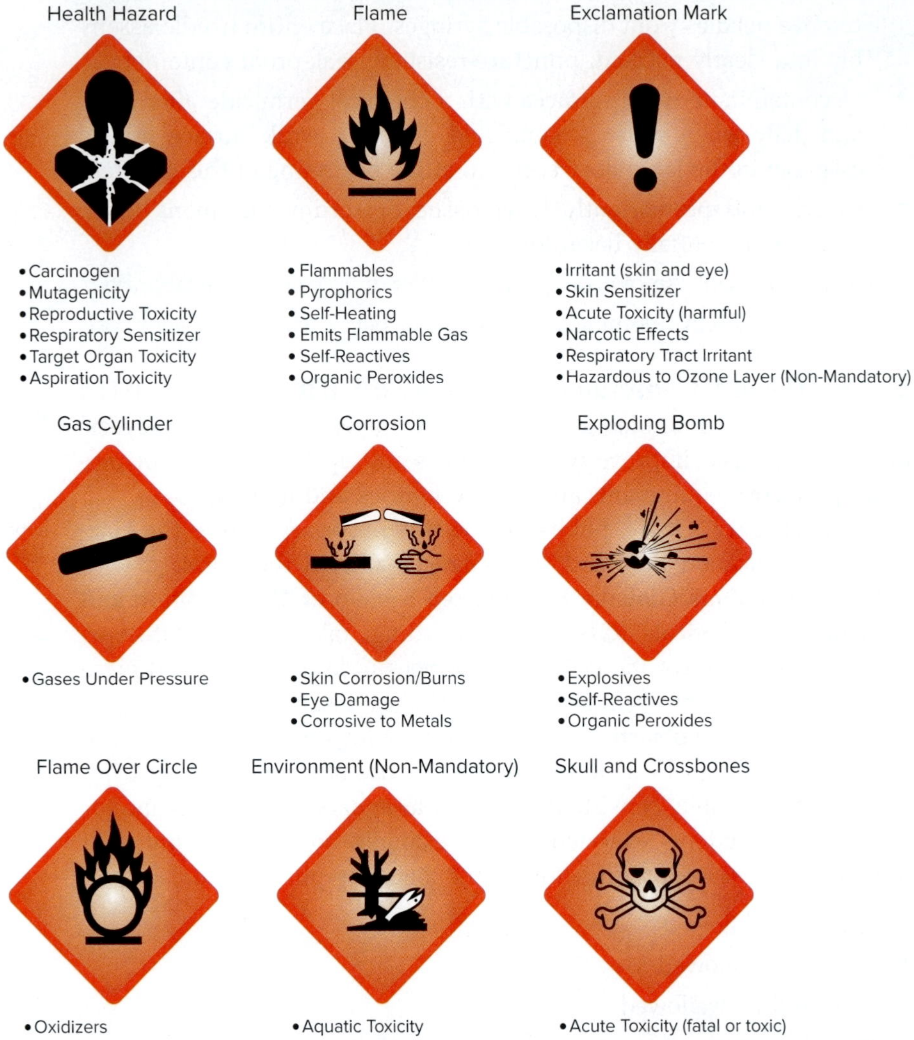

Source: www.osha.gov/Publications/HazComm_QuickCard_Pictogram.html.

Under the HCS, medical offices must have a written hazard communication program. A list of all office hazards must be compiled, posted on bulletin boards, and placed in a hazard communication manual. The list must include hazardous chemicals, hazardous equipment, and hazardous wastes. Hazards often found in the medical office include disinfectant sprays and lab reagents, electrical and mechanical equipment, and blood and body fluids.

Employers must obtain a Safety Data Sheet (SDS), formerly known as a Material Safety Data Sheet, for each hazardous chemical in use in the office. These sheets should be kept on file, and new ones should be placed in a binder where employees can readily review them. Manufacturers must supply SDSs when requested. Each hazardous product in use must have a hazard label, which is a condensed version of the SDS.

Employees must determine what hazardous chemicals are used, initial and date new SDSs as they are read, and initial and date records of safety training. Health care practitioners should see that a hazard communication manual is kept up-to-date and is accessible to all coworkers. Under the **General Duty Clause** of the HCS, any equipment that may pose a health risk is included as a hazard. This clause covers all areas for which OSHA has not developed specific standards and holds the employer ultimately responsible for the safety of employees: "Each employer shall furnish a place of employment which is free from recognized hazards that are causing or are likely to cause death or serious physical harm to his/her employees."

General Duty Clause
A section of the Hazard Communication Standard stating that any equipment that may pose a health risk must be specified as a hazard.

3. Chemical Hygiene Plan The Standard for Occupational Exposures to Hazardous Chemicals in Laboratories, or the **Chemical Hygiene Plan,** seeks to protect laboratory workers from harm due to hazardous chemicals. It is a written program that includes policies, procedures, and responsibilities designed to protect workers from hazards associated with the specific chemicals used in a particular workplace.

Chemical Hygiene Plan
The Standard for Occupational Exposures to Hazardous Chemicals in Laboratories that clarifies the handling of hazardous chemicals in medical laboratories.

4. Ionizing Radiation Standard A fourth OSHA standard, the Ionizing Radiation Standard, applies to all medical and dental offices that have X-ray machines. Requirements under this standard include:

- Preparing a survey of all types of radiation used, including X-rays
- Setting aside restricted areas where employees can limit exposures
- Providing personal radiation monitors such as film badges or pocket dosimeters for employees to wear
- Using caution signs to label those rooms and equipment where exposure could occur

5. Exit Routes Standard A fifth OSHA standard, the Exit Routes Standard, requires that safe and accessible building exits must be provided in case of fire or emergency. Basic responsibilities include providing enough exit routes for the number of employees in a space and posting a diagram of evacuation routes in visible locations.

6. Electrical standards OSHA electrical standards apply to electrical equipment and wiring in hazardous locations. Special wiring and equipment installation may be required if the facility uses flammable gases.

Every workplace must also post the state or federal OSHA poster explaining employees' rights to a safe workplace.

Medical and dental offices are currently exempt from maintaining an official log of reportable injuries and illnesses (OSHA Form 300) under the federal OSHA record-keeping rule, although they may be required to maintain records in some state plans. Employees in those states that have state OSHA plans should contact the state plan directly for more information. All employers, including medical and dental offices, must report any work-related fatality or the hospitalization of three or more employees in a single incident to the nearest OSHA office. Employees may call (800) 321-OSHA or the relevant state plan for assistance.

A guide for medical and dental office compliance with OSHA standards at www.osha.gov/Publications/OSHA3187/osha3187.html lists basic requirements of the Bloodborne Pathogens Standard. This is the most frequently requested and referenced OSHA standard affecting medical and dental offices. Some basic requirements of the OSHA Bloodborne Pathogens standard include:

- A written exposure control plan, to be updated annually
- Use of universal precautions
- Consideration, implementation, and use of safer engineered needles and sharps
- Use of engineering and work practices controls and appropriate personal protective equipment (gloves, face and eye protection, gowns)
- Offer no-cost hepatitis B vaccinations for employees at risk of exposure
- Require medical follow-up after an exposure incident
- Use of labels or color-coding for items such as sharps, disposal boxes and containers for regulated waste, contaminated laundry, and certain specimens
- Provide for the proper containment of all regulated waste
- Provide appropriate employee training

Medical Waste Tracking Act The federal law that authorizes OSHA to inspect hazardous medical wastes and to cite offices for unsafe or unhealthy practices regarding these wastes.

Medical Waste Tracking Act

By authority of the **Medical Waste Tracking Act,** OSHA may inspect hazardous medical wastes and will cite medical facilities for unsafe or unhealthy practices regarding these wastes. Hazardous medical wastes include but are not limited to blood products, body fluids, tissues, cultures, vaccines (live and weakened), sharps, table paper (with body fluids on them), gloves, speculums, cotton swabs, and inoculating loops.

A puncture-proof, leak-proof, approved sharps container must be provided for the disposal of sharp objects. Chemicals should be discarded in a glass or metal container. Flushable chemicals can be washed down the drain with large quantities of water. Other hazardous medical wastes must be contained in plastic, leak-proof biohazard bags. Incineration is often used to dispose of medical wastes. Reputable, licensed waste handlers should be used to handle this material.

Training

Under OSHA standards, each employer must have a written training program detailing how employees will be provided with information and training regarding hazards in the workplace. Training should include information about hazards in the work area, the location of the list of hazards and Safety Data Sheets, explanations of SDSs and the hazardous chemical labeling system, and any measures that employees can take to protect themselves against these hazards. Training logs should be kept, and employees who complete training should sign and date the log.

Current OSHA standards for health care settings may be obtained from the OSHA Web site at www.osha.gov.

Centers for Disease Control and Prevention (CDC) Guidelines

CDC guidelines have always recommended that health care practitioners wear gloves, eye masks, gowns, and other protective equipment when performing such tasks as capillary puncture, phlebotomy, pelvic exams, minor suturing, and throat culture. Health care workers should also wear protective equipment when performing tasks that do not involve direct contact with blood, body fluids, or tissue, in case of accidental exposure. These tasks include urinalysis, blood testing, examination of fecal occult blood, injections, positioning for X-rays, performing ultrasound and ECG tests, and examination of sweat, tears, and nasal secretions.

The CDC publishes a comprehensive online guide for all health care workers titled, *Guideline for Isolation Precautions: Preventing Transmission of Infectious Agents in Healthcare Settings,* available at http://www.cdc.gov/hipac/pubs.html. The document "is intended for use by infection control staff, health care epidemiologists, health care administrators, nurses, other health care providers, and persons responsible for developing, implementing, and evaluating infection control programs for health care settings across the continuum of care." It contains references to other guidelines and Web sites for more detailed information and for recommendations concerning specialized infection control problems, such as preventing surgical site infections; recommendations for the prevention, treatment, and control of tuberculosis; prevention of intervascular catheter infections; hand hygiene; and so on.

This Web site also includes a section on infection prevention and control recommendations for hospitalized patients with known or suspected Ebola virus infection.

The **Clinical Laboratory Improvement Act (CLIA)** of 1988, also called the Clinical Laboratory Improvement Amendments, replaced 1967 laboratory testing legislation that established standards for Medicare and Medicaid. The act established minimum quality standards for all laboratory testing and has been extensively amended since it was first written. The regulations define a laboratory as any facility that performs laboratory testing on specimens derived from humans for diagnosing, preventing, or treating disease or for assessing health. The law requires that laboratories obtain certification, pay applicable fees, and follow regulations concerning testing, personnel, inspections, test management, quality control, and quality assurance.

Clinical Laboratory Improvement Act (CLIA)
Also called Clinical Laboratory Improvement Amendments. Federal statute passed in 1988 that established minimum quality standards for all laboratory testing.

The Division of Laboratory Services, within the Survey and Certification Group under the Center for Medicaid and State Operations, has responsibility for implementing the CLIA program. The Federal Drug Administration has responsibility for some CLIA functions. More information about the Clinical Laboratory Improvement Act and its amendments is available online at www.cms.gov/clia/.

Check Your Progress

16. For the facility described in this chapter's opening scenario, which OSHA standards and/or CDC guidelines discussed earlier would apply?
17. What protective gear does the CDC recommend for laboratory employees?
18. What specific health care procedures and/or facilities does the Clinical Laboratory Improvement Act cover?
19. Are there penalties for violating any of the OSHA standards concerned with safety in the workplace? Explain your answer.

10.4 Workers' Compensation and Unemployment Insurance

WORKERS' COMPENSATION

workers' compensation
A form of insurance established by federal and state statutes that provides reimbursement for workers who are injured on the job.

Federal and state **workers' compensation** laws establish procedures for compensating workers who are injured on the job. The employer pays the cost of the insurance premium for the employee. These laws allow the injured worker to file a claim for compensation with the state or the federal government instead of suing. However, the laws require workers to accept workers' compensation as the exclusive remedy for on-the-job injuries. Federal laws cover the following employees: workers in Washington, DC; coal miners; maritime workers; and federal employees. State laws cover those workers not protected under federal statutes.

Workers who are injured on the job or who contract an occupational disease may apply for five types of state compensation benefits:

- Medical treatment, including hospital, medical, and surgical services; medications; and prosthetic devices
- Temporary disability indemnity, in the form of weekly cash payments made directly to the injured or ill employee
- Permanent disability indemnity, which can be a lump-sum award or a weekly or monthly cash payment
- Death benefits for survivors, which consist of cash payments to dependents of employees killed on the job
- Rehabilitation benefits, which are paid for medical or vocational rehabilitation

Employees who are injured on the job or become ill due to work-related causes must immediately report the injury or illness to a supervisor. An injury report and claim for compensation are then filed with the appropriate state workers' compensation agency. Forms from the attending or designated workers' compensation physician who examines and treats the employee must also be filed with the appropriate agency as proof of the employee's injury or illness.

A medical office employee may be responsible for filing the physician's report with the state workers' compensation agency. Requirements concerning waiting periods and other filing specifics vary with each state. When a claim is filed, all questions must be answered in full and as thoroughly as possible.

UNEMPLOYMENT INSURANCE

Unemployment insurance (sometimes called reemployment insurance) funds are managed jointly by state and federal governments. Under the Federal Unemployment Tax Act (FUTA), employers contribute to a fund that is paid out to eligible unemployed workers. Each state also provides unemployment insurance, and credit is given to employers against the FUTA tax for amounts paid to the state unemployment fund. The total cost is borne by the employer in all but a few states.

Out-of-work employees should contact a state unemployment office to determine whether they qualify for unemployment benefits. Online, fax, or in-person applications are accepted. Former employees are denied unemployment compensation for three main reasons: (1) They quit their jobs without cause, (2) they were fired for misconduct, or (3) they are unemployed because of a labor dispute. Independent contractors and self-employed individuals usually do not qualify for unemployment compensation.

A claimant may need:

- A Social Security number
- Driver's license or other state identification
- Wage records for the past 18 months, including all employers' names and addresses
- A statement of the reasons for leaving the job
- A declaration that he or she is available for work and willing to accept work

10.5 Hiring and the New Employee

When interviewing for a position or when asked to interview a job applicant, the health care practitioner must know the legal boundaries.

INTERVIEWS

Because of federal and state laws against discrimination in hiring, inquiries cannot be made concerning an applicant's

- Race or color
- Religion or creed
- Gender
- Family
- Marital status
- Method of birth control
- Age, birth date, or birthplace
- Disability
- Arrest record (with some exceptions in many states)
- Residency duration
- National origin (However, the Immigration Reform and Control Act of 1986 requires new employees to complete an I-9 form, intended to prevent the employment of illegal aliens.)
- General military experience or discharge
- Membership in organizations

Questions concerning one's Social Security number, qualifications (including license or certificate), and job experience are proper, and they should be answered as thoroughly and truthfully as possible. As part of the hiring process, applicants may be asked to take a physical examination.

During a job interview, applicants may refuse to answer a question that is clearly improper or not job-related, but this could cost them the job. The question "May I ask how this relates to the position?" is generally more acceptable than a blunt, "That question is illegal, and I don't have to answer it." Furthermore, the mere asking of an improper preemployment interview question does not in itself give an applicant grounds for a legal challenge if he or she is not hired.

The following guidelines can help those employees who are responsible for conducting preemployment interviews:

- Make a list of questions that relate specifically to the job description of the position to be filled and stick to them.
- Do not rush the interview or let it drag on beyond reasonable time limits.
- General questions that may prove helpful include these: What are your qualifications for this position? Why are you leaving your present position? Why do you want this job? What salary do you expect? When can you begin work? What are your professional strengths? What are your professional goals?
- Remain objective and listen well.
- End the interview on a positive note. Indicate when a decision will be made, and follow through on your promise to inform the applicant of your decision one way or the other.

BONDING

In some medical offices and other workplace locations where employees are responsible for collecting fees and handling financial matters, prospective employees may be asked whether they are bondable. An employer can purchase a surety bond for a specific amount from an insurance carrier. If a bonded employee should embezzle or otherwise abscond with funds, the employer can collect from the insurance carrier up to the amount of the bond. However, the employer must have filed a complaint against the alleged dishonest employee in order to collect on the bond. If the insurance company pays the bond, it will then seek to recover the amount from the offending employee.

BACKGROUND CHECKS

background check
The process of reviewing criminal and/or financial history to confirm information about an applicant for employment.

Employers may want to consider the backgrounds of applicants and employees. **Background checks** are becoming more common, particularly in health care. Employers may hire an outside firm to conduct both a financial and a criminal background check. Employers and the outside firms must comply not only with the various discrimination laws but also with the Fair Credit Reporting Act. The employee (current or prospective) must acknowledge that the check is going to occur. As an employer, you must comply with federal laws that protect applicants and employees from discrimination. The EEOC offers guidance in a joint publication with the Federal Trade Commission that may be found at www.eeoc.gov/eeoc/publications/background_checks_employers.cfm.

EMPLOYMENT PAPERWORK

Once employed, the new worker will be asked to provide certain information so that the employer may comply with federal and state regulations. Complete records for every employee must include:

- Social Security number
- Number of exemptions claimed

- Gross salary
- Deductions for Social Security, Medicare, and federal, state, and city taxes
- Withholding for state disability insurance, state unemployment tax, and health care plans, if applicable
- Properly completed I-9 form (This is proof of citizenship or the legal right to work in the United States.)

The law requires employers to withhold specified amounts from employees' pay and to keep records of and send these sums to the proper income tax center. The amount to be withheld is based on the employee's total salary, the number of exemptions he or she claims, marital status, and the length of the pay period involved.

Health care practitioners who are self-employed do not have to deduct withholding, but they must make quarterly city, state, and federal income tax payments. Self-employed individuals must also pay Social Security taxes (FICA) via a self-employment tax percentage that is higher than the rate paid by individuals who are not self-employed. The difference lies in the fact that a self-employed individual is making both the employer's and the employee's contribution.

Employers must provide each employee with a Form W-2, Wage and Tax Statement, by January 31 of each year. The W-2 shows the following information:

- Employer's tax identification number
- Employee's Social Security number
- Total earnings (wages and other compensation) paid by the employer
- Amounts deducted for income tax and Social Security
- Amount of advance earned income credit payment, if any

Check Your Progress

20. Distinguish between workers' compensation and unemployment insurance.
21. Is it permissible for an employer to ask a job applicant to take a physical exam? Why might such a requirement exist?
22. Place a check mark beside those questions that are considered illegal if asked in a preemployment interview.

    _______ Why are you leaving your present position?
    _______ Do you belong to a church?
    _______ What do you hope to achieve over the next 5 years?
    _______ How many children do you have, and how old are they?
    _______ Who will watch your children while you work?
    _______ Why do you want to work for us?
    _______ How many years' experience do you have as a medical assistant/dental assistant/physician assistant/nursing assistant?
    _______ Are you married?
    _______ Is your husband/wife employed, and if so, where?
    _______ What nationality are you?

Chapter Summary

Learning Outcome	Summary

LO 10.1 Identify federal laws regarding hiring and firing, discrimination, and other workplace regulation.	What issues have traditionally affected employees in the workplace?
	• Employment-at-will
	• Wrongful discharge
	• Just cause
	• Public policy
	What categories do federal and state laws generally address, regarding employees in the workplace?
	• Discrimination
	    • Being of a particular race, color, religion, or national origin; being male, female, or transgender
	    • Being over 40 years of age
	    • Having a history of a disability or having a disability that may be accommodated.
	    • Being pregnant
	    • Having a particular genetic disposition
	    • Joining a union or engaging in political activity
	• Wages and work hours
	    • Social Security
	    • Fair Labor Standards
	    • Equal pay
	    • Employee Retirement Income Security
	• Workplace safety
	• Medical leave

LO 10.2 Describe the Occupational Safety and Health Administration's (OSHA) top workplace priorities.	What are OSHA's workplace priorities? • Imminent danger situations • Investigation of workplace fatalities and worker hospitalization • Employee complaints of unsafe working conditions • Programmed inspections at high-hazard industries • Follow-up inspections
LO 10.3 Examine the role of health care practitioners in following OSHA, Centers for Disease Control and Prevention (CDC), and Clinical Laboratory Improvement Act (CLIA) standards for workplace safety.	What are the major OSHA standards? • Exposure to Occupational Bloodborne Pathogen Standard • Hazard Communication Standard • Chemical Hygiene Plan • Ionizing Radiation Standard • Exit Route Standard • Electrical Standard • Medical Waste Tracking Act • Training Plan What is one of the major roles of the CDC in protecting health care workers? • Preventing transmission of infectious agents What is the role of the Clinical Laboratory Improvement Act (CLIA) in quality laboratory testing? • Established minimum quality standards for all laboratory testing

LO 10.4 Summarize the purpose of workers' compensation laws and unemployment insurance.	What is the purpose of worker's compensation? • Five types of benefits for employees injured on the job Who manages unemployment insurance? • Individual states manage unemployment insurance.
LO 10.5 Determine the appropriate legal process for hiring employees and maintaining the required paperwork while a person is employed.	What should health care practitioners know about hiring for new employees? • Prohibited questions to ask job applicants • Guidelines for conducting interviews • Surety bond, if appropriate • Background check, if appropriate What is the minimum information necessary to complete the hiring process for tax purposes? • Social Security number • Gross salary • Deductions for state and federal taxes, Social Security, and Medicare • Deductions for health insurance or any other state-mandated deductions • Exemptions claimed • Properly completed I-9 form with proof of citizenship or legal right to work

Chapter 10 Review

Applying Knowledge

LO 10.1

1. Under the concept of employment-at-will, who has the right to terminate employment?
   a. The government
   b. Both the employer and the employee
   c. The business owner
   d. The employee's legal representative
2. When might an employee who is fired sue his or her former employer for wrongful discharge?
   a. Never
   b. Only 1 year after the discharge
   c. At any time if the employee was discharged for an illegal reason
   d. Six months after the discharge
3. Which of the following reasons for discharge is *not* illegal under antidiscrimination laws?
   a. The employee is too old.
   b. The employee joined a union.
   c. The employee has been unable to master the requirements of the job.
   d. The employee is too religious.
4. Which of the following common law concepts protects an employee who reports his employer's illegal chemical dumping activities?
   a. Employment-at-will
   b. Public policy

c. Wage and hours law

d. Antisexual harassment law

5. Which of the following federal laws protects employees from potential discrimination?

   a. Civil Rights Act of 1964

   b. Affirmative action

   c. Social Security Act

   d. ERISA

6. Which of the following federal laws protects employees from sexual harassment in the workplace?

   a. Equal Pay Act

   b. ERISA

   c. Civil Rights Act of 1964

   d. Social Security Act

7. Which of the following is *not* a form of sexual harassment in the workplace?

   a. A supervisor promises an employee a pay raise in exchange for sexual favors.

   b. A male employee makes unwelcome sexual advances to a male coworker.

   c. A female employee makes unwelcome sexual advances to a male coworker.

   d. A female supervisor hires a male assistant.

8. Which federal agency can be contacted to report charges or complaints of employment discrimination?

   a. Department of Labor

   b. Social Security Administration

   c. Equal Employment Opportunity Commission

   d. Internal Revenue Service

9. Which of the following employment issues do federal laws generally address?

   a. Employment discrimination

   b. Wages and hours

   c. Safety and welfare

   d. All of these

10. A form of sexual harassment that means "something for something" is called

    a. Right-to-know

    b. *Quid pro quo*

    c. ERISA

    d. *Res judicata*

11. Which of the following types of evidence may an employee produce to substantiate a wrongful discharge claim?

    a. Oral promises to the employee

    b. A written contract

    c. Company handbook

    d. All of these

LO 10.2

12. A right to know law is designed to protect
    a. Employers
    b. Government
    c. The public
    d. Employees

LO 10.3

13. What federal publication is the primary source for locating OSHA standards?
    a. Publication of Labor Statistics
    b. CDC list of OSHA regulations
    c. Web site of OSHA
    d. Workers' Compensation Guide
14. Which of the following does not govern work done in a clinical setting?
    a. Hazard Communication Standard
    b. Occupational Exposure to Bloodborne Pathogen Standard
    c. Needlestick Safety and Prevention Act
    d. Social Security Act
15. Which of the following is an OSHA regulation that applies to hazardous equipment in the workplace?
    a. Occupational Exposure to Bloodborne Pathogen Standard
    b. General Duty Clause
    c. Chemical Hygiene Plan
    d. None of these
16. Which of the following is *not* true of OSHA's Hazard Communication Standard?
    a. Requires medical offices to have a written hazard communication program
    b. Requires employers to obtain and post a Safety Data Sheet for each hazardous chemical in use in the workplace
    c. Has never been revised
    d. Requires a hazard communications manual be kept up-to-date and accessible to all employees
17. Safety for employees handling hazardous materials in the medical office requires employees to
    a. Wear protective equipment when handling hazardous materials
    b. Post Safety Data Sheets for hazardous chemicals in use
    c. Initial and date records of safety training
    d. All of these
18. The Clinical Laboratory Improvement Act (CLIA)
    a. Established minimum quality standards for all laboratory testing
    b. Has been extensively amended since it was first written
    c. Requires laboratories to obtain certification
    d. All of these

19. Which of the following helps control infections in the medical office?
  a. Wearing protective equipment when appropriate
  b. Disposing of sharps appropriately
  c. Cleaning/disinfecting work areas
  d. All of these

LO 10.4

20. Which laws allow an injured employee to file a claim with the state or federal government?
  a. Workers' compensation
  b. Needlestick Safety and Prevention Act
  c. General Duty Clause
  d. Clinical Laboratory Improvement Act
21. Which of the following is generally *not* a reason for an ex-employee to be denied an unemployment claim?
  a. Quit job without cause
  b. Fired for misconduct
  c. Quit due to sexual harassment
  d. Quit when spouse was transferred
22. Which of the following are generally *not* eligible for unemployment benefits?
  a. Women who quit to give birth
  b. Men who quit to care for young children
  c. Independent contractors and the self-employed
  d. Seasonal employees, such as construction workers

LO 10.5

23. Which of the following questions is illegal to ask a job applicant?
  a. Why did you leave your previous employment?
  b. Why do you want to work here?
  c. What are your 5-year employment goals?
  d. Do you have children?
24. A W-2 form typically does *not* include
  a. Change in employee's marital status
  b. Employer's tax identification number
  c. Total wages paid
  d. Employee's Social Security number
25. A type of insurance that allows employers to collect if employees embezzle or otherwise steal business funds is called
  a. Disability insurance
  b. Workers' compensation
  c. Unemployment insurance
  d. Surety bond

DO YOU KNOW THE LAWS?

Match each definition with the correct term by writing the letter in the space provided.

_____ 26. Established the EEOC.

_____ 27. Makes it illegal to discriminate because of pregnancy, childbirth, or related medical conditions.

_____ 28. Protects employees aged 40 or older.

_____ 29. Protects employees who engage in union or other organizational activities.

_____ 30. Regulates private pension funds and employer benefit programs.

_____ 31. Requires equal pay for equal work.

_____ 32. Ensures a safe work environment.

_____ 33. Regulates child labor and provides for minimum wages and overtime pay.

_____ 34. Provides for Medicare, unemployment insurance, disability, and OASI through FICA funding.

_____ 35. Protects individuals who are disabled or mentally ill.

_____ 36. Provides minimum federal standards for quality laboratory testing.

a. Wagner Act

b. Social Security Act

c. Fair Labor Standards Act

d. Equal Pay Act

e. Civil Rights Act of 1964

f. Age Discrimination in Employment Act

g. Occupational Safety and Health Act

h. Rehabilitation Act

i. Employee Retirement Income Security Act

j. Pregnancy Discrimination Act

h. Clinical Laboratory Improvement Act/Amendments

Ethics Issues Workplace Legalities

Use your critical thinking skills to answer the questions that follow each ethics issue.

Ethics ISSUE 1:

All ethical guidelines for health care practitioners remind them to be aware that even though sexually suggestive behavior may not have crossed the line legally, any form of sexual harassment or exploitation between medical supervisors and trainees, employers and employees, coworkers, or medical practitioners and patients is unethical.

Discussion Questions

37. You are a surgical technologist in a large hospital. Whenever you work with a certain surgeon, she tells off-color jokes to you and your coworkers, and makes suggestive comments to workers of the opposite sex. One coworker tells you that he might quit his job because he is married and the surgeon's behavior makes him so uncomfortable that he dreads coming to work. Is the surgeon's behavior illegal or simply in bad taste? Explain your answer.

38. Do you or your coworkers in the previous situation have grounds for a sexual harassment complaint? Explain your answer.

39. If you have determined that you do have a complaint, how would you proceed?

Ethics ISSUE 2:

Patients are often accompanied by third parties who play an important part in the health care practitioner–patient relationship. The health care practitioner interacts and communicates with these individuals and often is in a position to offer them information, advice, and emotional support. The more deeply involved the individual is in the clinical encounter and in medical decision making, the more troubling sexual or romantic contact with the health care practitioner would be. Key third parties include but are not limited to spouses or partners, parents, guardians, and proxies.

Source: AMA Code of Medical Ethics, E-8.14.

Discussion Questions

40. As a medical assistant, you have been present when a young, single father brings his infant in for checkups. The child is seriously ill, and the father begins consulting you about his emotional anguish. You are also single and sense an attraction. When the young man asks you out, should you accept? Explain your answer.

41. Do you believe ethical standards governing such relationships are stricter for health care practitioners than for other professions, such as law professors and students? In your view, is this as it should be? Explain your answer.

Ethics ISSUE 3:

Health care practitioners have legal and ethical responsibilities to follow laws and procedures that protect their safety and patient safety.

Discussion Question

42. Assume you are the medical technologist in the chapter's opening scenario and you observe that every urine specimen analyzed during a hectic morning has a high leukocyte count. You realize this is unusual, but you don't want to fall behind, and you do not report the anomaly to your supervisor. Have you acted ethically? Explain your answer.

Case Studies

Use your critical thinking skills to answer the questions that follow each case study.

LO 10.3

While many people think of the health care industry as "clean," medical providers continue to accidentally contract diseases from incidents in the workplace. For example, Sheila, an emergency room nurse with 15 years' experience, had just finished drawing blood from a patient when she disposed of the needle in the sharps container and felt a prick through her glove from a used needle that was hung up in the drop-down container lid. Several months later, Sheila learned that she had not only been infected with the human immunodeficiency virus but also the hepatitis C virus. Other diseases health care practitioners often contract through needlesticks include methicillin-resistant *Staphylococcus aureus*, hepatitis B, malaria, syphilis, herpes, and many less common diseases.

43. In your opinion, were there precautions that Sheila could have taken in the emergency room where she worked to prevent her accidental infection? Explain your answer.

44. What other common hazards do health care practitioners face in a medical office or other medical setting? How would you deal with each?

LO 10.4

You have recently graduated from a 2-year medical assistant program, have earned certification, and want to apply for the following advertised positions: (1) a CMA in a pediatric clinic and (2) a CMA/receptionist for a physician in private practice. Write letters of application for each position and a résumé to be included with the cover letters. Consider the following questions:

45. What information will you give about your educational, employment, and personal background?

46. If interviewed for the position, how will you follow up?

Internet Activities

LO 10.1, LO 10.3, and LO 10.5

Complete the activities and answer the questions that follow.

47. Visit the Web site for the Equal Employment Opportunity Commission (EEOC) at www.eeoc.gov. Find the EEOC's Twitter account. What issues are trending on the EEOC's Twitter account?

48. In the summer of 2016, ZIKA was a major concern as an infectious disease. Google ZIKA. Find out what the latest status is for protecting Americans from this mosquito-borne disease.

49. The state of Florida requires some health care workers to have a "Level II" background check. These checks are initiated by the prospective employer. Do an Internet search on the current Level II background check. What type of health care employers require a background check? As a health care student, did you have to have a background check before you started your clinical program?

Resources

LO 10.1

Liuzzo, Anthony L. *Essentials of Business Law.* New York: McGraw-Hill, 2010: employment-at-will, p. 445; workers' compensation, pp. 456–458; Occupational Safety and Health Act, Civil Rights Act of 1964, Age Discrimination in Employment Act, etc., pp. 458–462.

www.forbes.com/sites/danielfisher/2016/11/22/texas-judge-issues-nationwide-injunction-against-obamas-overtime-rule/#672029bc747f

www.eeoc.gov/laws/index.cfm

LO 10.2

Workplace priorites: www.osha.gov/OshDoc/data_General_Facts/factsheet-inspections.pdf

LO 10.3

Hazardous communication: www.osha.gov/Publications/HazComm_QuickCard_Pictogram.html

Health care practitioners: www.osha.gov/Publications/OSHA3187/osha3187.html

Infection control: www.cdc.gov/hicpac/recommendations/index.html

Bloodborne infections: www.cdc.gov/niosh/topics/bbp/

LO 10.5

www.eeoc.gov/eeoc/publications/background_checks_employers.cfm

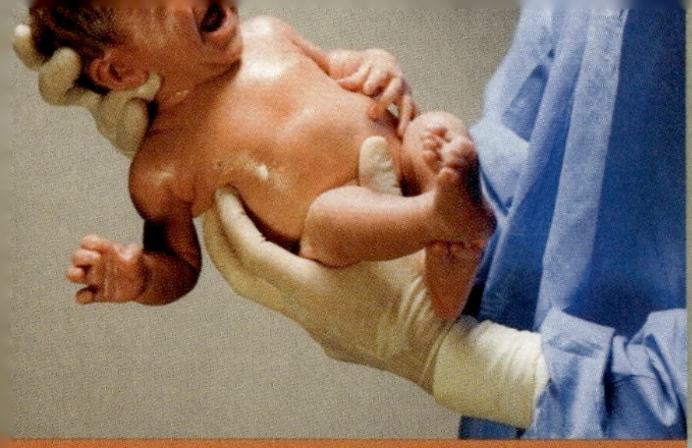

©Stephen Marks/Getty Images

11 The Beginning of Life and Childhood

Key Terms

artificial insemination
chromosome
clone
cloning
DNA (deoxyribonucleic acid)
emancipated minors
gene
gene therapy
genetic counselor
genetic discrimination
genetic engineering
genetics
genome
heredity
heterologous artificial insemination
homologous artificial insemination
Human Genome Project
infertility
in vitro fertilization (IVF)
mature minors
multipotent stem cells
mutation
parens patriae
pluripotent stem cells
safe haven laws
stem cells
surrogacy
surrogate mother
xenotransplantation

LEARNING OUTCOMES

After studying this chapter, you should be able to:

LO 11.1 Discuss family history as a predictor of disease risk.

LO 11.2 Identify appropriate uses for DNA testing, and explain how such tests might lead to genetic discrimination.

LO 11.3 Define *genetic engineering,* and explain why cloning and stem cell research are controversial issues.

LO 11.4 Explain three possible remedies for couples experiencing infertility problems.

LO 11.5 List those laws affecting health care that pertain especially to children's rights.

FROM THE PERSPECTIVE OF. . .

STEVE, a 32-year-old auto mechanic, lives in a large Midwestern city with Gloria, his fiancée. While growing up, he watched as his paternal grandfather, his maternal grandmother, his father's two brothers, and his mother's sister all developed Alzheimer's disease, the most frequent cause of dementia in older adults. In each case, the disease began with what appeared to be occasional memory loss—forgetting names, appointments, purses, and car keys—then progressed rather rapidly to forgetting how to perform routine tasks, such as making coffee, preparing a shopping list, or following a recipe. "I was riding with my granddad in his car one day when he signaled to make a left-hand turn across traffic and suddenly seemed confused about what to do next," Steve recalls. "I told him to step on the gas and get us across, and he made the turn, but after that, he quit driving."

Eventually, Steve's grandfather was placed in a skilled nursing facility, as were other members of his family who developed Alzheimer's disease as they aged.

"Now, I'm thinking of being genetically tested to see if I've inherited genes for Alzheimer's," Steve reveals. (The genetic test for Alzheimer's disease looks for variations of the apolipoprotein E—APOE—gene.) "I'm not sure I really want to know, but it seems likely that I could develop the disease, and if I knew, I could set aside some funds—maybe take out long-term care insurance—now, looking toward the day when I won't be able to care for myself."

From Steve's perspective, the knowledge that he could be genetically predisposed to developing a devastating disease is frightening, but on the other hand, such knowledge would give him time to prepare for the day when, if the disease develops, funds would be available for his care.

From Gloria's perspective, Steve's genetic test results, if negative for the variations of the APOE gene that predict the development of late-onset Alzheimer's, could allow her to view the future with less trepidation. Positive results, on the other hand, might allow her to prepare herself emotionally and financially for whatever Steve's future holds.

From a genetic counselor's perspective, Steve might benefit, in terms of peace of mind, from examining the pros and cons of predictive genetic testing.

11.1 Family History as a Predictor

You have no doubt noticed how certain physical characteristics run in families. For example, Jerry, who was in your fourth-grade class in elementary school, had red hair and freckles, exactly like his mother, father, and three siblings. And when you took piano lessons and struggled to learn your favorite songs, Brittany, the girl next door who was your age and took lessons from the same teacher, learned the most difficult Mozart concertos in half the time it took you to learn "Chopsticks." You thought it might have had something to do with the fact that her father and his two brothers were professional musicians.

Later in life, when your college friend developed breast cancer in her thirties, she told you she had feared such a diagnosis because her mother had also developed breast cancer before the age of 40. As an adult, you also learned that your father's parents fought the same battle he did with high blood pressure, and your mother and her sister worried about heart attacks because their mother died of a heart attack before she reached her sixties.

heredity
The process by which organisms pass genetic traits on to their offspring.

genetics
The science that accounts for natural differences and resemblances among organisms related by descent.

DNA (deoxyribonucleic acid)
The combination of proteins, called nucleotides, that is arranged to make up an organism's chromosomes.

chromosomes
Units within cell nuclei where genetic material is stored.

You know by now that the above examples reflect an individual's **heredity**—the process by which genetic traits are passed on to one's offspring. At this point in your life, you have also learned that **genetics** is the science that accounts for differences and resemblances among people—and other organisms—related by descent.

As a result of genetics research, improved science education, and extensive media coverage of genetics issues, most of the general population, and certainly anyone involved in providing health care, is now familiar with the term **DNA (deoxyribonucleic acid).** DNA makes up **chromosomes** (see Figure 11-1).

DNA and its partner in the chromosome replication process, RNA (ribonucleic acid), are nucleic acids made up of molecules called nucleotides. (RNA comes into play when DNA replicates itself. Its chemical composition is similar to but not exactly the same as that of DNA.) Each nucleotide that comprises DNA contains a phosphate group, a sugar group, and a nitrogen base. The nitrogen bases found in DNA are adenine (A), thymine (T), guanine (G), and cytosine (C). The order of the bases inside the DNA molecule forms the *genetic code* that relays DNA's instructions.

DNA was first isolated in 1868, but the structure of the molecule was not mapped out until 1953, when J. D. Watson and F. H. C. Crick proposed an arrangement that consists of a double helix (a ladderlike structure) of nucleotide chains coiled around the same axis. Pairs of the bases, represented by the letters A, T, G, and C, make up the "rungs" of the helix ladder. The order of these four chemicals functions as an alphabetic code, allowing organisms to create long, complicated codes.

gene
A tiny segment of DNA found on a chromosome within a cell's nucleus. Each gene holds the formula for making a specific enzyme or protein.

The entire DNA strand is billions of base pairs, or rungs, long. Fortunately, an organism does not need to read and interpret the entire DNA strand each time it needs to build proteins. Instead, the organism needs to access only a small part of the DNA, called a **gene,** to build the protein for which it carries the code. Some genes are only a few hundred base pairs long, whereas others may be several million base pairs long.

The relationship between the DNA one inherits from ancestors and diseases and other health problems that recur in families has been scientifically confirmed. Although there are many possible causes of human disease, family history is often one of the strongest risk factors for common disease complexes such as cancer, cardiovascular disease, diabetes, autoimmune disorders, and psychiatric illnesses. In addition to the inheritance of a complete set of genes from each parent that may or may not carry the code for disease, a person also inherits a vast array of cultural and socioeconomic experiences from family that minimize or maximize the risk for health problems.

Forty-six chromosomes (23 pairs) are found inside the nucleus of every human cell, except egg and sperm cells, which have 23 chromosomes each. We inherit half of our chromosome complement from our mother and half from our father. These 46 chromosomes carry the genes

FIGURE 11-1 DNA Is the Combination of Proteins Called Nucleotides That Make Up Each Human Chromosome.

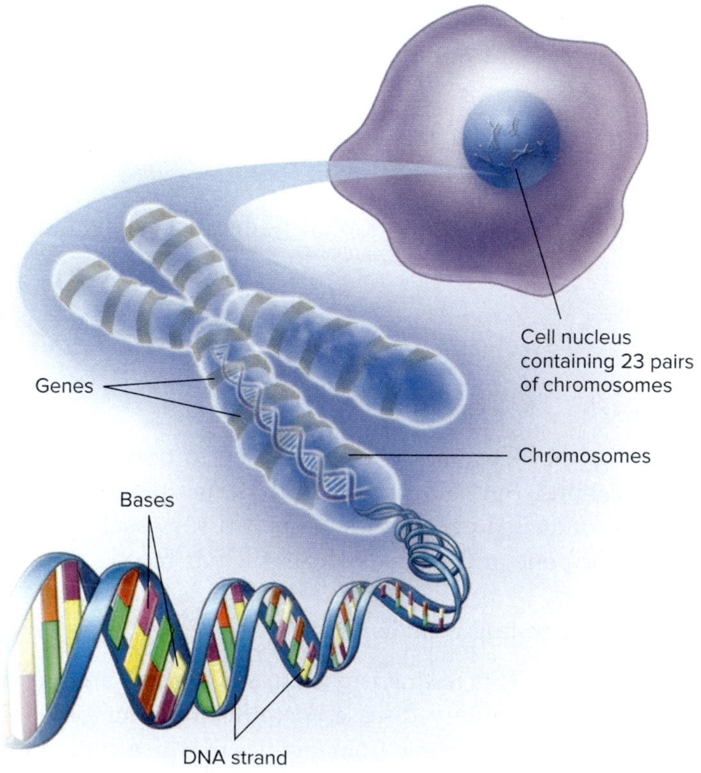

responsible for all our human characteristics, from eye, skin, and hair color to height, body type, and intelligence. Each gene is a tiny segment of DNA that holds the formula for making a specific enzyme or protein.

The genes that make up the human **genome**—all the genetic information necessary to create a human being—are responsible for all the cells, organs, tissues, and traits that make up each individual.

genome
All the DNA in an organism, including its genes.

The **Human Genome Project,** funded by the U.S. government, was started in 1990 to analyze the entire human genome. Scientists around the world who worked on the project set out to map all of the genes within the 23 pairs of human chromosomes. The project was scheduled for completion in 2003 but was finished ahead of time, in mid-2000. One surprising finding was that instead of a suspected 100,000 genes, humans have approximately 20,000 to 25,000 genes.

Human Genome Project
A scientific project funded by the U.S. government, begun in 1990 and successfully completed in 2000, for the purpose of mapping all of a human's genes. This Web site is an excellent resource:.www.genome.gov/25019879

Goals of the Human Genome Project that have largely been accomplished were to locate and map the location of each gene on all 46 chromosomes and to create a data bank of the information that would be available to all scientists or physicians who could use it. The scientists involved in the project also vowed to continue to examine the ethical, legal, and social issues originating with human genetics research and to train other scientists to use the technologies developed to improve human health. For detailed information about the project and its current status, visit www.genome.gov/10001772/all-about-the--human-genome-project-hgp/.

Check Your Progress

Give the term that is defined by each phrase.

1. The science that studies inherited traits.
2. The threadlike structures inside cell nuclei that are composed of DNA and carry an organism's genes.
3. A tiny segment of DNA that holds instructions for making a specific enzyme or protein.
4. All the genes necessary to replicate a human being.
5. A worldwide project to locate and map the location of all human genes.

11.2 DNA Testing

Our increasing knowledge about DNA has led to tests that have widespread applications. Specially trained technicians perform DNA tests. The tests are conducted on samples of solid tissues such as hair roots, skin, muscle, or bone and on body fluids such as blood, sweat, semen, or saliva.

Uses of genetic testing include:

1. *Predictive testing.* This testing is used to see if genes are present that could lead to hereditary diseases or other harmful genetic conditions. Individuals who come from families in which certain inherited diseases have appeared may opt for predictive genetic testing to confirm or rule out the presence of a disease-causing gene. For example, Huntington's disease (also known as Huntington's chorea) runs in families, but symptoms typically do not develop until individuals reach middle age. Because the disease is incurable, debilitating, and fatal, affecting the brain and the nervous system, adults with relatives who have developed the disease may opt to be tested to plan for any eventuality. (Steve, in the chapter's opening scenario, was considering predictive genetic testing to determine if his genome included variations of the APOE gene associated with the development of Alzheimer's disease.)
2. *Carrier testing.* Used to determine if individuals carry harmful genes that could be passed on to offspring.
3. *Prenatal testing.* This testing is used to identify genetic disorders in utero. Ultrasound, a noninvasive test used since the 1960s, allows for detecting some abnormalities in the fetus, but results must be confirmed with a diagnostic test. Amniocentesis, performed 15 to 20 weeks into pregnancy and also used since the 1960s, can identify chromosomal abnormalities, inherited diseases, and certain developmental defects, but the test involves withdrawing amniotic fluid via a needle extraction through the mother's abdomen and carries some risk to the fetus. Chorionic villus sampling, developed in the 1980s, involves inserting a needle through the pregnant belly or a catheter through the cervix to suction cells from the placenta. It is performed 10 to 13 weeks into a pregnancy and also carries some risk to the fetus. Since 2011, maternal blood tests have been developed for use

at 10 weeks' gestation or later that allow testing for chromosomal abnormalities with no risk to the fetus. Because maternal blood contains fetal DNA that has passed through the placenta, testing the mother's blood can reveal chromosomal abnormalities in the fetus.

4. *Preimplantation testing.* These tests look for harmful genes in embryos after artificial insemination but before implantation. They are usually offered to couples who have a reasonable chance of passing on harmful genes.
5. *Forensic testing.* Forensic testing is used in law enforcement to eliminate or designate suspects in a crime, identify homicide victims, or otherwise analyze DNA samples for law enforcement purposes.
6. *Tracing lineage.* This testing is used in determining parentage or other relationships within families.
7. *Newborn screening tests.* These tests are usually performed routinely to check for treatable, harmful genetic conditions or diseases, such as phenylketonuria (see Table 11-1).
8. *Diagnostic testing.* Health care practitioners can use DNA testing to confirm a diagnosis, including confirming or ruling out certain genetic diseases.
9. *Medical treatment determination.* These tests look for changes or variants in the genes that dictate how medications are processed to determine whether or not a certain medication will be effective in a specific patient, set the best dose for a specific patient, or determine for each individual tested if side effects from a medication are likely. While one's genome doesn't change, the test must be performed for each medication prescribed. Similarly, a cancerous tumor's DNA can sometimes be analyzed to determine which treatment will be most effective in stopping its growth. The science involved is called *pharmacogenetics* or *pharmacogenomics,* and it is discussed in more detail in Chapter 13.

GENETIC DISEASES

Permanent changes in DNA, or **mutations,** often cause genetic diseases. Mutations can involve one gene, as in sickle cell anemia, hemophilia, cystic fibrosis, Aicardi syndrome, and Huntington's disease, or they can involve more than one gene. When more than one gene is involved, environmental factors, such as the changes caused by aging, smoking, exposure to environmental toxins, or other factors, may trigger the onset of a genetic disease, as in cases of Alzheimer's disease, diabetes, obesity, and some forms of cancer. Another type of genetic disease can arise from abnormalities in the structure or number of whole chromosomes. Down syndrome, for example, results from an extra copy of chromosome 21.

mutation
A permanent change in DNA.

These mutations occur in nuclear DNA, but diseases can also result from mutations in mitochondrial DNA (mtDNA), which multicelled organisms inherit mostly from mothers. (Mitochondria exist outside cell nuclei but within cell membranes and are responsible for cell metabolism and respiration.) Mutations in mtDNA may contribute to the loss of neurons in Alzheimer's and Parkinson's disease, and have been associated with diabetes, autism, and a variety of metabolic disorders. Health care practitioners should refer any patient who wants to undergo genetic

genetic counselor
An expert in human genetics who is qualified to counsel individuals who may have inherited genes for certain diseases or conditions.

testing to a **genetic counselor.** Genetic counselors can explain test results and help patients deal with difficult questions concerning those results.

As DNA testing has become more widely available and more reliable, use of test results has become an important issue. For example, if a couple learns through amniocentesis that the fetus the mother is carrying will be born with Down syndrome, should they consider aborting the fetus? Should the young man who learns he has the gene for Huntington's disease opt not to marry to avoid taking the chance of passing the gene on to offspring? And will the woman in her twenties who learns she has one of two genes known to predispose her to breast cancer live her life any differently than she would have, had she not been tested?

DNA testing has also raised the issue of privacy. For instance, should employers and health and life insurance companies have access to DNA test results? How can individuals be certain that information about their genetic makeup is not shared with unknown sources?

Clearly, advances in genetics and genetic testing have led to difficult ethical, social, and medical questions for patients and their families and for health care practitioners.

Table 11-1 Genetic Diseases

The National Center for Biotechnology Information maintains a list of genetic diseases and tests at www.ncbi.nlm.nih.gov/gtr/. Tests for thousands of genetic diseases are now available. Some genetic diseases for which reliable tests are available include:

Aarskog syndrome: Linked to the X chromosome and found mostly in males (females may have a milder form); affects height, muscle and skeletal formation, and appearance of the face.

Aicardi syndrome: Found mostly in females; involves a gene on the X chromosome; the corpus callosum, which connects the right and left sides of the brain, is absent. Causes spasms in infants.

Alzheimer's disease: The most frequent cause of dementia in older adults that eventually leads to organ breakdown and death.

Cancer: Especially some types of breast, ovarian, and colon cancer.

Cystic fibrosis: Affects the mucus glands of the lungs, liver, pancreas, and intestines, causing progressive disability due to multisystem failure. There is no cure, and many individuals with the disease die young, often in their twenties and thirties.

Down syndrome: Causes learning disabilities, cognitive impairment, and other physical problems.

Duchenne muscular dystrophy: Causes rapidly worsening muscle weakness; usually appears before age 6.

Elliptocytosis: Red blood cells are abnormally shaped, causing fatigue, shortness of breath, an enlarged spleen in adults and jaundice in infants.

Fragile X syndrome: A rare condition causing learning disabilities and cognitive impairment.

Gaucher's disease: Affects fat metabolism.

Hemochromatosis: An iron storage disorder and the most commonly occurring inherited disease.

Huntington's disease, also called Huntington's chorea: An adult-onset, untreatable, ultimately fatal disease of the brain and nervous system.

Mucopolysaccharidosis: A metabolic disorder causing skeletal deformities and usually cognitive impairment.

Neurofibromatosis: Causes tumors that grow along the body's nerves and under the skin.

Phenylketonuria: A metabolic disorder for which all newborns are tested. It results in cognitive impairment if left untreated.

Sickle cell anemia: A malformation of the red blood cells most often diagnosed in African Americans.

Spinocerebellar ataxia: A rare disorder that eventually destroys the brain's cerebellum.

Tay-Sachs disease: A lipid metabolism disorder that affects some people of Jewish descent. Children with the disease seldom survive childhood.

GENETIC DISCRIMINATION

With the increased ability to identify genetic differences comes increasing concern for the proper use of such information. The term **genetic discrimination** describes the differential treatment of individuals based on their actual or presumed genetic differences.

genetic discrimination
Differential treatment of individuals based on their actual or presumed genetic differences.

Many people fear that participating in genetic research or undergoing genetic testing will cause them to be discriminated against based on their genetics. Such fears may keep patients from volunteering to participate in the research necessary for the development of new tests, therapies, and cures or may cause them to refuse genomics-based clinical tests. To address this, in 2008, the Genetic Information Nondiscrimination Act (GINA) was passed into law, prohibiting discrimination in the workplace and by health insurance issuers. In addition, there are other legal protections against genetic discrimination by employers, issuers of health insurance, and others.

In addition to GINA at the federal level and state laws against genetic discrimination, the Health Insurance Portability and Accountability Act (HIPAA), passed in 1996, prevents health insurers from denying coverage based on genetic information. HIPAA, however, applies only to individuals moving between group health insurance plans.

The Americans with Disabilities Act (ADA) of 1990, discussed in Chapter 10, also offers some protection against genetic discrimination in the workplace. It protects against discrimination those who have a genetic condition or disease, or are regarded as having a disability. Under a 1995 ruling by the Equal Employment Opportunities Commission, the ADA applies to anyone who is discriminated against on the basis of genetic information relating to illness, disease, condition, or other disorders. Furthermore, under the ADA, a person with a disability cannot be denied insurance or be subject to different terms or conditions of insurance based on disability alone, if the disability does not pose increased risks.

A major provision of the Patient Protection and Affordable Care Act of 2010 (referred to as ACA) was to establish "guaranteed issue." That is, insurance issuers must provide coverage for all individuals who request it. The law therefore prohibits issuers of health insurance from discriminating against patients with genetic diseases by refusing coverage because of preexisting conditions. ACA provides additional protections for patients with genetic diseases by establishing that certain health insurance issuers may only vary premiums based on a few specified factors, such as age or geographic area, thereby prohibiting the adjustment of premiums because of medical conditions.

11.3 Genetic Engineering

Our increased body of knowledge about DNA, chromosome structure, and the basis of heredity has allowed scientists to manipulate DNA within the cells of plants, animals, and other organisms to ensure that certain advantageous traits will appear and be passed on and that certain harmful traits are eliminated. This is called **genetic engineering.** Because the chemical composition of DNA is nearly identical throughout the plant and animal kingdoms, genes can often be interchanged among plants and animals to transfer desirable characteristics to different

genetic engineering
Manipulation of DNA within the cells of plants, animals, and other organisms through synthesis, alteration, or repair to ensure that certain harmful traits will be eliminated in offspring and that desirable traits will appear and be passed on.

species. Through this process, for example, genes from a species of Arctic flounder have been added to strawberry plants to make them better able to withstand cold temperatures. Genetic engineering has also created corn and soybean crops that are resistant to insect-borne diseases, "golden" rice with increased beta-carotene content, and bacteria that can devour oil spilled into oceans.

COURT CASE Genetic Information Lawsuit Settled

In January 2014, the U.S. Equal Employment Opportunity Commission (EEOC) announced in a press release that Founders Pavilion, a former Corning, New York, nursing and rehabilitation center, would pay $360,000 to settle a discrimination lawsuit brought by the EEOC.

The EEOC charged that Founders Pavilion requested family medical history as part of its post-offer, preemployment medical exams of applicants. The Genetic Information Nondiscrimination Act, passed by Congress in 2008 and enforced by the EEOC, prevents employers from requesting genetic information or making employment decisions based on genetic information.

The EEOC also alleged that Founders Pavilion fired two employees because they were perceived to be disabled, in violation of the Americans with Disabilities Act. According to the suit, Founders Pavilion also refused to hire or fired three women because they were pregnant, in violation of the Title VII of the Civil Rights Act of 1964 (Title VII).

The EEOC filed suit in the U.S. District Court for the Western District of New York after first attempting to reach a prelitigation settlement through its conciliation process.

As part of a five-year consent decree resolving the suit, Founders Pavilion will provide a fund of $110,400 for distribution to the 138 individuals who were asked for their genetic information. Founders Pavilion will also pay $259,600 to the five individuals who the EEOC alleged were fired or denied hire in violation of the ADA or Title VII.

Source: *EEOC v. Founders Pavilion, Inc.*, 13-CV-01438 EEOC Press Release: www.eeoc.gov/eeoc/newsroom/release/1-13-14.cfm.

LANDMARK COURT CASE Supreme Court Allows Patent for a Live, Human-Made Organism

After genetically engineering a bacterium capable of breaking down crude oil, Ananda Chakrabarty, who worked for General Electric, sought to patent his creation under Title 35 U.S.C. Section 101, which provides patents for people who invent or discover "any" new and useful "manufacture" or "composition of matter." On appeal from an application rejection by a patent examiner, the Patent Office Board of Appeals affirmed the patent rejection, stating that living things are not patentable under Section 101. When this decision was reversed by the Court of Customs and Patent Appeals, Sidney A. Diamond, commissioner of Patents and Trademarks, appealed, and the U.S. Supreme Court agreed to hear the case. The question debated was: Is the creation of a live, human-made organism patentable under Title 35 U.S.C. Section 101?

The Supreme Court said yes. In a 5-to-4 decision, the Court explained that while natural laws, physical phenomena, abstract ideas, or newly discovered minerals are not patentable, a live artificially engineered microorganism is. The creation of a bacterium that is not found anywhere in nature constitutes a patentable "manufacture" or "composition of matter" under Section 101. Moreover, the bacterium's human-made ability to break down crude oil makes it very useful.

Source: *"Diamond v. Chakrabarty." Oyez.* Chicago-Kent College of Law at Illinois Tech, n.d. November 17, 2016 *(www.oyez.org/cases/1979/79-136).*

LANDMARK COURT CASE

Supreme Court Decides the Issue of Patenting Genes

In June 2013, the U.S. Supreme Court decided a case brought by the Association for Molecular Pathology against Myriad Genetics, Inc. Myriad held patents for two of the genes associated with the development of breast cancer: BRCA1 and BRCA2. Ownership of these patents meant that research scientists and sometimes even physicians and their patients had to obtain Myriad's permission and, in most cases, pay fees to do research or testing involving the two genes. In its landmark decision, the Supreme Court ruled that genes cannot be patented because they are "naturally occurring" substances. However, artificial genes may meet requirements for developers to obtain patents.

The decision also emphasized, "[I]t is important to note what is *not* implicated by this decision. First, there are no method claims before this Court. Had Myriad created an innovative method of manipulating genes while searching for the BRCA1 and BRCA2 genes, it could possibly have sought a method patent. But the processes used by Myriad to isolate DNA were well understood and widely used by geneticists at the time of Myriad's patents."

Source: *Association for Molecular Pathology v. Myriad Genetics, Inc.*, 569 U.S. __ (2013).

However beneficial a genetic engineering result may sound, controversy is almost guaranteed when a new project is announced. Objections may be raised on the religious or moral grounds that humans simply should not tamper with the time-honored progression of life as dictated by nature. Or opponents may fear that the process will harm the environment by releasing genetically engineered superspecies that may crowd out naturally occurring species and lead to the eventual disappearance of many original organisms. Critics may also fear that the undisclosed addition of genes to plants or animals ingested by humans can have unforeseen effects. For instance, some fear that genes from peanut plants added to a product might cause harmful reactions in unsuspecting consumers who are allergic to peanuts.

In 2015, a bill was introduced in the U. S. House of Representatives amending the federal Food, Drug, and Cosmetic Act to prohibit the sale of food that has been genetically engineered or contains genetically engineered ingredients unless that information is clearly disclosed. As of mid-2016, the bill had not yet become law, but some food manufacturers were voluntarily certifying on their labels that a food contained no "genetically modified organisms (GMO)."

CLONING

One type of genetic engineering that is rapidly advancing is cloning. **Cloning** describes the processes used to create an exact genetic replica of another cell, tissue, or organism. The **clone** is produced asexually, from a single ancestor, and has the same genetic makeup as the original.

cloning
The process used to create an exact genetic replica of another cell, tissue, or organism.

clone
An organism produced asexually, from a single ancestor, that has the same genetic makeup as the original.

There are three different types of cloning:

1. *Gene cloning,* which produces exact copies of the segments of DNA called genes. There are two main reasons why geneticists want to clone genes. The first reason for cloning genes is to gain information

about the nucleotide sequence of the gene. A second reason is to manipulate a gene, either by altering its DNA sequence or by combining it with new DNA mixtures, which might mean placing the gene inside the DNA of a different organism. Both of these research objectives require having multimillion copies of genes available for study, and cloning is a way to ensure that exact replicas of the genes are produced.

2. *Therapeutic cloning,* which produces copies of embryonic stem cells with the professed purpose of repairing injured or diseased tissue in the human body. **Stem cells** are early embryonic cells and adult cells derived from certain tissues that have the potential to become any type of body cell. **Multipotent stem cells,** such as those found in adult blood-forming tissue, can become only a limited number of types of tissues and cells in the body. **Pluripotent stem cells,** found in embryonic tissue, can become almost all types of tissues and cells. Such cells have shown promise for treating patients with a wide variety of medical problems, such as Parkinson's, Alzheimer's, diabetes, strokes, burns, spinal cord injuries, and other neurological disorders. Most embryos used in stem cell research in the United States are the frozen products of in vitro fertilization that were not used to produce a pregnancy and are destined to be destroyed. Other stem cell cultures are grown specifically for research purposes and are scrutinized through government regulation.

stem cells
Cells that have the potential to become any type of body cell.

multipotent stem cells
Stem cells that can become a limited number of types of tissues and cells in the body.

pluripotent stem cells
Stem cells that can become almost all types of tissues and cells in the body.

3. *Reproductive cloning,* which produces copies of entire animals. The most famous clone was a Scottish sheep named Dolly. Dolly was created in 1996 from a single maternal cell and lived until 2003, when she was put down to prevent further suffering from a progressive lung disease. She had also developed arthritis, leading to speculation that she aged more quickly than normal.

   Scientists have since cloned more sheep, cattle, goats, mice, dogs, cats, monkeys, and pigs. Some lived normal life spans, while others, like Dolly, died young, suffering from conditions usually associated with aging.

   Genetically modified farm animals may be bred to develop a consistent source of prime, low-fat meat and other animal products, and some researchers hope cloning can lead to restoring endangered and extinct species. Animal cloning has also been done with human health and medical objectives in mind. For example, genetically modified mice are used extensively as models of human disease, including obesity, substance abuse, anxiety, cancer, and cardiovascular disease. Researchers may spend years developing a strain of mouse with the exact genetic mutations necessary to model a particular human disorder.

   Another objective of cloning genetically modified animals is to breed strains that can produce substances useful in medicine, such as insulin and growth hormone, or to clone animal tissues and organs for human medical use. For example, because pigs are similar to humans in organ size and other biological aspects, an objective in cloning them is to grow a potential source of organs and tissues for transplanting into human patients—a process called **xenotransplantation.**

xenotransplantation
Transplantation of animal tissues and organs into humans.

Many animal rights proponents object on ethical grounds to using animals in this way. They argue that animals should be allowed to exist in nature without being subjected to experiments for the benefit of humankind. Furthermore, other groups object to introducing animal cells into humans on ethical grounds and on grounds that the animal tissue can harm people.

Objections against animal cloning are sometimes also based on grounds that such experiments could lead to the cloning of humans, a process that is illegal in the United States and 30 other countries. Objections to human cloning based on animal biology and physiology include:

1. To date, animal cloning does not always yield viable offspring, with only one or two healthy animals resulting from approximately every 100 experiments.
2. Not only do most attempts to clone mammals fail, about 30 percent of clones born alive are affected with "large-offspring syndrome" and other debilitating conditions. Large-offspring syndrome occurs primarily in cloned lambs and calves that are the result of embryo manipulation. The process often creates oversized offspring due to deactivation of insulin-like growth factor 2 receptors, which would normally block the growth of cells at a certain point. When these receptors are deactivated, the embryos grow too large. Other symptoms can include enlarged hearts, immature lungs, and damaged kidneys.
3. Scientists do not yet understand the processes involved in reproductive cloning well enough to ensure success, and a large failure rate in human clones is unacceptable.
4. Like Dolly the sheep, many cloned animals have died prematurely from infections and other complications. The same problems would be expected to occur in human cloning.
5. Scientists do not know how cloning could impact mental development. While factors such as intellect and mood may not be important for a cloned cow or mouse, they are crucial for the development of healthy humans.

Ethical questions multiply when human cloning is discussed. Should trial and error over time be allowed when the objective is to create a healthy human baby? Besides the potential for physical problems over numerous tries, even if a viable human is finally produced, how would families handle the supercharged family dynamics that might result? For example, what if a couple divorces after a child has been cloned to resemble one parent? Will the other parent resent the child who looks so much like the divorced spouse? On a broader level, would cloning be reserved only for the wealthy who can afford the process and denied to all those in a society who cannot pay the fee?

Because such ethical questions would be difficult to resolve, most states have laws banning the cloning of humans, but to date, no federal law has been passed. The latest attempt at federal legislation was HR. 3498 the Human Cloning Prohibition Act of 2105, which was still in committee in mid-2016.

gene therapy
The insertion of a normally functioning gene into cells in which an abnormal or absent element of the gene has caused disease.

GENE THERAPY

Gene therapy is rapidly becoming an effective tool for correcting and preventing certain diseases. In fact, therapy for genetic disease is often very similar to therapy for other types of disorders, as in the following cases:

- Special diets can eliminate compounds that are toxic to patients. This applies to such diseases as phenylketonuria and homocystinuria.
- Vitamins or other agents can improve a biochemical pathway and thus reduce toxic levels of a compound. For example, folic acid reduces homocysteine levels in a person who carries the 5,10-methylenetetrahydrofolate reductase polymorphism gene.

Gene therapy may involve replacing a deficiency or blocking an overactive pathway. For instance, a fetus can sometimes be treated by treating the mother (e.g., corticosteroids for congenital virilizing adrenal hypoplasia) or by using in utero (inside the uterus) cellular therapy (e.g., bone marrow transplantation). Similarly, a newborn with a genetic disease may be a candidate for treatment with bone marrow or organ transplantation.

Genetic therapy may also involve the insertion of normal copies of a gene into the cells of persons with a specific genetic disease (this is called somatic gene therapy). Such somatic gene therapy has been undertaken for severe genetic disorders such as adenosine deaminase deficiency, an immunodeficiency that usually results in death during the first few months of life.

Germ-line gene therapy involves the correction of an abnormality in the genes of a sperm or egg but is presently considered an inappropriate way to deal with genetic diseases because of ethical issues, cost, lack of research in humans, lack of knowledge about whether or not changes would be maintained in the growing embryo, and the relative ease of treating the pertinent conditions somatically when needed.

Gene therapy could also involve turning off genes before their harmful properties can be expressed. For example, if the gene for Huntington's disease could be turned off before carriers reached adulthood, theoretically the disease could not develop.

The future of gene therapy is discussed in Chapter 13.

Check Your Progress

6. List five possible uses for genetic testing.
7. The process of manipulating the DNA of organisms to produce desired results is called ______________________.
8. Define *genetic discrimination.*
9. Define *cloning.*
10. Distinguish between multipotent and pluripotent stem cells.
11. What is the foremost objection to human reproductive cloning?
12. How might gene therapy be used to help a person born with a genetic disease?

11.4 Conception and the Beginning of Life

Fortunately, most couples who decide to have a child are able to conceive naturally, and most pregnancies proceed without problems. However, it is estimated that about 10 to 15 percent of reproductive-age couples in the United States will have difficulty conceiving. Of this percentage, either husband or wife will experience **infertility**—that is, the failure to conceive for a period of 12 months or longer due to a deviation from or interruption of the normal structure or function of any reproductive part, organ, or system.

infertility
The failure to conceive for a period of 12 months or longer due to a deviation from or interruption of the normal structure or function of any reproductive part, organ, or system.

INFERTILITY

When couples have reproductive difficulties and consult physicians who specialize in infertility problems, diagnoses are made and appropriate treatment recommended. Several options for infertile couples exist, depending on the type of fertility problem. Here are a few of the most common:

- **In vitro fertilization.** In this process, eggs and sperm are brought together outside the body in a test tube or petri dish. When fertilization takes place, the resulting embryo can then be frozen in liquid nitrogen for future use or implanted in the female uterus for pregnancy to occur.
- **Artificial insemination.** This process involves the mechanical injection of viable semen into the vagina. If a man's sperm cells are used to fertilize his partner's eggs, the process is called **homologous artificial insemination.** If the partner's sperm cells are not viable, a donor's sperm may be used to fertilize the woman's eggs. This is called **heterologous artificial insemination.**
- **Surrogacy.** If a woman cannot carry an embryo to term, the couple may elect to contract with a surrogate mother.

in vitro fertilization
Fertilization that takes place outside a woman's body, literally "in glass," as in a test tube.

artificial insemination
The mechanical injection of viable semen into the vagina.

homologous artificial insemination
The process in which a man's sperm is mechanically injected into a woman's vagina to fertilize her eggs.

heterologous artificial insemination
The process in which donor sperm is mechanically injected into a woman's vagina to fertilize her eggs.

SURROGACY

A **surrogate mother** is a woman who agrees to carry a child to term for a couple, often for a fee. If the surrogate is not genetically related to the embryo, the type of surrogacy is called *gestational* surrogacy. If the surrogate contributes eggs to produce the embryo or is related to either partner in the relationship, the type of surrogacy is called *traditional* surrogacy. (In one much-publicized case in the United States, a woman carried her own grandchild to term for her married daughter who was born without a uterus.) Traditional surrogacy differs from gestational surrogacy in that a traditional surrogate is genetically related to the fetus she carries.

Infertility treatments can cost several thousand dollars, with no guarantee of success. Most insurance plans do not cover expenses for infertility treatments or for contracting with a surrogate mother to bear a child. The law has been slow to catch up with technology, but many states have passed legislation regulating infertility clinics and surrogacy. Health care practitioners dealing with infertility should check state laws for current regulations.

Surrogacy
The process by which a woman becomes pregnant by artificial insemination or surgical implantation of a fertilized egg for the purpose of carrying a fetus to term for another woman..

surrogate mother
A woman who becomes pregnant, usually by artificial insemination or surgical implantation of a fertilized egg, and bears a child for another woman.

LANDMARK COURT CASE

Baby M—First Surrogacy Case

In 1985, a woman signed a contract agreeing to serve as a surrogate for a couple who could not conceive. She was then medically inseminated with the husband's sperm, and a pregnancy resulted. When the child was born in March 1986, the surrogate mother refused to give up the infant. The genetic father sued for violation of the surrogacy contract. The contract specified that the genetic father and his wife held custody and that the surrogate would terminate her parental rights. The trial court, considering the best interests of the child, affirmed the validity of the contract. In March 1987, an appellate court terminated the surrogate mother's parental rights and gave full custody of the then 1-year-old Baby M to her genetic father and his wife. The genetic father's wife legally adopted the baby.

Source: *In re Baby M*, 537 A.2d 1227, 109 N.J. 396 (1988).

LANDMARK COURT CASE

Gestational Surrogacy Contract Held Valid

A married couple was unable to have a child because the wife had undergone a hysterectomy. The wife's ovaries had not been removed, however, and could still produce eggs, so the couple opted for gestational surrogacy. They entered into a surrogacy contract with a woman who agreed to relinquish her parental rights after the child was born in exchange for a $10,000 fee and a paid life insurance policy. The wife's eggs were fertilized in vitro with the husband's sperm, and the resulting embryo was implanted into the surrogate's uterus. While she was still pregnant, the surrogate demanded immediate payment and threatened to not relinquish the child when it was born. The couple who had contracted with the surrogate filed a lawsuit seeking a legal determination that the surrogate had no parental rights to the baby. The surrogate countersued, and the court consolidated the two cases.

A trial court found for the married couple. It determined that the couple was the child's "natural parents" and held that the surrogate had no parental rights to the child. An appellate court and the state supreme court upheld this decision.

Source: *Johnson v. Calvert*, 5 Cal. 4th 84, 851 P.2d 776 (1993).

ADOPTION

Adoption is also an option for those couples who want to raise children. All 50 states have laws regulating adoption. Certain areas of federal law may also affect some aspects of the parent–child relationship established by adoption. For example, the Adoption Assistance and Child Welfare Act of 1980, the Child Abuse Prevention and Treatment and Adoption Reform Act, and the Indian Child Welfare Act all contain provisions that pertain to adoptive parents and their children.

Typically, any adult who shows the desire to be a fit parent may adopt a child. Depending on state law, both married and unmarried couples may adopt, and single people may adopt through a process called single-parent adoption. Some states list special requirements for adoptive parents, such as requiring an adoptive parent to be a specified number of years older than the child. There may also be state requirements concerning residency or the marital state of the prospective parent. Any adult who wishes to adopt will need to check state law before proceeding, and if potential adoptive parents use an adoption agency, they will also have to meet any agency requirements.

Some single individuals or couples may have a more difficult time qualifying as adoptive parents than others. For example, single men, gay singles, and homosexual couples may not specifically be prevented from adopting by state law, but they may have a more difficult time meeting state and agency requirements than married couples would.

All states strive to find placements that meet the best interest of the child, so in some cases, potential adoptive parents may be asked additional questions about lifestyle and why they want to adopt. (See "Best Interest of the Child Concept" for a more thorough explanation of "best interest of the child.")

Generally, couples can adopt a child of a different race. Adoptions of Native American children, however, are governed by the Indian Child Welfare Act, and the act's provisions outline specific rules and procedures that must be followed if the adoption of a Native American child is to be approved.

There are several different types of adoptions, depending on services used and whether or not a blood or marital relationship exists between adoptive parents and children:

- Agency adoptions occur when state-licensed and/or state-regulated public or private adoption agencies place children with adoptive parents. Charities or religious or social service organizations often operate private adoption agencies. Adoption agencies usually place those children who have been orphaned or whose parents have lost or relinquished parental rights through abuse, abandonment, or inability to support.
- Independent or private adoptions are arranged without the involvement of adoption agencies. Potential adoptive parents may hear of a mother who wants to give up her child, or they may advertise in newspapers or on the Internet to find such a mother. At some point in the process, an attorney must be involved to ensure the legality of the adoption. A few states prohibit independent adoptions. In those states where independent adoptions are allowed, they are usually strictly regulated.
- Identified adoptions are those in which adopting parents locate a birth mother or vice versa and then ask an agency to take over the adoption process. Prospective parents who find a birth mother willing to give up her child can bypass the long waiting lists that most agencies maintain for adoptions and can perhaps be better assured that the adoption will proceed in an orderly and legal fashion.
- International adoptions occur when couples adopt children who are citizens of foreign countries. In these procedures, adoptive parents must not only meet requirements of the foreign country where the child resides, they must also meet all U.S. state requirements and U.S. Immigration and Naturalization Service rules for international adoptions.
- Relative adoptions are those in which the child is related to the adoptive parent by blood or marriage. Stepparent and grandparent–grandchildren adoptions fall within this category.

11.5 Rights of Children

Common law has established the rights of parents to make health care decisions for minor children. In some circumstances, under the doctrine of ***parens patriae,*** literally "father of the people," the state may act as the parental authority. This doctrine is the legal principle that grants the

parens patriae
A legal doctrine that gives the state the authority to act in a child's best interest.

state the broad authority to act in the child's *best interest,* sometimes overriding parental decisions, and allows the state to remove abused or neglected children from the custody of offending parents.

BEST INTEREST OF THE CHILD CONCEPT

When alternatives are available for child placement or for determining medical treatment for minor children, the common standard is the "best interest of the child." In other words, which alternative will best safeguard the child's growth, development, and health? This standard is used in child placement situations. It is also used when legal authorities must work with health care practitioners to determine the least harmful and most appropriate treatment for an ailing child.

RIGHTS OF THE NEWBORN

Legally, the legal rights of newborns are the same as those of any other American citizen of any age. For newborns who are severely disabled, however, existing law provides for several treatment options. Under the federal Child Abuse Amendments (42 U.S.C. Section 5106g), if the parents agree, physicians may legally withhold treatment, including food and water, from infants who:

- Are chronically and irreversibly comatose
- Will most certainly die and for whom treatment is considered futile
- Would suffer inhumanely if treatment were provided

Treatment of newborns who are severely disabled raises many ethical questions. Should the federal government intrude into physicians' and parents' decisions with imposed regulations? Is it ever in an infant's "best interest" to die, or should medical treatment be administered regardless of the probable outcome? Is quality of life an issue that can ethically be considered? Who should decide among treatment options for newborns who are disabled if the parents are unwilling or unable to make such decisions?

ABANDONED INFANTS

An unfortunate fact of modern life is that there are too many stories in the news of mothers abandoning their infants shortly after giving birth by leaving them in dumpsters, by the roadside, in public restrooms, and so on, usually out of fear or desperation. As such abandonment numbers have increased, all 50 states have enacted **safe haven laws** that allow a parent to abandon a newborn at a safe location, usually within a specified time limit after birth, and without legal prosecution. State laws vary:

safe haven laws
State laws that allow mothers to abandon newborns to designated safe facilities without penalty.

- In some states, the baby can be handed over to a doctor or police officer, or left at a fire station or hospital.
- Some states do not entirely eliminate prosecution but will allow reduction in charges.
- In some states, the parent can remain anonymous, while in others, he or she must reveal their identity and give a medical history. In some states, medical histories can also be dropped off anonymously.
- Most states place limits on the ages of children who can be abandoned without prosecution for two reasons: To encourage parents determined to abandon their children to do so early, while the

children can receive adequate nutrition and medical care, and to prevent situations that occurred when safe haven laws were new in which parents have abandoned problem children of all ages to the care of the state.

- Most states specify which locations are considered safe havens to prevent parents from leaving infants on the steps of empty churches or in other locations where discovery and emergency care are unavailable.
- Safe haven providers are also required, under most state laws, to take the child into custody, provide medical care as necessary, and inform the abandoning parent, if possible, that he or she is relinquishing the child for adoption. Some state laws also require safe haven providers to try to determine the identity of the nonrelinquishing parent and to attempt to learn family and medical history information.

See www.childwelfare.gov/systemwide/laws_policies/statutes/safehaven.cfm for state-specific information about safe haven laws.

Since safe haven laws went into effect across the country, adoption experts have indicated that the laws have caused some undesirable results:

- If included in the law, a "no hassle" provision, which promises no prosecution for abandonment if the child has not been injured or abused, may discourage mothers from using established adoption and child welfare policies, while encouraging irresponsible and destructive behavior.
- The laws seem to some to be government statements that it's OK to abandon a baby.
- The abandoned children have little hope of learning family medical histories.
- The laws allow one parent to abandon a child, thus stripping the other parent of all rights.

The issue of abandonment also raises many ethical questions for society and for health care practitioners. Is the "safe haven" concept ethical—because prosecution is usually waived for parental abandonment under safe haven laws—or is it a form of child abuse and neglect? Should abandoned infants be eventually returned to the parents who abandoned them, or should such parents be forced to relinquish parental rights? What public health measures might help prevent such events from occurring?

Check Your Progress

13. Define *infertility.*
14. List and define three medical procedures that might be available to infertile couples.
15. Adoptions are regulated primarily by ______________.
16. Name four types of adoptions.
17. Under the federal Child Abuse Amendments, physicians may, with the consent of parents, withhold treatment for those infants who ______________.
18. What are safe haven laws designed to prevent?
19. What are the disadvantages of safe haven laws?

Source: Questions are from Eileen E. Morrison and Beth Furlong, *Health Care Ethics: Critical Issues for the 21st Century,* Jones and Bartlett, 2014, p. 125.

TEENAGERS

While common law has dictated that parents have a right to decide what medical care their young children receive, laws for older children differ from those for newborns. For example, states recognize that some older minors have the capacity to consent to their own medical care. For instance, teenagers considered mature or emancipated minors may give consent for medical treatment.

mature minors
Individuals in their mid- to late teens who, for health care purposes, are considered mature enough to comprehend a physician's recommendations and give informed consent.

Mature minors are individuals in their mid- to late teens who are considered mature enough to comprehend a physician's recommendations and give informed consent. Most states allow mature minors to seek medical treatment without the consent of a parent or guardian in certain critical areas, such as mental health, drug and/or alcohol addiction, treatment for sexually transmitted diseases, pregnancy, and contraceptive services.

emancipated minors
Individuals in their mid- to late teens who legally live outside parents' or guardians' control.

Emancipated minors legally live outside their parents' or guardians' control. A judge may issue an emancipation order at the request of parents or a minor child after certain important factors have been considered:

- Does the minor live at home with parents or other supervising adults, or is he or she living independently? If living at home, does he or she pay for room and board?
- Does the minor have a job, and does he or she spend his or her earnings without parental supervision?
- Does the minor pay his or her own debts?
- Is the minor claimed as a dependent on the parents' tax return?

The court may declare minors emancipated if one or more of the following criteria are met:

- They are self-supporting.
- They are married, provided the marriage is legal. In most states, persons must be at least 16 to marry and those under the age of 18 must have parental consent. Emancipation is not forfeited if the minor divorces or is separated or widowed.
- They are serving in the armed forces.

Emancipated minors do not usually gain all the rights of adults. Some limits, such as the legal age for purchasing alcohol or tobacco products, voting age, mandatory school attendance age (unless married), and other legal age restrictions, still apply.

Minors have the same constitutional rights as adults, including the right to privacy. This is especially relevant for the increasing numbers of adolescents in the United States who are sexually active. Many hesitate to seek birth control or family planning counseling if they must inform or seek consent from their parents.

No state explicitly requires parental involvement for a minor to obtain any of the services listed above. In some states, however, laws leave the decision about whether or not to inform parents that minor sons and daughters have received or are seeking contraceptives, prenatal care, or treatment for sexually transmitted diseases to the discretion of the treating physician, based on the best interest of the minor.

LANDMARK COURT CASE

Judge Rules That Minor May Consent to Her Own Medical Treatment

Nancy, a 17-year-old Kansas girl, gave permission for a doctor to transplant some skin from her wrist to her finger. Her mother later sued on Nancy's behalf, on the grounds that Nancy was a minor.

Nancy's mother had been hospitalized for major surgery. After the operation, Nancy accompanied her mother to her hospital room. A nurse asked Nancy to wait in the hallway. She didn't notice that Nancy's hand was resting on the wall near the door jamb, with her right ring finger in the space between the door and the jamb. As the nurse closed the door, Nancy cried out in pain. The door had closed on her finger, severing the tip.

Nancy was taken to the emergency room, where a doctor decided to graft a small piece of skin from Nancy's wrist over the raw tip of her finger. Nancy's mother was still recovering from her surgery, and it would be hours before she could give consent for her daughter's treatment. Nancy's parents were divorced, and her father lived in another city. To spare Nancy a long, uncomfortable wait, the emergency room physician called the girl's family physician and received his agreement that he should treat Nancy.

When Nancy's mother recovered, she sued the hospital, claiming that the nurse had been negligent in causing her daughter's injury and that the doctor had not obtained proper consent to treat her minor daughter.

The nurse was not found negligent. Regarding the question of consent, the Kansas Supreme Court ruled that Nancy "was of sufficient age and maturity to know and understand the nature and consequences of the 'pinch graft' utilized in the repair of her finger."

Source: *Younts v. St. Francis Hosp. and School of Nursing*, 205 Kan. 292, 469 P.2d 330, 338 (1970).

In addition to the ability to consent to these specific services, laws in some states give minors the right to consent to general medical and surgical care under some circumstances, such as being a parent themselves, being pregnant, or reaching a certain age.

Several states also allow minors who are parents to consent to medical care for their children. In many states, mothers who are minors may also legally place their children up for adoption without the consent or knowledge of the mothers' parents.

In many states, minors seeking an abortion must involve at least one parent in the decision. This means that teenagers who do not tell their parents about a pregnancy must either travel out of state or obtain approval from a judge—a process known as *judicial bypass*—to obtain an abortion. Currently, the trend is toward state and federal legislation making it increasingly difficult for minors to obtain an abortion without parental involvement.

For exact legal restrictions regarding minors, health care practitioners should check statutes in the states where they practice.

In certain cases, the legal right of a minor to decline medical treatment has been upheld.

COURT CASE Minor Appeals for Judicial Bypass to Obtain an Abortion

A 17-year-old high school senior, called "A. V. P." in her lawsuit, asked the court in her state to issue an order authorizing her to have an abortion without parental approval or notification. Her reasons were that her mother had banished her older sister from their home when she became pregnant, indicating that her mother would also banish her. Furthermore, she had received a college scholarship before her pregnancy that she would probably lose because she would have to forego college to support herself and her child. Additionally, A. V. P. said the father of her child severed their relationship upon learning of her pregnancy and would not help her support a child. She also told the court that she did not think she was emotionally or financially ready to care for a child and would not consider adoption because she had heard tales of adopted children being abused.

The court found that A. V. P. "presented herself as a responsible and mature young lady for her age" but denied her petition for an abortion without parental approval or notification because "[W]e believe that A. V. P. would benefit from consulting with her mother . . . and that this decision is too important to be made without the knowledge and advice of A. V. P.'s mother. . . ."

Source: State in Interest of A.V.P., 108 So.3d. 1204 (La. Ct. App. 2013).

COURT CASE Life-Saving Medical Treatment—Can A Minor Refuse Treatment?

In September 2014, a 17-year-old girl named Cassandra was diagnosed with Hodgkin's lymphoma. Cassandra did not want to undergo chemotherapy because she viewed the medicine as a poison. Along with her mother, Cassandra skipped several appointments with the oncologist. The odds of recovery from Hodgkin's lymphoma treated with a full course of chemotherapy are 80 to 85 percent. Her mother indicated that she supported Cassandra's decision. Neither Cassandra nor her mother cited religious reasons for refusing the treatment. The only reason Cassandra expressed for not having chemotherapy was that she did not want any poison in her system.

The Department of Children and Families (DCF) investigated, using information provided by Cassandra's doctors. Based on investigation findings, a trial court granted DCF temporary custody of Cassandra. An injunction was sought by the family's attorneys, but the court denied their request.

According to court documents, the teen started treatment in November but ran away. Under a second court order, Cassandra was removed from her home in December 2014. Without treatment, the doctors said, there was a near certainty of death within 2 years.

In early January 2015, the Connecticut Supreme Court determined Cassandra was not mature enough to make an informed decision and should continue to receive chemotherapy.

Cassandra was confined to a room at Connecticut Children's Medical Center with a staffer posted at the door to keep her from leaving. She was also not allowed a phone or other communication opportunities. She left the hospital in late April, reportedly cancer free.

According to the American Civil Liberties Union of Connecticut, which filed an amicus brief supporting the mature minor doctrine in Cassandra's case, six other states—Illinois, Maine, Tennessee, West Virginia, Michigan, and Massachusetts—and the District of Columbia have held or suggested that mature minors, like other competent people, have the right to consent to or forego medical treatment. Texas was the only state to reject the mature minor doctrine.

Source: In Re Cassandra C.* (SC 19426) Rogers, C. J., and Palmer, Zarella, Eveleigh, McDonald, Espinosa and Robinson, Js. Argued January 8—officially released January 8, 2015**

Check Your Progress

20. Define the term *mature minor.*
21. Name three criteria that may be considered to determine if a minor is to be declared emancipated.
22. What effect do the previous designations *mature minor* and *emancipated minor* have on a minor's health care decisions?
23. In what treatment areas are minors most likely to make their own health care decisions?

Chapter Summary

Learning Outcome	Summary
LO 11.1 Discuss family history as a predictor of disease risk.	Why does family history predict disease risk? • Because of what we now know about genetics and heredity How does the term *genetics* differ from the term *heredity?* • Genetics is the science that accounts for natural differences and resemblances among organisms related by descent. • Heredity is the process by which organisms pass on genetic traits to their offspring. What terms, integral to the study of genetics, are defined in this chapter? • DNA—deoxyribonucleic acid: The combination of proteins, called nucleotides, that is arranged to make up an organism's chromosomes • Chromosome: A microscopic structure found within the nucleus of all living cells that carries genes responsible for the organism's characteristics • Gene: A tiny segment of DNA that holds the formula for making a specific enzyme or protein • Genome: All the DNA in an organism, including its genes What is the Human Genome Project? • A scientific project funded by the U.S. government, begun in 1990 and successfully completed in 2000, for the purpose of mapping all of a human's genes.

LO 11.2 Demonstrate appropriate uses for DNA testing, and explain how such tests might lead to genetic discrimination.	What is DNA testing?
	• Testing one's DNA to discover one's genetic makeup
	What are the different types of DNA testing explained in this chapter?
	• Predictive
	• Carrier
	• Prenatal
	    • Amniocentesis—testing a sample of amniotic fluid for genetic or other conditions in a developing fetus—is a common prenatal test
	    • Chorionic villus sampling
	    • Maternal blood tests
	• Preimplantation
	• Forensic
	• Tracing lineage
	• Newborn screening
	• Diagnostic
	    • Medical treatment determination
	What is a mutation?
	• A permanent change in DNA
	What does a genetic counselor do?
	• Genetic counselors are qualified to counsel individuals before and after genetic testing.
	What is genetic discrimination?
	• Genetic discrimination is different treatment of individuals based on actual or presumed genetic differences.
	What federal laws are in place to protect Americans against genetic discrimination in health insurance and employment?
	• Genetic Information Nondiscrimination Act (GINA) of 2008
	• Health Insurance Portability and Accountability Act (HIPAA)
	• Americans with Disabilities Act (ADA)
	• Patient Protection and Affordable Care Act (ACA) of 2010

LO 11.3 Define *genetic engineering,* and explain why cloning and stem cell research are controversial issues.	What is genetic engineering?
	• Genetic engineering is the manipulation of DNA within an organism's cells through synthesis, alteration, or repair to ensure that certain harmful traits will be eliminated in offspring and that desirable traits will appear and be passed on.
	What is a clone?
	• An organism produced asexually, usually from a single cell of the parent.
	What is xenotransplantation?
	• Transplantation of animal tissues and organs into humans
	What are stem cells?
	• Cells that can become another type of body cell
	  • Multipotent: Adult cells that can become a limited number of types of tissues and cells
	  • Pluripotent: Embryonic cells that can become almost all types of tissues and cells
	What is gene therapy?
	• Treatment of harmful genetic diseases or traits by eliminating or modifying the harmful gene

LO 11.4 Explain three possible remedies for couples experiencing infertility problems.	What is infertility?
	• The failure to conceive for a period of 12 months or longer due to a deviation from or interruption of the normal structure or function of any reproductive part, organ, or system.
	What alternatives are available for infertile couples who want to become parents?
	• In vitro fertilization (IVF)
	• Artificial insemination
	  • Homologous: partner's sperm and woman's eggs
	  • Heterologous: donor sperm and woman's eggs
	• Surrogacy
	• Adoption

LO 11.5 List those laws affecting health care that pertain especially to children's rights.	Under what doctrine may the state act as a child's parental authority?
	• *Parens patriae*
	  • Best interest of the child concept
	When may physicians, with the parents' consent, legally withhold treatment and nourishment from a newborn who is severely disabled?
	• If the child is chronically and irreversibly comatose
	• If the child will most certainly die and treatment is considered futile
	• If the child would suffer inhumanely if treatment were provided
	What are safe haven laws?
	• Laws that allow mothers to abandon newborns to designated safe facilities without penalty
	How do mature minors differ from emancipated minors?
	• Mature minors: Individuals in mid- to late teens who are considered mature enough to comprehend a physician's instructions and give informed consent
	• Emancipated minors: Individuals in mid- to late teens who legally live outside parental or guardian control, usually through judicial decree, as long as the minor is
	  • Self-supporting
	  • Legally married
	  • Serving in the armed forces

Chapter 11 Review

Applying Knowledge

LO 11.1

1. Define *genetics.*
2. Define *DNA.*
3. *Heredity* is best defined as ________________________.
4. What is a *genome?*
5. Name two goals of the Human Genome Project.

LO 11.2

6. Susan's father developed Huntington's disease when she was 28. She is healthy but wants to be tested to see if she has the gene to develop the disease. What type of genetic testing will she have?
   a. Predictive genetic testing
   b. Diagnostic genetic testing
   c. Carrier genetic testing
   d. Preimplantation genetic testing
7. A permanent change in DNA is called a
   a. Gene
   b. Chromosome
   c. Mutation
   d. Genome
8. Which of the following is the least invasive and least risky test to determine if harmful genes are present in a fetus?
   a. Amniocentesis
   b. Maternal blood test
   c. Chorionic villus sampling
   d. Carrier DNA testing
9. In which of the following situations might DNA testing be indicated?
   a. A man involved in a paternity suit
   b. Parents who suspect they brought the wrong baby home from the hospital
   c. A woman who is a suspect in a murder
   d. All of these
10. *Genetic discrimination* is best described as
    a. A government-sponsored project
    b. A form of favoritism in employment
    c. Differential treatment of individuals based on their actual or presumed genetic differences
    d. None of these

LO 11.3 Match each definition with the correct term by writing the letter in the space provided.

_____ 11. An experimental treatment for hereditary diseases

_____ 12. The process that produced Dolly the sheep

_____ 13. Specialized cells considered most valuable for purposes of genetic manipulation

_____ 14. Those specialized cells that can become almost any kind of cell

_____ 15. Those cells that can become only one type of body cell

a. Multipotent

b. Stem cells

c. Gene therapy

d. Cloning

e. Pluripotent

LO 11.4

16. *Artificial insemination* may be an acceptable remedy for

a. Pregnancy

b. Infertility

c. Surrogacy

d. Cloning

17. Which of the following best defines *in vitro fertilization?*

a. The union of egg and sperm

b. The fusion of egg and cell nucleus

c. Fertilization taking place outside a woman's body

d. Cloning

18. Which of the following best defines *surrogacy?*

a. A woman bears a child for another woman.

b. A woman is artificially inseminated.

c. Fertilization takes place outside a woman's body.

d. None of these

LO 11.5 Match each definition with the correct term by writing the letter in the space provided.

_____ 19. The government serves as a child's parent.

_____ 20. The common standard when the government makes decisions for minor children.

_____ 21. Federal regulations concerning newborns who are severely disabled take their authority from which federal regulation?

_____ 22. State laws that allow a parent to abandon newborns to designated safe locations.

_____ 23. In the past, this has dictated that parents have a right to decide what medical care children receive.

a. Civil Rights Act

b. *Parens patriae*

c. Safe haven laws

d. Best interest of the child

e. Common law

f. Child Abuse Amendments

24. In most states, which of the following age groups can receive some types of medical care without parental permission?

a. Mature minors

b. Minors over age 14

c. Minors under age 18

d. None of these

25. Minors may be declared emancipated only if they
    a. Go to court and request emancipation
    b. Receive parental permission to request emancipation
    c. Are self-supporting
    d. None of these
26. Once declared emancipated, a minor can lose that status if he or she
    a. Was married but divorces
    b. Was in the military but is discharged
    c. Was self-supporting but loses a job
    d. None of these
27. A physician or other health care practitioner who treats a minor in a non emergency situation, without parental consent, risks being charged with
    a. Kidnapping
    b. Assault and/or battery
    c. Violating the Civil Rights Act
    d. No charges can ever be made

Ethics Issues The Beginning of Life and Childhood

Use your critical thinking skills to answer the questions that follow each ethics issue.

Ethics ISSUE 1:

A 56-year-old widowed woman is living alone but has always wanted to have a baby. She has read about reproductive technology and the methods used to help women conceive, and she formulates a plan and contacts a local for-profit fertility clinic. At the clinic, the woman tells her fertility doctor about her longing to have a baby. She says she realizes her eggs may be too old for her to conceive, so she suggests that donor eggs and donor sperm be used, but she wants to gestate the embryo herself, with the help of hormone treatments. She is financially secure and can pay cash for all treatments. Her plan for raising the child includes naming a 39-year-old nephew and his wife as parents if her child should become orphaned. She produces a letter of consent from her nephew and says she will draw up a will leaving her money to a trust fund for her child, to be administered by his adoptive parents if she does not survive to raise the child herself.

Discussion Questions

28. Because most women do not have their motives examined before they become pregnant, should the clinic consider the woman's motives and her plan before deciding to help her?
29. What unique risks do you think might affect this woman's pregnancy and the birth of her child, and should the clinic turn her down because of these risks?

Ethics ISSUE 2:

The ethics involved in using human embryos for cloning research are complicated. Some scientists claim a moral obligation to pursue such research, with the goal of creating compatible tissue for transplants or discovering genetic information that might cure presently incurable diseases. Other scientists see such research as morally wrong.

Discussion Questions

30. Do you think scientists have an ethical obligation to present all sides of the issue of cloning research to keep members of the public informed?
31. In your opinion, if cloning humans becomes possible, should autonomy play a role? If so, how?
32. If humans could be cloned, should their status in society be the same as noncloned humans?

Source: Questions are from Eileen E. Morrison and Beth Furlong, *Health Care Ethics: Critical Issues for the 21st Century,* Jones and Bartlett, 2014, p. 125.

Ethics ISSUE 3:

Predictive genetic testing is offered to asymptomatic adults even when there is no effective treatment. Testing of young people in similar circumstances is controversial, and guidelines recommend against it. Most young people seeking genetic testing want to know (or their parents want to know) if they have a genetic predisposition to develop Huntington's disease.

Discussion Questions

33. In your opinion, should immature young people—say under the age of 14—be genetically tested for adult-onset diseases that have no effective treatment or cure? Explain your answer.
34. Should mature young people who express a genuine desire to know be genetically tested for Huntington's disease or any other adult-onset disease for which there is no effective treatment? Explain your answer.

Case Studies

Use your critical thinking skills to answer the questions that follow each case study.

LO 11.1

All 50 states now have safe haven laws that allow mothers to leave unwanted newborns (usually up to the age of 72 hours) to the care of a safe haven provider. Such an act relieves the mother of any criminal liability but also relieves her of her parental rights to the child. In some states, the mother may be required to provide her name and family history (although some states will guarantee this information remains confidential). Note that mothers will forfeit their rights to anonymity and criminal liability if they have abused or otherwise neglected the child up to the time of abandonment. Mothers also have the right to be informed by safe haven staff that by surrendering the child, they are releasing the child for adoption and that they have the right to petition the court in the appropriate state (within a set time period, such as 28 days) to regain custody.

In most states, a child-placement agency must make "reasonable efforts" to identify and locate the nonrelinquishing parent (typically, the father) by posting notice in a publication such as a newspaper in the county where the child was surrendered.

Source: http://family.findlaw.com/adoption/safe-haven-laws.html.

35. What ethical questions are raised by safe haven laws?
36. In your opinion, are fathers' rights adequately served, both legally and ethically, by safe haven laws?

LO 11.4

As reproductive technology advanced, headlines announcing "Couple Battles over Frozen Embryos" became more and more commonplace. For example, in the 1980s, a man went to court and succeeded in preventing his ex-wife from using their frozen embryos to become pregnant. He maintained that after he and his wife had divorced, he no longer wanted to become a parent and should not be forced to do so against his will.

In 1998, a divorced woman in New Jersey won a legal battle with her ex-husband over custody of seven frozen embryos the couple had created in vitro while still married. The wife wanted to have the embryos destroyed, while the ex-husband argued his right to adopt his own embryos to be implanted in a future partner or donated to an infertile couple.

And in 2016, a famous actress was sued by a right to life group who wished to obtain her frozen embryos that were part of a divorce battle.

37. In your opinion, should frozen embryos be considered property to be awarded during a divorce? Why or why not?
38. Should a man who loses custody of frozen embryos in a lawsuit be responsible for child support if his ex-wife is implanted with the embryos and becomes pregnant at a later date? Explain your answer.
39. Should the husband or wife who wins custody of frozen embryos be allowed to destroy them, against the wishes of the ex-husband or ex-wife? Why or why not?

Internet Activities

LO 11.3 and LO 11.5

Complete the activities and answer the questions that follow.

40. Visit the Web site for the Human Cloning Prohibition Act of 2015 at www.congress.gov/bill/114th-congress/house-bill/3498/text. What is the current status of this bill? Has human cloning been in the news recently? If so, how?
41. Visit the Web site for the Genetically Engineered Food Right-to-Know Act at www.congress.gov/bill/114th-congress/house-bill/913. What is the current status of this bill? Have genetically engineered foods been in the news lately? If so, how?
42. Use the search terms [Your State] and "safe haven laws" to determine the law in your state. Are safe havens defined? Is an age limit designated for abandoned infants? Does the law specify that reasonable attempts will be made to find fathers?

Resources

LO 11.1

Genetics: https://ghr.nlm.nih.gov/gene/APOE

Nucleotide: www.ncbi.nlm.nih.gov/nuccore

Human Genome Project: www.genome.gov/10001772/all-about-the--human-genome-project-hgp/

LO 11.2

Genetic testing: www.ncbi.nlm.nih.gov/gtr/

Genetic discrimination: www.genome.gov/10002077/genetic-discrimination/

LO 11.3

Cloning: https://medlineplus.gov/cloning.html

www.genome.gov/25020028/cloning-fact-sheet/

Human Cloning Prohibition Act: www.congress.gov/bill/114th-congress/house-bill/3498/text

Genetically Engineered Food Right-to-Know Act: www.congress.gov/bill/114th-congress/house-bill/913

www.fda.gov/Food/GuidanceRegulation/GuidanceDocumentsRegulatoryInformation/LabelingNutrition/ucm059098.htm

LO 11.5

http://family.findlaw.com/adoption/safe-haven-laws.html

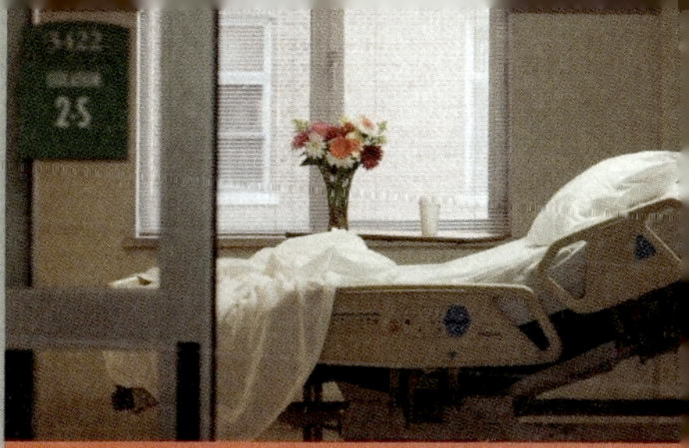

©David Sacks/Getty Images

12

Death and Dying

LEARNING OUTCOMES

After studying this chapter, you should be able to:

LO 12.1 Summarize attitudes toward death and criteria for determining death.

LO 12.2 Describe the legal documents used in end-of-life decisions.

LO 12.3 Identify health care services for terminally ill patients.

LO 12.4 Describe the right-to-die movement.

LO 12.5 Identify the major features of organ donation in the United States.

LO 12.6 List the various stages of grief.

Key Terms

active euthanasia
advance directives
brain death
coma
curative care
do-not-resuscitate (DNR) order
durable power of attorney
health care power of attorney
hospice
involuntary euthanasia
living will
National Organ Transplant Act
palliative care
passive euthanasia
Patient Self-Determination Act
persistent vegetative state (PVS)
terminally ill
Uniform Anatomical Gift Act
Uniform Determination of Death Act
Uniform Rights of the Terminally Ill Act
voluntary euthanasia

FROM THE PERSPECTIVE OF. . .

ANGELA HAS BEEN A REGISTERED NURSE FOR 22 YEARS. Just as some hospital nurses are drawn to surgery, the emergency room, or the intensive care unit, Angela prefers hospice and palliative care. "Broadly speaking," Angela explains, "medicine is about repairing, extending, and medicating, while end-of-life care is more about the patient as an individual, about basic human needs. In addition, it isn't just the patient you are caring for; you are caring for the entire family group—everybody needs you.

"We live in a time when death has been removed from family and home for the most part," Angela continues, "and people generally have less understanding of the process than a hundred years ago. . . . The family most often feels helpless and confused. The hospice nurse is able to help not just the patient but the family, too, through a sad and often frightening time."

Sometimes family members are hesitant about approaching a dying loved one. For example, Angela remembers a situation where the mother of two siblings in their thirties was dying. "When I arrived, they were practically plastered against the walls of the room, clearly unsure of what they should be doing." Angela encouraged the two family members to come to their mother's bedside and comfort her. "The son pulled a chair to the side of the bed and held his mother's hand. The daughter climbed onto the bed and cradled her mother. . . . I like to think that because I urged them to take a more active part in her passing that they found comfort after their mother was gone."

Angela also recalls a patient in his eighties whose 32 family members joined him in his hospice room. "It was almost a living wake. They talked for hours about his life and the experiences they had each shared with him. They laughed and they cried, and it was wonderful. This sharing in their loved one's death was a beautiful experience for those left behind, and I hope it helped him in some way as well."

From Angela's perspective as a hospice nurse, the end of a life is a time when family members can come together to comfort their dying loved one and one another. She sees her job as a facilitator for this natural process.

From the perspective of the individual who is dying, the nearness of family members is comforting, as well as the presence of a nurse who is not uncomfortable with end-of-life issues.

From the perspective of surviving family members, Angela has heard many times that her attitude—don't be afraid to comfort your loved one—gave them the courage to participate in the process and comforted them after the death occurred.

12.1 Attitudes toward Death and the Determination of Death

ATTITUDES TOWARD DEATH AND DYING

Prior to the twentieth century, death was an intimate experience for most families. Antibiotics and chemotherapies had not yet been discovered; genetically engineered drugs, organ transplantation, and life-support machines were still science fiction; and infectious diseases periodically decimated populations. Nearly every husband and wife, mother and father, brother and sister had lost a loved one. Loved ones customarily died at home, surrounded by family members who bade them good-bye and then mourned their passing with funeral rituals and rites, including the following:

- Black has long been worn by undertakers, mourners, and pallbearers to show grief. In ancient times, it was also used as a disguise to protect against malevolent spirits that might be lurking nearby.
- An early custom for mourners was to go barefoot and to wear sack-cloth and ashes. This was said to discourage the dead from becoming envious as they might be if mourners appeared at funerals wearing new clothes and shoes.
- Pagan tribes began the custom of covering the face of the deceased with a sheet because they believed that the spirit of the deceased escaped through the mouth. They often held the mouth and nose of a sick person shut, hoping to retain the spirit and thus delay death.
- In earlier times, traffic was halted for a funeral procession because any delay in transporting a soul might turn it into a restless ghost, reluctant to pass over into the next world.
- Wakes held today come from the ancient custom of keeping watch over the deceased, hoping that life would return. In England, the dead were always carried out of the house feet first; otherwise, their spirits might look back into the house and beckon family members to come with them.
- Pagan beliefs concerning funeral wreaths held that the circle formed by the wreath would keep the dead person's spirit within bounds.
- The firing of a rifle volley over the deceased is similar to the tribal practice of throwing spears into the air to ward off spirits hovering over the deceased.
- In the past, holy water was sprinkled on the body to protect it from demons.

By the late twentieth century, individuals were more likely to die in the hospital, at least in the Western world. Once admitted to hospitals, the dying were isolated from family members and surrounded by machines designed to prolong life as long as possible. Consequently, modern technology has effectively hidden death from view, but in so doing, it has also made the end of life a fearful prospect.

Technology in the twenty-first century has allowed patients to prolong their lives. Prescription drugs alleviate pain and may also be used to painlessly end patients' lives. Artificial respirators allow physicians to prolong life, often for substantial periods. Targeted treatments are extending life but not necessarily the quality of life. According to research done by the Pew Research Center in 2013, approximately 31 percent of Americans believe that everything possible should be done to prolong life, regardless of the circumstances. In 1990, only about 15 percent of the American public believed that everything possible should be done to save the life of the patient in all circumstances (see Figure 12-1).

About a third of those people surveyed indicated that regardless of the pain, everything possible should be done in end-of-life treatment (see Figure 12-2).

Attitudes toward death and dying vary with individuals, of course, but as each of us ages, we will likely begin to think of our own mortality and

FIGURE 12-1 Allowing One to Die

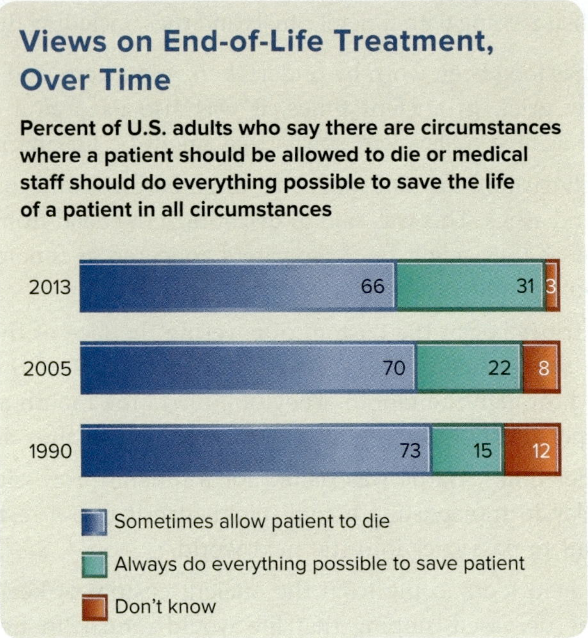

Source: PEW Research Center.

FIGURE 12-2 Preferences for Treatment at End-of-Life

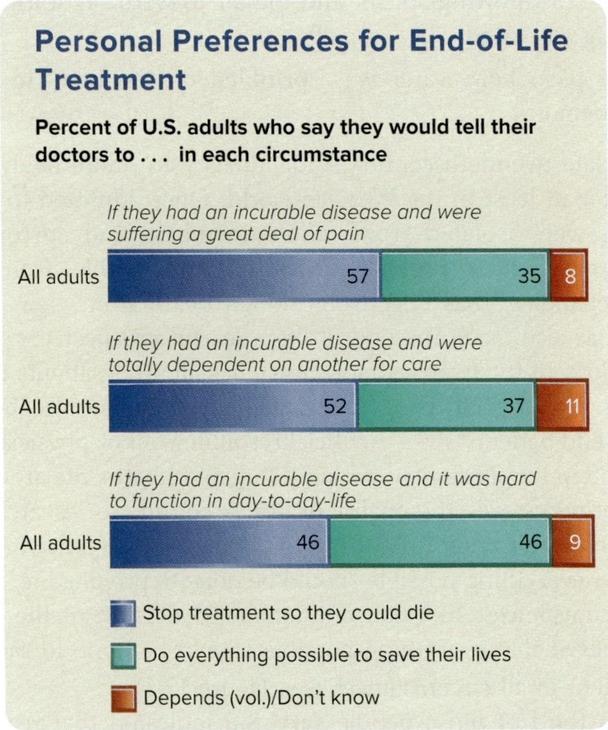

Source: www.pewforum.org/2013/11/21/views-on-end-of-life-medical-treatments/#an-aging-america-with-limited-attention-to-preparation-for-dying.

perhaps to wonder how the end will come. Will I die alone in an impersonal, clinical hospital environment? Will my health care providers be so committed to preserving life that they delay my dying to an irrational degree? Will I suffer in pain? Will I feel a sense of tasks left unfinished and goals left unrealized, or will I experience a peaceful letting go?

Because the fears associated with death and dying are universal, health care practitioners should evaluate their own attitudes to effectively and compassionately respond to dying patients and their families.

DETERMINATION OF DEATH

Modern medical technology and life-support equipment may keep a person's body "alive"—the heart may beat and blood may circulate—long after the brain ceases to function. This makes it difficult in some cases to determine the moment when death actually occurs. For this reason, in 1981, a **Uniform Determination of Death Act** was proposed by the President's Commission for the Study of Ethical Problems in Medicine and Biomedical Research working in cooperation with the American Bar Association, the American Medical Association, and the National Conference of Commissioners on Uniform State Laws. The National Conference of Commissioners on Uniform State Laws has no legislative authority. Acts that the commissioners propose must still be approved by state legislatures, and that is sometimes difficult to accomplish. States have their own criteria for determining when death actually occurs, but most have adopted the act's definition of **brain death** as a means of determining when death actually occurs:

Uniform Determination of Death Act
A proposal that established uniform guidelines for determining when death has occurred.

brain death
Final cessation of bodily activity, used to determine when death actually occurs; circulatory and respiratory functions have irreversibly ceased, and the entire brain (including the brain stem) has irreversibly ceased to function.

- Circulatory and respiratory functions have irreversibly ceased.
- The entire brain, including the brain stem, has irreversibly ceased to function.

When the brain is injured or shuts down due to lack of oxygen, a patient may appear near death when, in fact, he or she is in a **coma**, which is a condition of deep stupor from which a patient cannot be roused by external stimuli. Patients can and do recover from comas, as opposed to a persistent vegetative state. A **persistent vegetative state (PVS)** exists as a result of severe mental impairment, characterized by irreversible cessation of the higher functions of the brain, most often caused by damage to the cerebral cortex. In a PVS, only involuntary bodily functions are present, and there exists no reasonable expectation of regaining significant mental function.

coma
A condition of deep stupor from which the patient cannot be roused by external stimuli.

persistent vegetative state (PVS)
Severe mental impairment characterized by irreversible cessation of the higher functions of the brain, most often caused by damage to the cerebral cortex.

Before pronouncing an unresponsive and unconscious patient dead, physicians may perform a series of tests to determine whether death has occurred. Death is indicated if the following signs are present. The patient:

- Cannot breathe without assistance
- Has no coughing or gagging reflex
- Has no pupil response to light
- Has no blinking reflex when the cornea is touched
- Has no grimace reflex when the head is rotated or ears are flushed with ice water
- Has no response to pain

Today, the declaration of death occurs only when the last signs of brain and respiratory activity are gone. (An electroencephalogram, nuclear scan, or cerebral angiogram may be administered to test for brain activity.) Technically, death results from lack of oxygen. When deprived of oxygen, cells cannot maintain metabolic function and soon begin to deteriorate.

AUTOPSIES

After a patient is declared dead, family members (next of kin) may be asked to consent to an autopsy. An autopsy is a postmortem examination to determine cause of death and/or to obtain physiological evidence when necessary. Autopsies performed in hospitals may confirm or correct clinical diagnoses, thus providing a measure of quality assurance. Autopsy results can also highlight those cases in which diagnoses tend to be incorrect or treatments tend to be ineffective, thereby adding to scientific knowledge and revealing areas that need further study. In cases of suspicious deaths, autopsy results can provide information to help law enforcement authorities, such as cause and time of death. (Legal requirements concerning autopsies are discussed in Chapter 9.)

While autopsies must be performed in cases in which the death is suspicious or due to homicide, the number of autopsies performed in all other deaths each year has steadily declined. One reason that fewer autopsies are performed today is cost—insurance companies and government health care programs usually do not pay for autopsies. (However, when patients die in hospitals, often an autopsy can be performed free of charge.) Some clinicians argue that technological advances have made clinical diagnoses more accurate, so that postmortem diagnoses are less essential. Another reason for the decline in autopsies is that in many smaller hospitals, pathologists are not readily available.

Furthermore, even though autopsies can yield information that may clarify causes of death, reveal genetic disease that runs in families, or reassure survivors that their loved ones could not have been saved, when an autopsy is not mandated by law, family members are often reluctant to give consent. They may feel that their loved one has "suffered enough," that the physician already knows the cause of death, or that the procedure would interfere with viewing of the body during funeral rites. Health care practitioners may believe that these perceptions of autopsies are inaccurate, but they must remain sensitive to the beliefs and emotions of surviving family members.

Check Your Progress

1. Briefly explain how attitudes toward death and dying in the United States have changed over the years.
2. The ____________, while not a law, was proposed as a universal means of determining when death actually occurs.
3. Distinguish between *coma* and *persistent vegetative state.*
4. Define *brain death.*
5. Name six signs for which physicians may test that indicate death has occurred.
6. Identify at least one reason that autopsies have steadily declined.

12.2 Legal Documents for Terminally Ill Patients

PLANNING AHEAD

In today's health care environment, individuals are well advised to be prepared for the time when they or their legal representatives may have to make decisions about medical treatment, including the use of life-sustaining measures. To address this concern, the federal **Patient Self-Determination Act** was passed in 1990 and took effect December 1, 1991. The act requires hospitals and other health care providers to provide written information to patients regarding their rights under state law to make medical decisions and execute **advance directives.** (Advance directives include the living will, durable power of attorney, and health care power of attorney.) The act also provides that:

- Health care providers will document in the patient's medical record whether he or she has executed an advance directive.
- Providers may not discriminate against an individual based on whether or not he or she has executed an advance directive.
- Providers must comply with state laws respecting advance directives.
- Providers must have a policy for educating staff and the community regarding advance directives.

Congress's action in passing this law was due, in large part, to the *Nancy Cruzan* case, decided by the U.S. Supreme Court in June 1990.

As a result of the Patient Self-Determination Act, patients are encouraged to execute living wills or durable powers of attorney while still able to do so and before life-sustaining measures become necessary for life to continue.

Patient Self-Determination Act
A federal law passed in 1990 that requires hospitals and other health care providers to provide written information to patients regarding their rights under state law to make medical decisions and execute advance directives.

advance directive
A written statement of a person's wishes regarding medical treatment, often including a living will or power of attorney or both. These documents are done to make sure the patient's wishes are carried out should the person be unable to communicate them to a doctor.

LIVING WILL

A **living will** directly provides instructions to physicians, hospitals, and other health care providers involved in a patient's treatment. It may detail circumstances under which treatment should be discontinued, such as coma, brain death, or a terminal condition. It may also detail which treatments or medications to suspend (for example, invasive surgery, artificial nutrition or hydration, and measures that serve no purpose except to delay death) and which to maintain (for example, kidney dialysis and drugs for pain). In addition, it may list which "heroic measures" (for example, emergency surgery and cardiopulmonary resuscitation) should and should not be used. A living will may also indicate preferences regarding organ donation, autopsy, and alternative treatments. Living wills may designate an agent to carry out these wishes if the patient is incapable of making decisions.

All 50 states accept the validity of living wills, although they also specify various requirements that must be met. Standard state forms may be obtained from a number of sources for completion by individuals and their attorneys.

Generic living will forms may also be obtained from various sources, but users should be aware of any state-specific requirements. Some states

living will
An advance directive that specifies an individual's end-of-life wishes.

honor out-of-state advanced directives; however, some do not, so it is important that a patient is familiar with the specific law in his or her state of residence. Copies of completed forms should be given to designated family members or agents and may be filed with medical records upon a patient's admission to the hospital.

DURABLE POWER OF ATTORNEY

durable power of attorney
An advance directive that confers upon a designee the authority to make a variety of legal decisions on behalf of the grantor, usually including health care decisions.

The **durable power of attorney** is not specifically a medical document, but it may serve that purpose. It confers upon a designee the authority to make a variety of legal decisions on behalf of the grantor. It takes effect when the grantor loses the capacity to make decisions through either unconsciousness or mental incompetence. The document may place limits on the rights and responsibilities of the designee (usually an attorney or a spouse), and it may give specific instructions regarding the grantor's medical and other preferences. Standard forms are available and are governed by state law.

HEALTH CARE POWER OF ATTORNEY

health care power of attorney
A legal document that specifically identifies a person to take responsibility for a patient's health care decisions when the patient is not able to do so.

A **health care power of attorney** is a state-specific, end-of-life document. Depending on the state, the representative(s) designated may be called a health care agent, health care proxy, health care surrogate, health care representative, health care attorney-in-fact, or a patient advocate.

With a health care power of attorney, individuals specify their wishes and designate an agent to make medical decisions for them in the event that they lose the ability to reason or communicate. As with the living will, this document outlines specific types of care and treatment that should be permitted or excluded. It also carefully outlines the specific responsibilities and authority of the representative. Some states prohibit attending physicians, hospital employees, or other health care providers from serving as representatives, unless related to the patient by blood. Patients should name one or more alternates in case the primary representative cannot serve when called (see Figure 12-3).

DO-NOT-RESUSCITATE (DNR) ORDER

do-not-resuscitate (DNR) order
Order written at the request of patients or their authorized representatives that cardiopulmonary resuscitation not be used to sustain life in a medical crisis.

The **do-not-resuscitate (DNR) order** is a medical order written by a physician when requested by the patient. The order instructs health care providers not to do cardiopulmonary resuscitation (CPR) if a patient's heart stops beating or the patient's breathing stops. It is only used in an emergency and does not include instructions for treatments. The physician writes the order only after talking with the patient (if possible), the health care representative, or the patient's family. The information is placed on the patient's chart at the health care facility. Most states also recognize a state-authorized DNR bracelet. Each state has its own approved form. An example from the state of Florida may be found at www.floridahealth.gov/licensing-and-regulation/trauma-system/_documents/dnro-form-multi-lingual2004bwyw.pdf.

FIGURE 12-3 Health Care Power of Attorney

I, ______________________________, designate and appoint:

Name: ______________________________

Address: ______________________________

Telephone Number: ______________________________

to be my agent for health care decisions and pursuant to the language stated below, on my behalf to:

(1) Consent, refuse consent, or withdraw consent to any care, treatment, service or procedure to maintain, diagnose or treat a physical or mental condition, and to make decisions about organ donation, autopsy and disposition of the body;

(2) Make all necessary arrangements at any hospital, psychiatric hospital or psychiatric treatment facility, hospice, nursing home or similar institution; to employ or discharge health care personnel to include physicians, psychiatrists, psychologists, dentists, nurses, therapists or any other person who is licensed, certified or otherwise authorized or permitted by the laws of this state to administer health care as the agent shall deem necessary for my physical, mental and emotional well-being; and

(3) Request, receive and review any information, verbal or written, regarding my personal affairs or physical or mental health including medical and hospital records and to execute any releases of other documents that may be required in order to obtain such information. In exercising the grant of authority set forth above my agent for health care decisions shall:

The powers of the agent herein shall be limited to the extent set out in writing in this durable power of attorney for health care decisions, and shall not include the power to revoke or invalidate any previously existing declaration made in accordance with the natural death act.

The agent shall be prohibited from authorizing consent for the following items:

The durable power of attorney for health care decisions shall be subject to these additional limitations:

This power of attorney for health care decisions shall become effective immediately and shall not be affected by my subsequent disability or incapacity or upon the occurrence of my disability or incapacity.

Any durable power of attorney for health care decisions I have previously made is hereby revoked. This durable power of attorney for health care decisions shall be revoked in writing, executed and witnessed or acknowledged in the same manner as required herein.

Executed this ______________________________, at ______________________________

____

(Signature of principal)

State ____________ County ____________ S.S. No. ____________

This instrument was acknowledged before me ____________ (date) by ____________ (name)

____

(Signature of notary public)

Check Your Progress

7. What purpose do advance directives serve?
8. Distinguish between a living will and a durable power of attorney.
9. Distinguish between a health care power of attorney and a durable power of attorney.
10. How must health care practitioners proceed if a patient has a do-not-resuscitate order in place?
11. Generic living will forms are acceptable legal documents if they are _____ _______.

12.3 Health Care Services for Terminally Ill Patients

PALLIATIVE CARE VERSUS CURATIVE CARE

palliative care
Treatment of a terminally ill patient's symptoms to make dying more comfortable; also called comfort care.

curative care
Treatment directed toward curing a patient's disease.

When it becomes evident that a patient's disease is incurable and death is imminent, **palliative care** may serve the dying patient better than **curative care.** Curative care consists of treatments and procedures directed toward curing a patient's disease. Palliative care, also called comfort care, is directed toward providing relief to terminally ill patients through symptom and pain management. The goal is not to cure but to provide comfort and maintain the highest possible quality of life. Going beyond relief of disease symptoms, palliative care includes relief of emotional distress and other problems, so that a patient's last months and days may be as comfortable as possible.

Palliative care has emerged as a way to help patients with serious illnesses live a more comfortable and fulfilling life, whether their diseases are terminal or not. For example, through palliative care:

- A 90-year-old stroke patient with limited mobility is able to continue living independently in his home.
- An ovarian cancer patient is more comfortable and can actually continue working as she undergoes aggressive chemotherapy treatment.
- A lung cancer patient receives counseling about his disease and help in navigating the complex U.S. health care system.

Survey data from 2013 (Dumanovsky, 2013) indicates that 90 percent of hospitals with 300 beds or more reported palliative care programs. Smaller hospitals reported fewer programs, with only 56 percent of hospitals with less than 300 beds reporting palliative care programs. Both not-for-profit and public hospitals were more likely to have a palliative care program.

Palliative care is not the same as hospice care, which is limited to terminally ill patients (see the next section).

The Center to Advance Palliative Care, based in New York, provides information to help patients and their families receive care that addresses all of the patient's needs. (Visit the center's Web site at www.capc.org for information about goals and services.)

HOSPICE CARE

hospice
A facility or program (often carried out in a patient's home) in which teams of health care practitioners and volunteers provide a continuing environment that focuses on the physical, emotional, and psychological needs of the dying patient.

Terminally ill patients are often referred to facilities or agencies that provide **hospice** care. A hospice in medieval times was a way station for travelers. The first hospice organization opened in the United States in 1974. The industry has seen a great deal of growth since then. According to the National Hospice and Palliative Care Organization, there were approximately 6,100 hospices across all 50 states, the District of Columbia, and U.S. territories in 2014. Approximately 1.6 million patients received care in that same year.

In the United States, hospice care may be provided in facilities built especially for that purpose, in hospitals and nursing homes, or at home. (Angela, in the chapter's opening scenario, practices in a hospital. The floor she supervises is designated a hospice.) Hospice care focuses on relieving pain, controlling symptoms, and meeting emotional needs and personal values of the terminally ill, instead of targeting the underlying disease process. The hospice philosophy also recognizes that family members and other caregivers deserve care and support, continuing after the death of the patient. Hospice programs ease dying; they do not support active euthanasia (a Greek term meaning "good death") or assisted suicide.

Bereavement services are also available through hospice care to help patients discuss such issues as preparing a will and planning a funeral, and to help surviving family members cope with grief and loss after the patient dies. Hospice programs generally provide bereavement services through discussion groups, follow-up visits from hospice personnel, and sometimes referrals to appropriate mental health professionals.

Most in-home hospice programs are independently run in a fashion similar to visiting nurse or home health care agencies. Patients receive coordinated care at home by multidisciplinary teams composed of physicians, nurses, social workers, home health aides, pharmacists, physical therapists, clergy, volunteers, and family members. Hospice teams meet regularly to work on patients' needs concerning pain and other serious symptoms, depression, family problems, inadequate housing, financial problems, or lack of transportation. The team then expands, amends, or otherwise revises each patient's care plan, as necessary.

For patients to be eligible for hospice care, physicians usually must certify that they are not expected to live beyond 6 months. Hospice care is generally reimbursed by Medicare, Medicaid, and many private insurance companies and managed care programs.

END-OF-LIFE DISCUSSIONS WITH HEALTH CARE PROVIDERS

While modern medicine has effectively delayed the moment of death, in many cases, it has dealt less conscientiously with compassionate, comfort care for **terminally ill** patients: those who are not expected to live beyond 6 months, usually because of a chronic illness that has progressed beyond effective treatment or for which there is no cure. Physicians and other health care practitioners may struggle with providing the appropriate conversations with patients and their families.

terminally ill
Referring to patients who are expected to die within six months.

Physicians and other health care practitioners are trained to save lives. Discussions about death and dying had been left to family and faith-based leaders. However, the need for practitioner involvement has been recognized.

Medical schools are now required to teach end-of-life care. While the requirement by the Liaison Committee on Medical Education is not specific, it is estimated that medical students now get 14 hours of training, usually as part of another course (National Academies Press, 2015).

In early 2016, the American Association of Colleges of Nursing (AACN) announced its new set of competencies and recommendations for palliative care education in undergraduate nursing. There are 17 palliative care competencies that student nurses should achieve before graduation.

Advanced registered nurse practitioners (ARNP) may earn certificates in palliative care in several universities across the country. The National Association of Social Workers offers a certification at master's level for social workers. Both certificates require continuing education units, as well as experience in palliative care.

In 2006, a medical board subspecialty in hospice and palliative care was approved by the American Board of Medical Specialties. Physicians must first be board certified in a specialty such as internal medicine, pediatrics, surgery, family medicine, or several others. A complete list is available at www.aahpm.org. After completing required education courses, completing a one-year fellowship, and passing an exam, a physician can be board certified in hospice and palliative care. The American Academy of Hospice and Palliative Care has certified 6,952 physicians in this area. Some experts estimate that twice that many will be needed in the United States.

In January 2016, Medicare began reimbursing physicians for having a conversation with patients about advance directives.

In early 2016, the John A. Hartford Foundation, Cambia Health Foundation, and California HealthCare Foundation commissioned Perry Undem Research/Communication to conduct a national survey of primary care physicians and specialists who regularly see patients 65 and older. The survey explored current experiences billing Medicare for these conversations as well as motivations and barriers to having these conversations. The findings of the survey, released in April 2016, indicate:

- Approximately half (46 percent) of the physicians reported that they frequently or sometimes feel unsure of what to say.
- Less than one-third (29 percent) of the physicians reported any formal training on talking with patients and their families about end-of-life care.
- Most of the physicians (95 percent) say they support the new Medicare reimbursement for conversations with patients about advance directives. And three-quarters (75 percent) of the physicians say the benefit will make them more likely to talk with older patients about advance planning.
- While 99 percent of physicians indicated that it was important for health care providers to have conversations with patients about advance directives, only 29 percent of physicians report that a formal system exists in their practice or system for assessing end-of-life wishes and goals of care.
- There is no place in their electronic health record indicating if a patient has an advance care plan, according to 24 percent of the physicians surveyed.
- Physicians who have had training in end-of-life discussions find the conversations rewarding. Those with training are more confident about what to say in these conversations.

Source: www.jhartfound.org/blog/talking-with-patients-about-end-of-life-care-new-poll-reveals-how-physicians-really-feel/.

Despite a conscious effort to improve training and attitudes regarding dying patients, end-of-life care remains one of the most emotional issues for health care practitioners.

Check Your Progress

12. Distinguish between *palliative care* and *curative care*.
13. Define *hospice*.

Indicate with a "C" or a "P" whether each of the following actions constitutes a form of curative care or palliative care.

_______ 14. Allowing a patient who is terminally ill with lung and stomach cancer to self-administer morphine patches as needed for pain relief

_______ 15. Administering radiation treatments after breast cancer surgery

_______ 16. Surgical severing of certain nerves to relieve suffering for a patient terminally ill with cancer of the spine

_______ 17. Counseling a terminally ill patient and his or her family concerning funeral arrangements and other end-of-life decisions

_______ 18. Administering antibiotics to cure an infected tooth

_______ 19. Cosmetic surgery for a teenaged patient whose face was burned in a fire

20. What are the requirements for an ARNP to earn a certificate in palliative care?
21. What are the major concerns physicians have in talking with patients about advanced directives and other end-of-life care?

12.4 The Right to Die Movement

Americans have long been concerned that advancing medical technology may allow health care practitioners to delay death beyond the point where any quality of life can be maintained or a cure realized, thus depriving individuals of the right to die as they wish. This concern led to the first living will, created and made available to the public by attorney Luis Kutner, who founded the Euthanasia Society. Kutner's goal was to help dying people exercise their rights to control end-of-life medical care.

The right to die first became a matter for the courts to deliberate in 1976, with the death of Karen Ann Quinlan.

The *Quinlan* case raised important questions in bioethics, euthanasia, and the legal rights of guardians. The case resulted in the development of formal ethics committees in hospitals, long-term care facilities, and hospices. It also called attention to the need for advance health directives.

Another landmark case in the right to die movement involved Nancy Cruzan, a 26-year-old woman who was severely injured in a car crash.

While these landmark legal cases furthered certain right to die arguments, other events in the nation's history have also furthered the cause. Here is a timeline:

- 1946—Committee of 1776 Physicians for Legalizing Voluntary Euthanasia is formed in New York state.
- 1967—Attorney Luis Kutner and members of the Euthanasia Society (later called Choice in Dying and then Partnership for Caring; both organizations now defunct) devise the original living will.

- 1973–American Hospital Association creates the Patient's Bill of Rights. (To date, attempts to pass a federal Patient's Bill of Rights have consistently failed.)
- 1976–California's Natural Death Act, the nation's first right to die statute, is signed into law.
- 1977–Laws dealing with the refusal of treatment are passed in Arkansas, Idaho, Nevada, New Mexico, North Carolina, Oregon, and Texas.
- 1984–The District of Columbia and 22 states have statutes that recognize advance directives.
- 1989–The **Uniform Rights of the Terminally Ill Act** serves as a guideline for state legislatures in constructing laws addressing advance directives.

Uniform Rights of the Terminally Ill Act
A 1989 recommendation of the National Conference of Commissioners on Uniform State Laws that all states construct laws to address advance directives.

- 1990–Congress passes the Patient Self-Determination Act, the first federal act concerning advance directives.
- 1990–Jack Kevorkian, MD, assists Janet Adkins in committing suicide by using a lethal injecting machine. Dr. Kevorkian participated in several assisted deaths.
- 1992–Pennsylvania becomes the fiftieth state to enact advance directive legislation.
- 1992–Oregon voters pass a Death with Dignity Act that allows physician-assisted suicide, becoming the first state law to allow physician-assisted suicide. Voters in Oregon confirmed this vote again in 1997.
- 1997–The U.S. Supreme Court holds that state bans on physician-assisted suicide do not violate the U.S. Constitution. The Court leaves the decision up to each state on whether to ban physician-assisted suicide.
- 1997–By this date, 35 states have enacted statutes expressly criminalizing assisted suicide; 9 states criminalize assisted suicide through common law.
- 2001–The California Supreme Court clarifies the right to die in a decision that states the right to die does not extend to people who are conscious and in a twilight state, are unable to communicate or care for themselves, and have not left formal written directions for health care.
- 2006–In 2003, the federal government files suit against the state of Oregon, stating that because federal drug laws do not permit or condone physician-assisted suicide, the Oregon law was illegal. In 2006, in a 6-3 decision, the U.S. Supreme Court held that the federal government did not have the authority to prosecute a state's physicians.
- 2008–Via voter initiative, Washington state passes the Death with Dignity Act, effective in 2009.
- 2009–The Montana Supreme Court rules that physicians may assist patients in ending their lives by prescribing lethal medication that the patient self-administers (Rights of the Terminally Ill Act interpretation).

- 2013—Vermont becomes the third state to implement a Death with Dignity Act (the first to initiate the act through legislation, as opposed to a voter initiative). Four states now allow physician-assisted suicide.
- 2014—The New Mexico Supreme Court rules physician-assisted suicide is illegal in New Mexico.
- 2016—California's End of Life Option Act takes effect in June 2016.
- 2016—In November 2016, Colorado became the sixth state to approve a Death with Dignity Act.
- 2017—In February 2017, a Death with Dignity Act went into effect in Washington D.C.

LANDMARK COURT CASE

Right to Die Precedent

In 1976, the parents of Karen Ann Quinlan, then 22, obtained permission from a New Jersey court to remove their daughter from a respirator. Karen Ann had been in a persistent vegetative state for several months after allegedly ingesting an unknown combination of alcohol and drugs. Karen Ann's father, as her legal guardian, had asked her physicians to remove the respirator believed to be sustaining her life. The physicians refused, and the Quinlans sued for their daughter's right to die. A lower court held for the physicians, but on appeal, judges allowed Karen Ann's respirator to be disconnected. She continued to live via a feeding tube, but died in June 1985 of pneumonia, at the age of 31.

Source: In re Quinlan, 70 N.J. 10, 49, 355 A.2d 647, 668 (1976).

LANDMARK COURT CASE

Legal Struggle to Remove Feeding Tube

On January 11, 1983, Nancy Beth Cruzan was driving alone when she lost control of her older model car that had no seat belts. Nancy was thrown from the car and landed face down in a water-filled ditch. When emergency medical technicians (EMTs) arrived, Nancy had no vital signs, but the EMTs resuscitated her. After about 2 weeks, Nancy had not awakened, and her condition was diagnosed as persistent vegetative state following irreversible brain damage. Physicians inserted a feeding tube for Nancy's long-term care.

After 4 years with no improvement, Nancy's parents asked to have the feeding tube removed. The hospital demanded a court order, and a 3-year legal battle ensued. The trial court ruled that the feeding tube could be removed, based on testimony given by one of Nancy's friends that she would not want to live on artificial life support. The Missouri State Supreme Court reversed the trial court's ruling, holding that the lower court did not meet the *clear and convincing evidence* standard. The case reached the U.S. Supreme Court, where justices affirmed the Missouri State Supreme Court ruling and recognized that the right to refuse medical treatment is guaranteed by the U.S. Constitution. The case was sent back to the trial court for the purpose of gathering clear and convincing evidence that Nancy Cruzan would not have wanted to live in a persistent vegetative state. Three of Nancy's friends testified as to her wishes, and the court ruled that this met the clear and convincing evidence standard and that the feeding tube could be removed. This decision was also appealed, but the appeal failed to change the court's ruling, and Nancy's feeding tube was removed in December 1990. She died 11 days later.

Source: Cruzan v. Director, Missouri Department of Health, 497 U.S. 261 (1990).

EUTHANASIA AND PHYSICIAN-ASSISTED SUICIDE

In the United States, there has been much debate over whether or not physicians should play a role in ending a terminally ill patient's life. Mercy killing of the hopelessly ill is known as euthanasia. Four types of euthanasia may occur:

active euthanasia
A conscious medical act that results in the death of a dying person.

passive euthanasia
The act of allowing a dying patient to die naturally, without medical interference.

voluntary euthanasia
The act of ending a dying patient's life by medical means with his or her permission.

involuntary euthanasia
The act of ending a terminal patient's life by medical means without his or her permission.

- **Active euthanasia** is a conscious medical act that results in the death of a dying patient.
- **Passive euthanasia** is the act of allowing a patient to die naturally, without medical interference.
- **Voluntary euthanasia** requires the patient's consent or that of his designated representative to use medical means to end the patient's life.
- **Involuntary euthanasia** is the act of ending a patient's life by medical means without the consent of the patient or the patient's representative.

According to some polls, there is growing support for physician-assisted euthanasia. It is often referred to as physician-assisted suicide. It is, at its very least, a difficult issue. As mentioned earlier in the chapter, there are several ways a patient can make clear his or her health wishes through advance directives. However, as of late 2016, only six states (Oregon, Washington, Vermont, Montana, California, and Colorado) have laws allowing physician-assisted suicide. These laws are referred to as "Death with Dignity," "End of Life Options," "Patient Control at the End of Life," or "Rights of the Terminal Ill." The term *suicide* is not used. Advocates of allowing a terminally ill patient to ask for assistance in dying refer to the process as physician-assisted death.

According to the organization Death with Dignity, the laws or court decisions allow "qualified mentally competent, terminally ill adults to request a prescription medication for the purpose of hastening their death" (www.deathwithdignity.org). The decision on the part of the patient is voluntary. There are strict eligibility requirements and safeguards. It is the patient who takes the medication prescribed. Physicians cannot legally perform lethal injections, mercy killing by other means, or active euthanasia.

Oregon's law was first passed passed in 1992. However, it was not effective until 1997 due to lawsuits. Through 2015, 1,545 Oregon citizens have had prescriptions written under the law, and 991 patients have died from ingesting the prescribed medications. In Washington, where the law was effective in 2009, there have been 938 prescriptions written and 917 patients have died either naturally or from ingesting the medications.

There are many sides to the debate over physician-assisted death. Some advocates believe a person has the right to control his or her own life, including choosing to end it. Others see the question from a quality-of-life perspective. That is, when one suffers from an incurable, debilitating, and/or painful disease, he or she should have the right to end the suffering.

Those who argue against physician-assisted suicide also hold a variety of opinions. Some simply say that killing a human being is always wrong. Others cite the Hippocratic oath as evidence that physicians are always bound to protect life and, therefore, should not be asked to assist a suicide. Opponents also claim that the potential for abuse is too great.

LANDMARK COURT CASE

Right to Die or the Right to Live?

In 1990, 27-year-old Terri Schindler Schiavo suffered an apparent heart attack at her home in Florida. Emergency medical technicians restored a heartbeat, but Terri remained comatose at first, then later semicomatose. Terri's husband, Michael Schiavo, was appointed her guardian, and she was placed in a long-term care facility, where she was finally diagnosed as being in a persistent vegetative state.

In 1992, Michael Schiavo sued Terri's physician for malpractice and was awarded $600,000. Terri was awarded $1.4 million and $250,000 in separate medical malpractice trials.

In 1993, Michael Schiavo refused medically recommended rehabilitative therapy for Terri, and her parents intervened. Bob and Mary Schindler, Terri's parents, petitioned the court to remove Michael Schiavo as Terri's guardian. A judge denied the guardianship petition. In 1997, a judge approved Michael Schiavo's petition to remove the tubes delivering Terri's hydration and nutrition. Terri seemed semiconscious, and her parents insisted she might be successfully rehabilitated.

In 1998, the court appointed a guardian *ad litem* to investigate Terri's case. The guardian *ad litem* recommended against removing Terri's feeding tubes and was dismissed for bias. In 2001, the court ordered the feeding tubes removed, despite physicians' testimonials that Terri was not in a PVS and could swallow. Many physicians also testified that Terri was in a PVS. In April of that year, Terri's feeding tubes were removed, but in light of new evidence, a new judge ordered feeding restored.

Court battles continued, with Michael Schiavo petitioning the court to end Terri's life and her parents counterpetitioning to keep Terri alive. Finally, in October 2003, the Florida legislature passed a law—"Terri's Law"—allowing then-Governor Jeb Bush to issue an executive order to let Terri continue to receive nutrition and hydration. The law was repealed in September 2004.

In March 2005, Michael Schiavo won court approval to have his wife's feeding tube removed. Terri died 13 days later, on March 31, 2005, after having been in an apparent PVS for 15 years. An autopsy performed in June 2005 confirmed that Schiavo was in a persistent vegetative state.

Source: *Schindler v. Schiavo*, Florida Supreme Court, 900 So.2d 554 (2005).

For example, if physician-assisted death is sanctioned, will relatives of wealthy patients advocate for their deaths? Does serious illness alter mental states so that these patients cannot be trusted to make such decisions rationally? Will quality-of-life issues take precedence in deciding who should take advantage of statues that regulate physician-assisted suicide?

The debate over physician-assisted death will continue for years to come, but until legal issues are settled, health care practitioners are reminded that, legally and ethically, they are bound to consider existing law and the welfare of patients.

Check Your Progress

22. How were decisions in the *Quinlan, Cruzan,* and *Schiavo* cases significant in the right to die movement?
23. Define *euthanasia.*
24. How does passive euthanasia differ from active euthanasia? Is either process legal in the United States?
25. How does voluntary euthanasia differ from involuntary euthanasia? Is either process legal in the United States?
26. In your opinion, is any death with dignity act ethical? Explain your answer.

12.5 The National Organ Transplant Act

National Organ Transplant Act
Passed in 1984, a statute that provides grants to qualified organ procurement organizations and established an Organ Procurement and Transplantation Network.

Passed in 1984, the **National Organ Transplant Act** addresses the severe shortage of organs available for transplantation. It provides funds for (1) grants to qualified organ procurement organizations (OPOs) and (2) the establishment of an Organ Procurement and Transplantation Network (OPTN) to assist OPOs in the distribution of unused organs outside their geographical area.

The Organ Procurement and Transplantation Network maintains the only national patient waiting list. It is a unique public/private organization that links all the professionals involved in the organ donation and transplantation system. OPTN goals are to:

- Increase the the number of transplants.
- Provide equity in access to transplants.
- Improve wait-listed patient, living donor, and transplant recipient outcomes.
- Promote living donor and transplant recipient safety.
- Promote the efficient management of the OPTN.

Source: https://optn.transplant.hrsa.gov/governance/about-the-optn/vision-goals/.

The United Network for Organ Sharing (UNOS), based in Richmond, Virginia, administers the OPTN under contract with the Health Resources and Services Administration of the U.S. Department of Health and Human Services.

According to UNOS, there is always a shortage of organs available for transplantation. In fact, every 10 minutes in the United States, another person needing an organ is added to the list. On average, 22 people die each day waiting for a transplant, and one donor can possibly save up to eight lives.

Information on organ donation, including a link to register as an organ donor in your state, is available at www.organdonor.gov/index.html. Organ procurement organizations nationwide coordinate donor information through OPTN. The Association of Organ Procurement Organizations (www.aopo.org) provides a list of organizations at the local level in each state.

ORGAN DONOR DIRECTIVES

Patients may also want to make clear to hospital personnel that they wish to donate organs for transplantation or medical research in the event of their death. This can be accomplished in several ways:

- Some states allow licensed drivers to fill out organ donation forms on the back of their licenses.
- Nondrivers or residents of states where driver's licenses do not include this information may carry an organ donor card in their wallets, specifying their desire to donate organs (Figure 12-4).
- Organizations such as the National Kidney Foundation, the United Network for Organ Sharing (UNOS), and the Living Bank provide donor registration materials in response to requests.
- In addition to having an organ donor card, patients should make clear to family members their wishes regarding organ donation in the event of their death.

FIGURE 12-4 Sample Uniform Donor Card

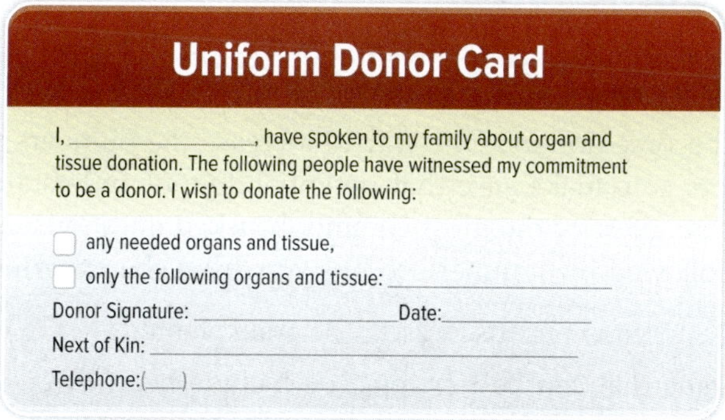
Uniform Donor Card

I, _______________, have spoken to my family about organ and tissue donation. The following people have witnessed my commitment to be a donor. I wish to donate the following:

☐ any needed organs and tissue,

☐ only the following organs and tissue: _______________

Donor Signature: _______________ Date: _______________

Next of Kin: _______________

Telephone:(____) _______________

THE UNIFORM ANATOMICAL GIFT ACT

In 1968, the **Uniform Anatomical Gift Act** (UAGA) was approved by the National Conference of Commissioners on Uniform State Laws for the purpose of allowing individuals to donate their bodies or body parts, after death, for use in transplant surgery, tissue banks, or medical research or education. The UAGA was revised in 2006. The act was not officially enacted as law, but states accepted it because it made certain provisions uniform throughout all states. Many states have enacted the 2006 act with minor changes. Major provisions include the following:

Uniform Anatomical Gift Act A recommendation of the National Conference of Commissioners on Uniform State Laws, which all states accepted, allowing individuals to donate their bodies or body parts, after death, for use in transplant surgery, tissue banks, or medical research or education.

- Any person 18 years of age or older who is of sound mind may make a gift of his or her body, or certain bodily organs, to be used in medical research or for transplantation or storage in a tissue bank.
- The 2006 revisions added a provision allowing a parent of a minor, a guardian of an individual, or an agent acting under a health care power of attorney to make an anatomical gift during the life of the child, ward, or principal.
- Donations made through a legal will are not to be held up by probate.
- Except in autopsies, the donor's rights override those of others.
- Survivors may speak for the deceased if arrangements were not made prior to his or her death (provided the deceased did not express an objection to donation before his or her death).
- Physicians who rely on donation documents for the acceptance of bodies or organs are immune from civil or criminal prosecution. However, if the physician (or hospital) knows the deceased was opposed to donation or if, in the absence of prior arrangements, survivors express an objection, then the donation should be refused.
- Hospitals, surgeons, physicians, accredited medical or dental schools, colleges and universities, and tissue banks or storage facilities may accept anatomical gifts for research, advancement of medical or dental science, therapy, or transplantation.
- The time of death of the donor must be established by a physician who is not involved in transplanting the donor's designated organs, and the donor's attending physician cannot be a member of the transplant team.
- Donors may revoke the gift, and gifts may be rejected.

FREQUENTLY ASKED QUESTIONS ABOUT ORGAN DONATION

Because there are more people waiting for organ transplants than there are organs available, individuals are encouraged to designate their willingness to become donors. One way to increase the numbers of possible organ donors is to make sure that potential donors understand the process. Here are a few of the most commonly asked questions about organ donation, followed by summarized answers from the experts:

Q: What organs and tissues can be transplanted?

A: Organs that can be transplanted include heart, liver, kidney, pancreas, lung, stomach, and small and large intestines. Other tissues often transplanted include bone, corneas, skin, heart valves, veins, cartilage, and other connective tissues.

Q: Is the donor or the donor's family responsible for paying for transplantation of donated organs?

A: No. Costs are borne by the recipient or his or her insurance plan, when applicable.

Q: If a prospective, designated donor is injured in an accident, will the attending doctors allow that person to die in order to harvest donated organs?

A: Absolutely not. A willingness to donate organs in no way compromises the medical care provided to accident victims. The organ procurement organization is notified that organs are available only after a patient is declared dead, and the transplant team is not notified until surviving family members have consented to the donation.

Q: How old or young can a donor be?

A: Donors range from newborns to the elderly.

Q: If a person donated an organ, would the recipient and/or the recipient's family learn the donor's identity and contact the donor or his or her family?

A: A donor's name is released to recipients only if the recipient asks for the information and the donor's family agrees.

Q: Are organs transplanted only after a prospective donor has died?

A: Not necessarily. Voluntary transplants from living donors to living recipients may also take place. For example, kidneys, lungs, skin, and other tissues are successfully transplanted from compatible living donors to recipients.

Q: May a family member who is an acceptable medical match for a recipient refuse to donate an organ to a relative in need of a transplant?

A: Of course. No laws exist that would compel a person to donate an organ against his or her will, regardless of relationship to the intended recipient.

Q: If I, as a willing organ donor, sign the back of my driver's license indicating that I am a donor and then die, can my relatives legally "undo" my wishes?

A: No. A signed declaration on the back of a driver's license still is legally effective to authorize donation in every state in the United States. Moreover, the relevant laws specify that the consent of the donor's relatives is not needed in such circumstances. However, prospective organ donors should also make their wishes known to family members while they are able, because in spite of their having signed a card, if relatives protest the donation, fear of bad publicity regarding organ donation will likely prevent the donation from occurring.

Check Your Progress

27. What law made organ donation possible in the United States?
28. In your opinion, why is there a shortage of transplant organs in the United States?
29. What suggestions do you have for alleviating the shortage of transplant organs?
30. What is UNOS, and what is its function?
31. A widely circulated urban legend tells of a person who has a sexual tryst with a stranger and awakens in a bathtub minus a kidney. Why do you know the story is untrue?

12.6 The Grieving Process

Regardless of our personal philosophy and belief system concerning death and dying, we are all destined to experience the loss of an acquaintance, a friend, or a loved one. At that time, we need to grieve. Unfortunately, in our modern-day culture, we are often uncertain of how to deal with grief in our own lives or how to help someone else who is grieving. The following facts and guidelines can help us respond helpfully to others.

WHAT IS GRIEF?

Grief is the human reaction to loss. Individuals may grieve over a divorce, the loss of a job, or relocation, but grief after the death of a loved one is undoubtedly the most painful. Patients who are diagnosed with a terminal illness also experience profound grief. The grieving process is different for each individual who experiences it, but, over time, some similarities have been observed.

STAGES OF GRIEF

The late Elisabeth Kübler-Ross, MD, recognized for many years as an authority in the field of death and dying, was the first to list and describe the coping mechanisms of people who grieve. Such individuals experience five stages of grief, she maintained, not necessarily in any particular order, before coming to terms with the death of a loved one or the prospect of imminent death.

Stage 1. This first stage is identified with feelings of denial and isolation. This is the it-can't-be-true stage in which patients believe the physician's diagnosis must be a mistake or relatives informed of a loved one's death deny that the person is gone. They may suggest that X-rays or results of blood tests were somehow mixed up or that identities of accident victims were somehow mistaken. Denial is usually a temporary state, claims Kübler-Ross, and is soon replaced by partial acceptance. A terminally ill patient seldom continues to deny his or her disease until death comes, and grieving relatives realize all too soon that a loved one has, in fact, died.

Stage 2. When denial can no longer be maintained, the patient or grieving relative progresses to anger, rage, and resentment. "Why me?" is the typical reaction. Patients are angry over the "betrayal" of once-healthy bodies and the loss of control over their lives. Grieving relatives may feel anger toward a God that took the loved one away. Even the terminally ill family member may feel the same anger at God for leaving others behind to bear the pain of loss. Anger is a normal reaction to death and may be expressed in different ways. For example, a bereaved person may yell at others or withdraw in sullen silence.

Stage 3. Grieving individuals next respond with attempts at bargaining and guilt. Just as children continue to ask for a favor after parents have said no, patients may ask for "just enough time to see my daughter married" or "one more week at work before I have to quit." Something in the human psyche seems to believe, if only for a short time, that if we are "good," the "bad" will be taken away or postponed.

A corresponding experience for individuals grieving the loss of a loved one is guilt. The bereaved person may somehow feel responsible for the death, especially if the relationship with the deceased was not good. He or she might be tortured by thoughts of how things might have been different if only the loved one had lived.

Stage 4. The fourth stage involves depression or sadness, which is the most expected reaction to loss. Patients coping with terminal illness may face not only physical pain and debilitation but also loss of financial security and inevitable changes in lifestyle—all of which can cause them to feel that their situation is hopeless. Individuals grieving the loss of a loved one may see no point in going on.

During this state, bereaved persons may cry frequently or may be unable to cry at all, expressing their grief in body language—downcast eyes, shuffling steps, and stooped shoulders. Daily routines may be difficult or impossible to maintain. If depression continues for a prolonged period of time, health care providers, family members, or friends should help the bereaved person seek professional counseling.

Stage 5. Finally, those experiencing the grieving process reach a stage of acceptance. At this point, the person has finally accepted his or her loss. Terminally ill patients have come to terms with dying, and bereaved persons have accepted that the loved one is gone. For example, patients may write wills, complete advance directives, or plan funerals. A grieving spouse may finally decide to remove a deceased partner's clothing from a shared closet or to convert his or her office to a spare bedroom. Grieving family members can now move on to the growth stage in which they adjust daily routines or become involved in new activities and relationships.

Although the stages of grief have been universally observed, each person dealing with loss grieves differently. Bereaved persons may not show their grief. A stage may be skipped or returned to repeatedly during the grieving process. A combination of all of the emotions just described may be felt at the same time.

Roberta Temes, PhD, also describes her perception of the distinctive behaviors of grief in her book *Solace: Finding Your Way Through Grief and Learning to Live Again* (Amazon Books, 2009). She discusses three stages as significant as one grieves:

1. Numbness, characterized by mechanical or rote functioning and social isolation
2. Disorganization, where feelings of loss are so painful and disorienting one can't make plans or decide what to do next
3. Reorganization, a return to one's previous, more normal and functional way of life

While no one list of the stages of grief is useful for everyone, most touch on the types of behavior mentioned previously, which many people have experienced or observed at times of loss.

On the other hand, in *The Truth about Grief* (Simon & Schuster, 2011), Ruth Davis Konigsberg emphasizes that Kübler-Ross based her theory solely on interviews with terminally ill patients and she was concerned primarily about the patients' feelings about their own approaching deaths. She did not ask them about her now famous stages of grief because she conceived of the five stages later, after she had conducted the interviews. When Kübler-Ross's book was a surprise best seller, Konigsberg asserts, it marked the beginning of a new approach to death and dying, which "helped shatter the stoic silence that had surrounded death since World War I, and her ideas certainly raised the standard of care for dying people and their families. But she also ushered in a distinctly secular and psychological approach to death, one in which the focus shifted from the salvation of the deceased's soul . . . to the quality of his or her last days."

While Kübler-Ross's stages of grief have been applied to a wide range of experiences of loss, Konigsberg writes that they have also fostered certain misconceptions about grief, such as the following, as summarized in the January 24, 2011, edition of *Time:*

1. A person who has experienced loss or is facing death does not always grieve in stages. Rather, the person experiences "a grab bag of symptoms that come and go and, eventually, simply lift."
2. Expressing grief helps some who experience it but not all. In fact, a study published in the *Journal of Consulting and Clinical Psychology* in 2008 followed more than 2,000 people immediately after the events of 9/11 and for 2 more years, and found that some people who did not express their initial reactions showed fewer signs of distress later on.
3. When an individual loses his or her spouse, grief hits women harder than men. Several studies have shown that widows may show higher

incidents of depression than widowers, but relatively speaking, men suffer more from the loss of a spouse.

4. Grief may never end. Researchers have found that the worst of grief is usually over within about 6 months. Thoughts and memories of those lost linger, of course, but the actual pain of loss does subside.
5. Counseling always helps those who grieve. Just as individuals grieve in different ways, for different lengths of time, some may find that counseling shortens the grieving period, while others come to terms with grief on their own.

Check Your Progress

The following questionnaire is intended to generate discussion. Check each statement that tells how you feel. There are no correct or incorrect answers.

_______ 32. I feel uncomfortable talking to someone who is dying.

_______ 33. I do not know what to say to a person who is dying.

_______ 34. I would not want to tell a patient that he or she has a terminal condition.

_______ 35. I think I can help a dying patient be more comfortable with his or her impending death.

_______ 36. I am afraid of becoming too attached to a dying patient, and as a result, I will not be able to control my feelings.

_______ 37. I do not think a person should be told that his or her condition is terminal because doing so adds to his or her suffering.

_______ 38. I do not think death should be discussed in the presence of children.

_______ 39. I The thought of being around a dying person makes me uncomfortable.

_______ 40. I think elderly people are the most fearful of death.

_______ 41. Being around a dying person reminds me that someday I, too, will die.

Source: Adapted from W. Worden, *Grief Counseling and Grief Therapy* (New York: Springer, 1982).

The message for health care practitioners is to remain flexible in their expectations of other people's grief. That is, to realize that every person grieves in his or her own way, and some are resilient enough to get through grief on their own, while others may benefit from a combination of the helpful measures outlined in this chapter.

FINDING SUPPORT

People who are grieving can find support from a variety of sources. They can read books on the subject, attend a bereavement support group sponsored by a hospital or hospice, visit a counselor, talk with a member of the clergy, or talk with family members and friends.

Health care practitioners can be excellent sources of support for terminally ill patients and their families. Talking and listening are the most helpful activities others can perform, the experts advise. Do not force a conversation, but make yourself available to talk. Do not respond in kind if patients are angry and resentful. Talking about distress helps relieve it, and sensitive listening is effective in itself. The following list of recommendations for talking to a dying patient is adapted from *"I Don't Know What to Say . . . ": How to Help and Support Someone Who Is Dying* (Little, Brown, 1989), by oncologist Dr. Robert Buckman:

- Pay attention to setting. Sit down, relax, do not appear rushed, and act as though you are ready to listen.
- Determine whether or not the patient wants to talk. Ask, "Do you feel like talking?" before plunging into conversation.
- Listen well, and show that you are listening. Pay attention to the patient's words, without the distraction of planning your next remark.
- Encourage the patient to talk by saying, "What do you mean?" or "Tell me more."
- Remember that silence and nonverbal communication, such as grasping a hand or touching a shoulder, are also effective.
- Do not be afraid to describe your own feelings. It is permissible to say, "I find this difficult to talk about" or even, "I don't know what to say."
- Make sure you haven't misunderstood. You can ask, "How did it feel?" or say, "You seem angry."
- Do not change the subject. If you are uncomfortable, admit it. Don't try to distract the patient by changing the subject to something less threatening, such as the weather.
- Do not give advice early. The time may come when the patient asks for your advice, but it is usually not prudent to offer unsolicited advice because it stops the dialogue.
- Encourage reminiscence. Sharing memories can be a wrenching experience, but it can also encourage patients to look positively at the past.
- Respond to humor. Humor allows patients to express fears in a non-threatening way. Do not try to cheer someone up with your own jokes, but if patients want to tell jokes or funny stories, humor them.

In short, the more you try to understand the feelings of others, the more support you will be able to give.

Chapter Summary

Learning Outcome	Summary

LO 12.1 Summarize attitudes toward death and criteria for determining death.	Which Western rituals surrounding death have survived to the present?
	• Mourners wearing black
	• Halting traffic for a funeral procession
	• Wakes
	• Firing a rifle volley over the deceased
	• Funeral wreaths
	What is the Uniform Determination of Death Act?
	• A federal proposal that defines brain death as a means of determining when death actually occurs:
	  • Circulation and respiration have irreversibly ceased.
	  • The entire brain, including the brain stem, has irreversibly ceased to function.
	What is the difference between a coma and a persistent vegetative state?
	• Coma: A condition of deep stupor from which the patient cannot be roused by external stimuli
	• Persistent vegetative state (PVS): Severe mental impairment characterized by irreversible cessation of the higher functions of the brain, most often caused by damage to the cerebral cortex
	What tests may be performed to determine if death has occurred?
	• Cannot breathe without assistance
	• No coughing or gagging reflex
	• No pupil response to light
	• No blinking reflex when cornea is touched
	• No grimace reflex when head is rotated or ears are flushed with ice water
	• No response to pain

LO 12.2 Describe the legal documents used in end-of-life decisions.	What is the Patient Self-Determination Act? • A federal act that requires hospitals and other health care providers to give written information to patients regarding their rights under state law to make medical decisions and to execute advance directives What are the four types of advance directives? • Living will: An advance directive that specifies a patient's end-of-life wishes • Durable power of attorney: An advance directive that gives a designee authority to make a variety of legal decisions for a patient, including health care decisions • Health care power of attorney: A durable power of attorney for health care decisions only • Do-not-resuscitate (DNR) order: A written medical order written by a physician when a patient specifies that he or she does not wish to be resuscitated if his or her heart stops
LO 12.3 Identify health care services for terminally ill patients.	What is the difference between palliative care and curative care? • Palliative care: Treatment of a patient's symptoms to make him or her more comfortable—also called comfort care • Curative care: Treatment directed toward curing a patient's disease What is a hospice? • A facility or program in which health care practitioners and volunteers provide a continuous environment that focuses on the physical, emotional, and psychological needs of the dying patient What is meant by the phrase *terminally* ill? • A patient has 6 months or less to live.

Are physicians and nurses required to have training in palliative care?

- Medical school students have some training in end-of-life care.
- Physicians may earn a board-certified subspecialty in palliative care.
- Bachelor-prepared nurses have 17 competencies in end-of-life care that must be completed to graduate.

LO 12.4 Describe the right-to-die movement.

What is the Uniform Rights of the Terminally Ill Act?

- A 1989 federal proposal to guide state legislatures in constructing laws concerned with advance directives.

What is euthanasia?

- Mercy killing of the hopelessly ill
  - Active euthanasia: A conscious medical act that results in the death of a dying person
  - Passive euthanasia: Allowing a dying patient to die without medical interference
  - Voluntary euthanasia: Requires the patient's consent or the consent of the patient's legal representative to implement
  - Involuntary euthanasia: The use of medical means to end a dying patient's life without his or her consent

What is a death with dignity law in the United States?

- A death with dignity law allows for a qualified mentally competent terminally ill adult to request a prescription medication from their physician for the purpose of hastening their death.

What states have approved physician-assisted death as of 2016?

- Oregon
- Washington
- Vermont
- Montana
- California
- Colorado

LO 12.5 Identify the major features of organ donation in the United States.

What is the National Organ Transplant Act?

- A 1984 federal law that provides grants to qualified organ procurement organizations and that established an Organ Procurement and Transplantation Network (OPTN)
  - Established the United Network of Organ Sharing (UNOS) to administer the OPTN. The UNOS:
    - Increases the effectiveness and efficiency of organ sharing and equity in the national system of organ allocation.
    - Increases the supply of donated organs available for transplant.

What is the Uniform Anatomical Gift Act?

- A federal proposal that states enact laws allowing anyone 18 or older of sound mind to make a gift of his or her body or certain organs for use in medical research, transplantation, or storage in a tissue bank. A parent of a minor, a guardian of an individual, or an agent acting under a health care power of attorney to make an anatomical gift during the life of the child, ward, or principal may also make an anatomical gift. The act recommends that:
  - Donations made through a legal will are not to be held up by probate.
  - Except in autopsies, the donor's rights override those of others.
  - Survivors may speak for the deceased if no arrangements for donation were made prior to death, provided the deceased did not express an objection to donation before death.
  - Physicians who rely on donation documents for the acceptance of bodies or organs are immune from civil or criminal prosecution.
  - Hospitals, surgeons, physicians, accredited medical or dental schools, colleges and universities, and tissue banks or storage facilities may accept anatomical gifts for research, advancement of medical or dental science, therapy, or transplantation.

	• Time of death of the donor must be established by a physician who is not involved in transplanting the donor's designated organs, and the donor's attending physician cannot be a member of the transplant team. • Donors may revoke the gift, and gifts may be rejected.
LO 12.6 List the various stages of grief.	What is grief? • The human reaction to loss What are Elizabeth Kübler-Ross's stages of grief? • Denial • Anger • Bargaining • Depression • Acceptance What are Roberta Temes's stages of grief? • Numbness • Disorganization • Reorganization

Chapter 12 Review

Applying Knowledge

LO 12.1

1. Before the twentieth century, death most likely occurred
   a. In a hospital
   b. In a hospice
   c. At home
   d. At work
2. The purpose of the Uniform Determination of Death Act was to
   a. Define guidelines for determining when death actually occurs
   b. Teach caregivers how to prepare patients for death
   c. Teach caregivers how to use technology to prolong life
   d. None of these
3. The Uniform Determination of Death Act defines __________ as a means of determining when death actually occurs.
   a. Cessation of breathing
   b. Brain death
   c. Blood pressure reading
   d. Cessation of ability to speak
4. *Coma* is best defined as
   a. A deep sleep
   b. Severe mental impairment
   c. A deep stupor from which the person cannot be roused by external stimuli
   d. Cessation of all brain function

5. Persons said to be in a *persistent vegetative state*

   a. Cannot breathe on their own

   b. Can be aroused by external stimuli

   c. Have severe brain damage

   d. Are in a deep coma

6. Before pronouncing a nonresponsive and unconscious patient dead, physicians may perform certain tests. Which of the following is *not* a condition denoting death has occurred?

   a. Cannot breathe without assistance

   b. Cannot stand unaided

   c. Has no coughing or gagging reflex

   d. Pupils' lack of response to light

7. Recent reports indicate a decline in the number of nonmandatory autopsies performed in hospitals. Which of the following is a probable reason for the decline?

   a. Fewer patients are dying.

   b. Family members of deceased patients are often reluctant to give permission for an autopsy.

   c. No one wants to perform them.

   d. The law does not allow hospitals to perform autopsies.

LO 12.2

8. If one has 6 months or less to live, he or she is said to be

   a. Under palliative care

   b. Eligible for curative care

   c. Terminally ill

   d. Not eligible for hospice care

9. The general term used to describe documents serving to appoint an individual, chosen by the patient, to represent the patient's health care interests is

   a. Advance directive

   b. Curative care directive

   c. Palliative care directive

   d. Guardian *ad litem*

10. An authorization in advance to withdraw artificial life support is

    a. Assault

    b. Battery

    c. An advance directive

    d. Uniform Anatomical Gift directive

11. The Patient Self-Determination Act does *not* provide for

    a. Documenting the existence of an advance directive in the patient's medical record

    b. Nondiscrimination regarding whether or not a patient has an advance directive

    c. Compliance with state laws respecting advance directives

    d. Legal prosecution of health care practitioners who influence a patient's decision in preparing an advance directive

12. A form of advance directive that allows hospital patients to tell health care practitioners not to revive them if breathing stops is called a

    a. Durable power of attorney

    b. Will

    c. Do-not-resuscitate (DNR) order

    d. Summons

LO 12.3

13. Care provided to relieve pain and make a patient's last days as comfortable as possible is referred to as

    a. ICU care

    b. Palliative care

    c. Curative care

    d. Hospital care

14. The training of medical students about palliative care is

    a. Not done

    b. Is a separate course in every medical school

    c. Is covered, but every medical school does it differently

    d. Is not taught until the student becomes an intern

15. Undergraduate nursing students

    a. Receive no training in palliative care

    b. Are not required to take a palliative care course until graduate school

    c. Have 17 competencies in palliative care they must demonstrate

    d. May take a course in counseling as an elective

16. Hospice care is found

    a. Only in hospitals

    b. Only in special facilities

    c. Only as home care

    d. In all of the above locations

LO 12.4

17. Landmark events in the right to die movement include

    a. The *Karen Ann Quinlan* case

    b. The *Nancy Cruzan* case

    c. The *Terry Schiavo* case

    d. All of these

18. Physician-assisted death is legal

    a. In all 50 states

    b. Presently, only in six states

    c. Only when the patient agrees to be euthanized

    d. Never

19. Advocates of allowing a terminally ill patient to ask for assistance in dying refer to the process as

   a. physician-assisted death

   b. physician-assisted suicide

   c. involuntary euthanasia

   d. passive euthanasia

20. How many times did Oregon voters pass a Death with Dignity Act?

   a. One

   b. Two

   c. Three

   d. Only once, then the legislature acted

LO 12.5

21. Which recommendation paved the way for organ transplantation in the United States?

   a. Uniform Patient Self-Determination Act

   b. Uniform Rights of the Terminally Ill Act

   c. Uniform Anatomical Gift Act

   d. Uniform Death with Dignity Acts

22. Which legislation established organ procurement and transplantation networks in the United States?

   a. Uniform Rights of the Terminally Ill Act

   b. Death with Dignity Acts

   c. DNR order

   d. National Organ Transplant Act

23. Which of the following is true of organ transplants?

   a. Organ donors or their families must pay if a transplant occurs.

   b. Only individuals under the age of 55 can serve as organ or tissue donors.

   c. Prospective donors should inform family members of their wishes.

   d. Only family members can donate certain organs for transplantation.

24. The Uniform Anatomical Gift Act does *not* include the provision(s) that

   a. Persons 18 and older and of sound mind may donate organs and tissues for transplantation

   b. Donations made through a will are not to be held up in probate

   c. Organs are not accepted from patients over 60 years of age

   d. Except in autopsies, the donor's rights override the rights of others

LO 12.6

25. Which of the following best describes grief?

   a. An emotion one feels when loss has occurred

   b. The wish to die

   c. An emotion that should be denied

   d. None of these

26. Dr. Elisabeth Kübler-Ross's five stages of coping with a death or with a terminal illness do *not* include which of the following?
    a. Acceptance
    b. Bargaining
    c. Depression
    d. All of these are included
27. Which of the following is *not* true of the stages of grief?
    a. All grieving people progress through the stages in order.
    b. Grieving people may not experience one or more of the stages of grief.
    c. A person may experience the second stage of grief before the first or the third stage before the second.
    d. A person may go back and forth among the stages until resolution is accomplished.
28. Which of the following behaviors is probably most helpful to a dying person?
    a. Ignoring the fact that the person is dying
    b. Avoiding any discussion of future events
    c. Giving the person your attention and listening well
    d. Telling jokes

Ethics Issues Death and Dying

Use your critical thinking skills to answer the questions that follow each ethics issue.

Ethics ISSUE 1:

An understanding of the principles that underlie biomedical ethics is important in addressing the issues that confront health care practitioners and their patients at the end of life. The ethical principles include autonomy (the patient's right to self-determination), beneficence (acting in the patient's best interest), nonmaleficence (do no harm), justice (determine what is fair and just), and fidelity (truthfulness and faithfulness).

Discussion Questions

29. Assume you are an emergency medical technician (EMT) responding to a 911 call at a grocery store. An elderly shopper has collapsed, and she is unconscious on the floor when you arrive. Her vital signs are weak. The woman is placed in the ambulance, where she arrests. You notice that the woman is wearing a bracelet that says "DNR," and a quick check of her purse reveals a signed and witnessed DNR order. What do you do?
30. An 80-year-old woman has suffered a massive heart attack and is on a ventilator in the hospital's intensive care unit. She apparently has no advance directive. Her three daughters arrive from different areas of the United States and express their opinions about their mother's medical care. One daughter says her mother would "not want to be kept alive" in her present state, while a second, more aggressive daughter demands that "everything" be done to keep her mother alive. The third daughter expresses no opinion. In your opinion, what should be done?

Ethics ISSUE 2:

In some states, state law allows EMTs to do what is right for the patient when transporting them for care. In other states, the law may say EMTs must obey the patient's instructions, regardless of what those instructions are.

Discussion Questions

31. As an EMT in a state where the law says you must do what is right for the patient, you are transporting a patient with chest pain, and you decide to transport her to a hospital with heart catheterization capabilities, even though the patient has expressed a desire to go to a less well-equipped hospital in the area. Legally and ethically, how will you respond?

32. You are an EMT in a state where state law says the patient has the last word. The patient has been injured in a car accident, and you want to take him to a hospital with a level 1 trauma center, but he says no, take him to a different hospital, without a level 1 trauma center. Legally and ethically, what will you do?

Ethics ISSUE 3:

As a health care practitioner, you are committed to acting in the patient's best interest, and you believe that the wishes of patients in end-of-life situations should be followed. Furthermore, professional codes of ethics generally state that the social commitment of health care practitioners is to sustain life and relieve suffering and that when the performance of one duty conflicts with the other, the preferences of the patient should prevail.

Discussion Questions

33. As a nurse, you are assigned to help care for a middle-aged patient with a terminal, end-stage disease. He is in pain but has asked that pain medication not be administered, so he can keep his mind clear. He has also expressed a fear of addiction. You know that the patient could be relieved of his pain if he would only agree to be medicated. What will you do?

34. A young mother who was severely injured in a car accident is brought into the hospital trauma center where you work. She belongs to the Jehovah's Witnesses church and emphatically states that she refuses to have a blood transfusion. You know she risks death without a transfusion, but she believes her decision is a matter of her salvation. As a member of the patient's health care team, what will you do?

35. The female patient in the car accident scenario is unconscious, but her husband makes her wishes known regarding blood transfusions. Can you accept the husband's decision on the patient's behalf? Explain your answer.

Ethics ISSUE 4:

Health care practitioners are ethically bound to respond to the needs of the patient at the end of life, but they are also ethically bound to practice fidelity.

Discussion Question

36. When asked in a survey if they would ever withhold the truth about a terminal or preterminal diagnosis from a patient in order to keep his or her spirits up, physicians' responses were:

    "Most of the time, I tell them exactly as it is; they need to know the truth, and who am I to judge what they should or shouldn't know? However, if the patient is very frail emotionally and physically and has a very supportive family, I may not."

    "It's not about hiding information. It's learning how to talk to patients and giving bad news in the best way possible. All the information should be given, but any positive that exists should be also talked about."

    "The truth, delivered with compassion, is a gift."

    "I think patients deserve total honesty from their physician. They want to know."

    "An elderly patient who is senile will not understand, benefit, or prepare, so it is senseless to inform them. However, a family member, next of kin, or whoever is the health proxy will be notified."

    Which of the preceding statements most closely matches your opinion? Explain your answer.

Ethics ISSUE 5:

Your elderly aunt has asked you to take on her health care power of attorney. She makes the request while she is healthy and able to make her own decisions. You agree and sign the appropriate legal papers. She tells you at this time that she never wants "heroic measures" to be undertaken to save her life if her quality of life would suffer.

Discussion Questions

37. Five years later, your aunt is 86 and suffering from diabetes, coronary problems, and dementia. While in a long-term care facility, your aunt suffers a severe heart attack and is transported to the local hospital's emergency room. She is conscious when she reaches the emergency room, and when the attending physician asks her if she wants "all measures taken to preserve her life," she says yes. When you arrive at the hospital, your aunt is comatose and has been placed in the intensive care unit. Her physician says she cannot recover, but he could transport her to a larger hospital where physicians could "try" a pacemaker. How will you respond?
38. What ethical issues will influence your decision?

Case Studies

Use your critical thinking skills to answer the questions that follow each case study.

LO 12.4

39. The state you live in passed a Death with Dignity law a year ago. Your 75-year-old grandmother's physical health has continued to deteriorate. Her physician recently told her that she probably has 6 to 8 months to live and that she will be partially paralyzed within 2 months and completely paralyzed within 4 months. She confides in you that she really would like to "end it all" and take advantage of the Death with Dignity law. How are you going to proceed? Will you proceed differently if you know that your father (your grandmother's son) is very opposed to the death with dignity process?

LO 12.5

40. Your 14-year-old nephew is in need of a new kidney. It is determined that you are a perfect match for a transplant. What will you consider before making a decision?

Internet Activities

LO 12.2, 12.4, and 12.5

Complete the activities and answer the questions that follow.

41. Visit the Web site for Caring Connections at www.caringinfo.org. Download a living will and a health care power of attorney form from at least two states. Compare the two states' forms. How do they differ? How are they the same?
42. How many states are considering death with dignity type laws? Have any of the six states that have approved death with dignity type laws changed them? There are several Web sites that will provide you with accurate information.
43. Visit the Web site https://optn.transplant.hrsa.gov/. Determine how many people are waiting for transplants, how many have had transplants so far in the year, and how many donors there have been in the same time period. What organs are most often transplanted? What organs are least often transplanted? Why is there such a big difference?

Resources

LO 12.1

Guidelines for brain death www.neurology.org/content/74/23/1911.full.html#sec-21

LO 12.2

DNR orders

www.floridahealth.gov/licensing-and-regulation/trauma-system/_documents/dnro-form-multi-lingual2004bwyw.pdf

https://medlineplus.gov/ency/patientinstructions/000473.htm

Living wills

www.pbs.org/now/shows/541/living-wills.html

www.mayoclinic.org/healthy-lifestyle/consumer-health/in-depth/living-wills/art-20046303

LO 12.3

Dumanovsky Tamara, Augustin Rachel, Rogers Maggie, Lettang Katrina, Meier Diane E., and Morrison R. Sean. The growth of palliative care in U.S. hospitals: A status report. *Journal of Palliative Medicine 19*(1): 8–15. December 2015. doi:10.1089/jpm.2015.0351.

Committee on Approaching Death: Addressing Key End of Life Issues, Institute of Medicine. *Dying in America: Improving Quality and Honoring Individual Preferences Near the End of Life.* Washington (DC): National Academies Press, 2015, Chapter 4, Professional Education and Development. Available from: www.ncbi.nlm.nih.gov/books/NBK285682/

Talking about death

www.jhartfound.org/blog/talking-with-patients-about-end-of-life-care-new-poll-reveals-how-physicians-really-feel/

www.pewforum.org/2013/11/21/views-on-end-of-life-medical-treatments/#an-aging-america-with-limited-attention-to-preparation-for-dying

www.pewforum.org/2013/11/21/to-end-our-days/

www.jhartfound.org/news-events/news/advance-care-planning-poll

www.jhartfound.org/images/uploads/resources/ConversationStopperPoll_Press_Release.pdf

http://files.kff.org/attachment/topline-methodology-kaiser-health-tracking-poll-september-2015

www.todaysgeriatricmedicine.com/news/ex_062613.shtml

www.huffingtonpost.com/2013/11/21/death-america-pew-research_n_4312321.html

Hospice care

www.nhpco.org/sites/default/files/public/Statistics_Research/2015_Facts_Figures.pdf

www.cdc.gov/nchs/fastats/hospice-care.htm

https://optn.transplant.hrsa.gov/governance/about-the-optn/vision-goals/

http://healthaffairs.org/blog/2014/09/09/improving-access-to-high-quality-hospice-care-what-is-the-optimal-path/

Certifications/Training in palliative care

http://aahpm.org/certification/subspecialty-certification

www.aacn.nche.edu/news/articles/2016/elnec

http://hpcc.advancingexpertcare.org/competence/aprn-achpn/

http://aahpm.org/certification/subspecialty-certification

www.aacn.nche.edu/elnec

LO 12.4

www.doh.wa.gov/YouandYourFamily/IllnessandDisease/DeathwithDignityAct

www.pewresearch.org/fact-tank/2015/10/05/california-legalizes-assisted-suicide-amid-growing-support-for-such-laws/

https://public.health.oregon.gov/ProviderPartnerResources/EvaluationResearch/DeathwithDignityAct/Pages/ar-index.aspx

LO 12.5

https://optn.transplant.hrsa.gov/

LO 12.6

Konigsberg, Ruth Davis. *The Truth about Grief.* New York: Simon & Schuster, 2011.

Konigsberg's book synopsized in *Time,* January 24, 2011, pp. 42–46.

Kübler-Ross, Elisabeth. *On Death and Dying.* New York: Scribner, 1969.

Temes, Roberta. *Solace: Finding Your Way through Grief and Learning to Live Again.* New York: Amazon Books, 2009.

Worden, W. *Grief Counseling and Grief Therapy.* New York: Springer, 1982.

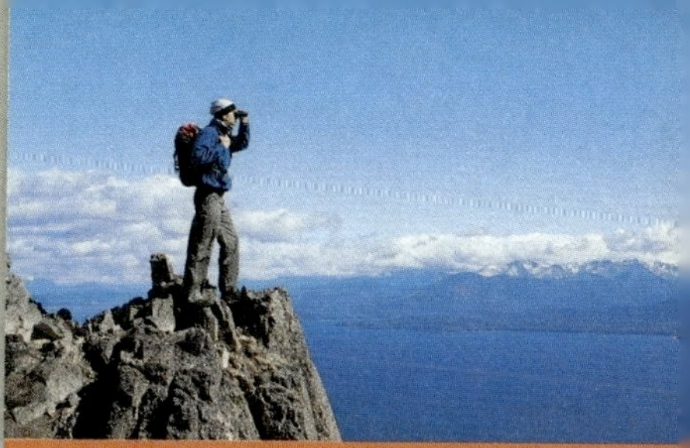

©Javier Pierini/Getty Images RF

Health Care Trends and Forecasts

13

Key Terms

- access
- Agency for Healthcare Research and Quality (AHRQ)
- birth rate
- cost
- fertility rate
- genomics
- gross domestic product (GDP)
- life expectancy
- life span
- personalized medicine
- pharmacogenomics
- proteomics
- quality
- stakeholders
- well-being

LEARNING OUTCOMES

After studying this chapter, you should be able to:

LO 13.1 Identify the expectations of the major stakeholders in the U.S. health care system.

LO 13.2 Describe the major factors influencing the cost of health care.

LO 13.3 Examine the major components of both access and quality in health care.

LO 13.4 Discuss those trends in medical research and treatment that may affect the delivery of health care in the future.

FROM THE PERSPECTIVE OF. . .

WHEN STEVE, a speech pathologist and gerontologist, meets with his group, they sometimes build a swimming pool—virtually, not literally. They discuss such steps in the process as: What are the pool's dimensions? How much dirt, in cubic feet, will we have to move? How much cement will we need? How many gallons of water will the pool hold? On days when they aren't building swimming pools, Steve's group may be reviewing little-known countries and areas in the world, such as Uruguay or the Ivory Coast.

Steve helps rehabilitate people recovering from head injuries who come to him as a result of on-the-job accidents, car crashes, adverse drug reactions, strokes, West Nile virus, Legionnaires disease, rodeo or sports mishaps, and other occurrences that result in brain injury. A neuropsychologist evaluates the individuals and draws up individual therapy plans and goals. The therapy is intense, Steve says, and repetitive. Because the brain is "an intricate little piece of equipment, no two cases of brain injury are alike in more than one or two functional aspects." But "we generally work on cognitive skills, such as listening, learning, and memory." For example, one of Steve's people had trouble remembering the names for everyday items. When asked to name a door, she could recall *hinge* and *knob* but not the more common *door*. Until, that is, Steve asked her for directions to an office in the building and she said, "You go through this door. . . ."

Steve celebrates successes with his people—no matter how small—but many times wishes doctors had referred brain-injured individuals earlier. "For too long, the general consensus has been based on a false assumption that injuries to the brain are incurable and the consequences permanent." While it is true that the site of the damaged tissue remains permanently in place, he says, "the brain has the remarkable ability to find neural pathways around the damaged tissue and recover lost functioning."

From Steve's perspective, brain-injured people should begin therapy as quickly as possible, and it's never too late to start therapy.

Too often from a physician's perspective, brain injuries cause permanent loss of function.

From an injured person's perspective, therapy may be tedious, but regaining lost function is often possible and always worth the struggle.

As you have progressed through *Law & Ethics for Health Professions,* you have gained knowledge about legal issues affecting every health care practitioner. You have also learned that in addition to the law, ethics play a crucial role in health care decisions. This final chapter outlines major concerns all Americans have with the country's health care system and offers a glimpse of possibilities for the future.

13.1 The Stakeholders

Those who have a vested interest in the health care industry in the United States and in any efforts to reform the industry are called **stakeholders.** The many health care stakeholders also have certain expectations and concerns that can align with or conflict with those of other

stakeholders
Those who have a vested interest in the health care industry in the United States, and in any efforts to reform the industry.

groups of stakeholders. Stakeholders include, but are not limited to, the following:

1. **Consumers—the patients and their families.** The patients who use health care services will always be at the head of the list of stakeholders. When health problems arise, patients want readily available and excellent health care, delivered by compassionate, skilled practitioners, at affordable prices. When receiving health care insurance from employers, employees want employers to provide a variety of health care insurance options, with features that can be customized to fit individual needs and with low out-of-pocket cost to the employee.
2. **Employers.** Because employers often provide health care benefits for employees, they hope to contract with health care providers who can deliver quality services at a reasonable cost. Employers want to maintain or lower the cost of their contribution to employees' health care. They want the employee to seek only needed care, follow providers' instructions, and recover quickly to full utility. They also want patients to reduce their health risk behaviors, that is, improve diet and exercise habits as recommended for healthy living, and to refrain from using alcohol in excess and from smoking.
3. **Health care facilities and practitioners.** As the providers of health care services, facilities such as hospitals, skilled nursing care organizations, physicians' practices, medical and dental clinics, laboratory and radiology services, rehabilitation hospitals, and many others engaged in providing some aspect of health care influence the quality, range, and cost of health care services provided.

   Health care practitioners tend to view quality in a technical sense: Were diagnoses correct? Did patients receive the appropriate therapies? What was the resulting health outcome for patients? Providers want to give patients the best service possible, using the most accurate and modern tests and treatments, which are also likely the most expensive. Providers also want to offer preventive care, which insurance companies (payers) may not cover.

   Health care facilities such as hospitals, clinics, group medical practices, skilled nursing organizations, and other entities, and health care payers such as managed care organizations (HMOs may also be service providers, for example, Kaiser Permanente), private insurance companies, and other insurance organizations are further classified as for-profit or nonprofit. For-profit companies are generally founded to generate income for an individual or individuals and their employees or their shareholders. For-profit companies provide health care services and products, just as nonprofit health care companies do. Both profit and nonprofit companies work toward having a positive income at the end of a year. The for-profit health care company may distribute that income to its owners or shareholders. The nonprofit, by law, must recycle the income back into the company's mission and activities.
4. **Federal, state, and local governments.** As one of the primary payers for health care, governments are near the top of the list of health care stakeholders. In the United States, the federal government helps pay the cost of health care services through provisions of the Patient Protection and Affordable Care Act (ACA) by helping lower-income enrollees in insurance exchanges pay for insurance and through

Medicare, Medicaid, Federal Employees Health Benefits Program, Military Health System, Veterans Health Administration, Indian Health Service, State Children's Health Insurance Program, and other programs. State governments also fund certain health care programs, including the state share of Medicaid, health benefits for public employees, and health care for persons with mental illness and developmental disabilities. At the city and county levels, local governments provide many health care services, often for vulnerable populations. Such services include locally owned and operated hospitals, free or pay-as-you-can medical clinics, employee and retiree health insurance, public health services, and the local share of Medicaid. Governments want people to have easily accessible quality health care at affordable costs. They also want people to take advantage of sources of information about how to achieve and maintain a healthy lifestyle, which involves choosing a healthy diet, exercising regularly, abstaining from illegal drugs, not smoking, and not using alcohol to excess. Governments have a vested interest in population health and, therefore, want all individuals to obtain recommended immunizations, get regular physicals, dental exams and other exams as necessary, and make every effort to follow a healthy lifestyle. Disparities in access to health care in the United States and the rising cost of health care products and services have often made these goals difficult to achieve.

5. **Private insurers.** Before managed care plans, private health insurance policies were traditionally written as third-party indemnity health insurance. Many of the Blue Cross Blue Shield indemnity plans were nonprofits. These were straightforward fee-for-service plans, with patients seeing any physician that accepted the insurance. Beginning in the late 1980s, managed care plans were developed to help reduce health care costs. As described in Chapter 3, managed care organizations are corporations that link health care financing, administration, and service delivery. This business model establishes a network of providers and coordinates patient care among its providers and hospitals. These plans usually limit the services subscribers may receive under the plans. These plans are sold to companies purchasing health insurance for their employees. They may also be sold in the ACA network of insurers.

   Private health insurers, whether indemnity plans or managed care plans, may be for-profit organizations, with the focus on the bottom line. Or if the private insurer/managed care plan is a nonprofit organization, it must also provide good reimbursement for providers, but any extra money is turned back into the provision of covered services after accounting for all costs.

6. **Volunteer facilities and agencies that provide health care or influence health care policies.** Disaster relief agencies and nongovernmental volunteer organizations that provide health care or funds for health care are also important stakeholders in the national health care system. Depending upon the organization, the focus is primarily on providing immediate, expert, cost-effective care to improve the health of patients in need.

7. **Health care practitioner training institutions.** Any training institution that prepares health care practitioners to administer health care

has a huge stake in the health care system and influences the system proportionately, according to the quality and quantity of practitioners they prepare. Training institutions want to attract students who will become competent, compassionate health care providers, and they hope to encourage others to attend their respective institutions.

8. **Professional associations and other health care industry organizations.** While each state's medical practice acts mandate licensing and/or certification for certain health care practitioners, professional associations and other industry organizations also establish and monitor health care practitioner ethics and offer advice and support for members of their diverse groups. This group of stakeholders strives to attract members to their organizations for the purpose of disseminating information, furthering education, or otherwise contributing to members' professional practice. Members of the organizations want to receive professional news and support without cost or for reasonable membership fees.
9. **Biotechnology companies.** Biotechnology companies, many of which are publicly traded on the stock market, are for-profit enterprises that research and develop treatments and cures for diseases and other medical conditions by applying technical advances in biology and other life sciences. While much of their research is applied to biologically based medicines (often constructed using an organism or an enzyme), their scope is much broader than health care, often involving agriculture. Such companies may or may not be owned by major pharmaceutical groups. Biotechnology companies are in business to earn a profit, so their aim is to offer products consumers will buy.
10. **Pharmaceutical companies.** Pharmaceutical companies are also for-profit enterprises, many of which are publicly traded on a stock exchange. Areas of health care involvement for pharmaceutical companies have always included research and development of chemically derived medications for specific disease protocols, but their business goals are to show a profit and to increase the wealth of stockholders. The profit incentive for pharmaceutical companies is often at odds with patients, health care providers, government payers, and insurance companies, which want to purchase effective drugs at affordable prices.
11. **Companies related to health care.** Companies that help manage the for-profit business of health care and companies making products to help patients engage in certain health care activities on their own, such as tracking fitness levels, following healthy diets, monitoring blood sugar, or performing other tasks between physician visits, also have a vested interest in the health care system. This group of health care stakeholders is in the business of selling products or services for a profit; therefore, they want to receive the highest possible price for their products, while recruiting new customers and retaining current customers. Consumers buying products or services from these businesses hope to receive maximum benefits at reasonable prices.

Key issues of concern to stakeholders within the American health care system are *cost, access,* and *quality*. The next two learning outcomes discuss these three important issues.

Check Your Progress

1. Name the top three stakeholders in the country's health care system.
2. Why are the top three stakeholders placed as 1, 2, and 3?
3. Give two examples of how one stakeholder group's expectations for health care conflict with those of another stakeholder group.
4. What are three major areas of concern for all health care stakeholders?

13.2 Cost of Health Care

cost
The amount individuals, employers, state and federal governments, HMOs, and insurers spend on health care in the United States.

access
The availability of health care and the means to purchase health care services.

quality
The degree of excellence of health care services offered.

Key issues of concern to stakeholders within the American health care system are ***cost, access,*** and ***quality***.

Cost refers to the amount individuals; employers; local, state, and federal governments; managed care organizations; private insurers; and other stakeholders spend on health care in the United States. As explained in the section entitled "Access," the number of people who have **access** to health care services—that is, the number of people for whom the services are available and for which they as consumers can pay—also helps determine cost. In addition, the cost of health care services also directly affects the **quality**, or degree of excellence, of health care services offered. Access and quality are discussed in LO 13.3.

THE NATION'S HEALTH CARE DOLLAR

In 2016, according to data provided by the Centers for Medicare and Medicaid Services, growth in health care spending for the United States was projected to average 5.6 percent from 2015–2025, hitting $3.35 trillion, or $10,345 per person by the end of 2016. The coverage expansion that began in 2014 as a result of the Affordable Care Act continued to have an impact on the growth of health care spending in 2015 and 2016. Additionally, faster growth in total health care spending in 2015 and 2016 was driven by stronger growth in spending for private health insurance, hospital care, physician and clinical services, and the continued strong growth in Medicaid and retail prescription drug spending. The overall share of the U.S. economy devoted to health care spending was 17.8 percent in 2015, up from 17.4 percent in 2014 and expected to rise to 19.9 percent by 2025.

Although we talk about health care's "cost for the country," ultimately, American taxpayers and consumers pay all health care costs. The nation's health dollar comes from the taxes and insurance premiums we pay, as well as from our co-payments (that part of health care charges we pay before insurance kicks in) and out-of-pocket expenditures (health care costs that insurance does not reimburse). Health care dollars are taken from consumers and move to providers through several routes, as illustrated in Figure 13-1.

The biggest funder of the nation's health care dollar, making up 74 percent, is health insurance. The category "health insurance" includes

FIGURE 13-1 The Nation's Health Care Dollar: Calendar Year 2015, Where It Came From

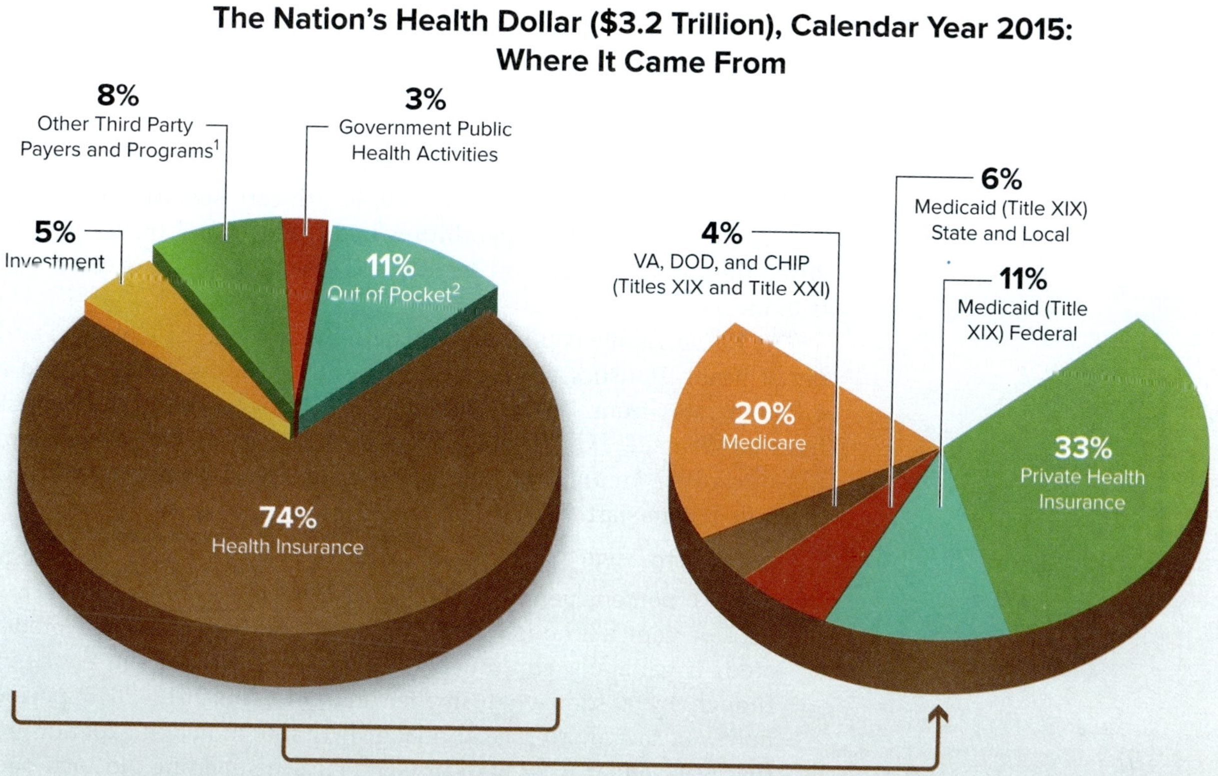

[1]Includes worksite health care, other private revenues, Indian Health Service, workers' compensation, general assistance, and maternal and child health, vocational rehabilitation, Substance Abuse and Mental Health Services Administration, school health, and other federal and state local programs.

[2]Includes co-payments, deductibles, and any amounts not covered by health insurance.

NOTE: Sum of pieces may not equal 100 percent due to rounding.

Source: Centers for Medicare & Medicaid Services, Office of the Actuary, National Health Statistics Group. www.cms.gov/Research-Statistics-Data-and-Systems/Statistics-Trends-and-Reports/NationalHealthExpendData/Downloads/PieChartSourcesExpenditures2015.pdf.

private health insurance purchased from companies offering policies; Medicare, a federal government health care program; Medicaid, funded by both state and federal governments; and other funders categorized as health insurance providers, including the Veterans Administration, Department of Defense (military health care), Children's Health Insurance Program, and other government contributors.

Medicaid and Medicare share about 37 percent of the cost when the health care dollar is split. Who pays for those receiving health care through those programs? All of us do through the taxes we pay. Medicare is paid for by a payroll tax on both the employer and the employee. Medicaid revenues come from both state and federal general taxes. This is represented in Figure 13-1 by the smaller pie graph on the right. Private insurance makes up 33 percent of this slice of the dollar, with the total share of the health insurance dollar now totaling 74 percent of the nation's health care dollar, as mentioned above.

The 11 percent "out-of-pocket" share of the health care dollar represents paying for services not covered by a health plan or insurer in the form of patients' co-payments and fees paid for products and services not reimbursed by insurance. For example, an insurance plan mandates paying $50 for a doctor visit before insurance payments kick in (co-payment), or a patient must pay the entire fee for services, such as a chiropractor, alternative medicine practitioner, or dental work, because these providers or services are not included in a health plan's list of approved fees.

Figure 13-2 illustrates how the nation spent the $3.2 trillion in health care expenses in 2015. In 1970, health care spending was $74.6 billion. By 2000, health expenditures had reached $1.4 trillion, and in 2015, the amount spent on health had doubled, to more than $3.2 trillion.

The Kaiser Family Foundation's Health System Tracker looks at a variety of health statistics, including how health spending has increased at different rates from 1970 to 2016. The following are some highlights from its Web site: http://www.healthsystemtracker.org/chart-collection/u-s-spending-healthcare-changed-time/?_sft_post_tag=health-spending#item-start

- From 1970–1980, the average annual growth in the U.S. economy was 9.2 percent per year, compared to health spending growth of 12.2 percent. Although health spending growth has since moderated, it generally continued to outpace growth of the economy, though by a somewhat smaller margin. The 2010–2013 period, however, saw an average annual growth rate in health expenditures that was similar to growth in GDP. Health spending did pick back up in 2014 and 2015 with the coverage expansions of the Affordable Care Act.
- On an average per-person basis and in constant dollars (dollars adjusted for inflation), health spending has increased from $1,734 per person in 1970 to $9,523 in 2014, just over a five-fold increase. However, an average per person is not necessarily a good number on which to judge health care expenditures.
- A small portion of the population accounts for a large share of health care spending in a year. In 2013, 50 percent of the *total* U.S. population accounted for 97 percent of the health care spending. Individual health care needs vary over the life span. People with serious or chronic illnesses, along with the elderly, often require more and higher-cost health services than those who are younger or otherwise need fewer and less costly services.
- The share of household budgets devoted to health expenditures has increased about 18 percent from 2002–2012. The majority of the increase can be attributed to spending on insurance premiums.
- National health care spending may also be analyzed by looking at the share of the nation's economy devoted to health care. The **gross domestic product (GDP)** is the total value of goods and services provided by a country during one year. In 1970, the United States devoted 6.9 percent of its GDP to total health spending through public and private funds. By 2014, the amount spent on health had increased to 17.5 percent of GDP.

gross domestic product (GDP)
The total value of goods produced and services provided in a country during one year.

FIGURE 13-2 The Nation's Health Care Dollar: Calendar Year 2015, Where It Went

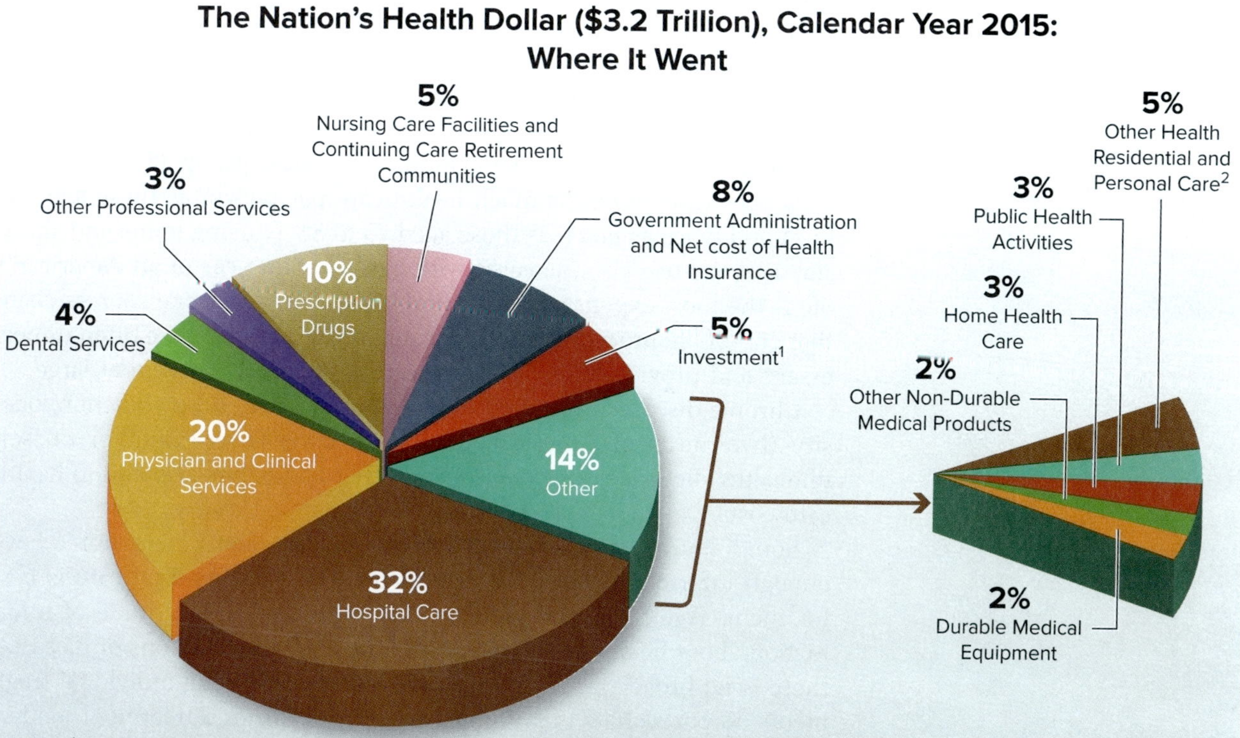

[1]Includes Noncommercial Research (2 percent) and Structures and Equipment (3 percent).

[2]Includes expenditures for residential care facilities, ambulance providers, medical care delivered in non-traditional settings (such as community centers, senior citizens centers, schools, and military field stations), and expenditures for Home and Community Waiver programs under Medicaid.

NOTE: Sum of pieces may not equal 100 percent due to rounding.

Source: Centers for Medicare & Medicaid Services, Office of the Actuary, National Health Statistics Group. www.cms.gov/Research-Statistics-Data-and-Systems/Statistics-Trends-and-Reports/NationalHealthExpendData/Downloads/PieChartSourcesExpenditures2015.pdf.

THE RISING COST OF HEALTH CARE

A consolidated list gleaned from a review of several organizations' surveys of health care costs—Kaiser Health News, the Bipartisan Policy Center, Becker's Hospital Review, and the Alliance for Health Reform—includes the following as contributors to increases in health care costs:

Fee-for-service reimbursement. Under current payment processes, facilities and practitioners are reimbursed for every service they provide, which often leads to a focus on volume instead of on care. The trend mandated by recent health care legislation is for payment to be based on quality and efficacy of care, rather than on the number of procedures and services provided—a change that could help lower health care costs in the future.

Fragmentation in payment and care delivery. Because patients often lack access to ongoing care and because different care providers often treat the same patient with little consultation, unnecessary care and errors often result. In addition, payment sources may fail to catch repetition of tests and other services to the same patient, thus overpaying for the same services.

Administrative burden on providers, payers, and patients. The long list of available health insurers and their complex billing processes cost the U.S. health care system billions in wasted costs every year and cost patients hours of time and frustration as they try to navigate the complicated system.

Aging population, rising rates of chronic disease, and lifestyle factors and personal health choices. According to Health Services Research, a department within the National Center for Biotechnology Information, after the first year of life, health care costs are lowest for children, rise slowly throughout adult life, and increase markedly after age 50. Annual costs for the elderly are approximately four to five times those of people in their early teens. Personal health expenditure also rises sharply with age within the Medicare population. The oldest group (85 and older) consumes three times as much health care per person as those aged 65 to 74 and twice as much as those aged 75 to 84. Nursing home and short-stay hospital use also increases with age. The last year of an American's life is the most expensive for medical treatment, and some sources claim that end-of-life procedures and repeated hospitalizations are often unnecessary and provide little value to the patient and the system at large.

Chronic diseases caused by smoking, alcoholism, drug addiction, obesity (two-thirds of American adults are either overweight or obese), unhealthy diets, lack of exercise, and other bad habits also add to health care costs.

Some sources also say average health care consumers don't have enough information to make decisions about what medical care is best for them. While it's true patients can find online a multitude of information about health in general and about specific conditions or diseases, there is no broad standard for evaluating or comparing individual treatments. Reports show that even when evidence finds a treatment ineffective or even harmful, it can take a long time for that information to actually change how practitioners practice or what patients request.

Advances in medical technology. According to several sources, new medical technology accounts for between 38 and 64 percent of increasing health care costs. New computer-aided diagnostic and therapeutic equipment is costly to acquire and use, and unnecessary duplication of expensive medical equipment, as when nuclear imaging equipment is found in every hospital, has also added to health care costs.

Patient expectations are often also a factor because patients may often believe that the most advanced (and usually most expensive) care is also the best in quality or is a better guarantee of a cure, when research has not borne out these conclusions in certain situations.

Tax treatment of health insurance. Before the 2010 passage of the Affordable Care Act, the majority of people with health insurance got it through their jobs. The employer-provided insurance system was set up so that the amount employers paid toward coverage was tax deductible for the business and tax exempt to the worker, thus encouraging more expensive health plans with richer benefits. Coverage design also played a role: Low deductibles or small office co-payments could encourage overuse of care. Increasingly, however, with implementation of the ACA, employers are moving toward higher-deductible coverage as a way to slow premium growth and require workers to pay more toward the cost of care.

Changing trends in health care market consolidation and competition for providers and insurers. Mergers and partnerships among medical providers and insurers are often in the news. While such consolidation may improve efficiency and help lower prices in a specific market, it can also have the opposite effect: lowering competition and driving up prices.

Higher physician, facility, and drug costs. Health care facilities and practitioners are consistently raising prices in concert with higher prices charged for supplies, products, and services such as utilities, labor, and other contingencies.

While medication makes up just about 10 percent of the total U.S. health care bill, costly new therapies to treat diseases such as hepatitis C and cancer are in use. Many drugs lost patent protection over the last five years, which in the past has meant cheaper generic drugs took their place, resulting in huge savings for buyers of medications. However, increasingly expensive new drugs, instead of cheaper generics, have replaced those drugs losing patents, thus ending that trend.

The health care legal and regulatory environment, including medical malpractice and fraud and abuse laws. Malpractice premiums, jury awards, and defensive medicine are often included as causes for increases in health care spending. Defensive medicine refers to the practice of prescribing unnecessary tests or treatment out of fear of facing a lawsuit. The many frauds perpetrated to obtain payments from health care payers also add to health care costs.

COSTS FOR INDIVIDUALS

The Patient Protection and Affordable Care Act of 2010 established "shared responsibility" among federal and state governments, employers, and individuals for ensuring that all Americans have access to affordable, quality health care. Because health care affordability is most often determined by access to private health insurance or government-assisted payment, such as Medicare or Medicaid, the ACA's primary goal was to increase access to insurance. Accordingly, the ACA initially prohibited insurance companies from refusing coverage for preexisting conditions and mandated extended coverage of children to age 26. Additional provisions of the ACA enacted in 2014 prohibited insurers from denying coverage or setting rates based on health status, medical condition, claims experience, genetic information, evidence of domestic violence, or other health-related factors. Insurance premiums were to vary only by family structure, geography, actuarial value, tobacco use, participation in a health promotion program, and age (by not more than three to one).

This attempt to ensure coverage for everyone, no matter how ill or otherwise likely to use health care services, was to be anchored at the younger, healthier end of the demographic scale by signing up 18- to 34-year-olds who had previously not carried health insurance because they were less likely to need health care services. To encourage younger, healthier people to enter the health insurance pool, the ACA required that every adult over 18 not covered by parents' health insurance buy insurance or pay a fine.

Penalties for not obtaining health insurance were relatively low for the first two years after the ACA was enacted. But as of 2016, those who had no health insurance but opted out of buying policies would have to pay a fine of either 2.5 percent of their annual household income or a flat fee of $695 per adult and $347.50 per child, whichever was higher. The Court Case in this section illustrates the requirement. Fines were to be collected after income taxes for 2016 were filed by deducting what was due for refusing health insurance from tax refunds. Whether or not the reduction in tax refunds would be enough over time to force previously uncovered individuals to buy health insurance remains to be seen as the ACA remains in force.

Federal tax credits and subsidies have been available since the ACA was enacted to cover the cost of health insurance for lower- and middle-income individuals entering the insurance market. In 2014, state- and federally administered health insurance marketplaces were established to provide additional access to health insurance coverage with insurance premium subsidies for low- and middle-income people. States were given the option of participating in a federally subsidized expansion of Medicaid eligibility. In mid-2016, according to the Kaiser Family Foundation, 32 states and the District of Columbia had adopted Medicaid expansion. In addition to Medicaid expansions, also in 2016, according to the National Academy for State Health Policy, there were 13 state-based health insurance exchanges, 25 federally facilitated marketplaces, and various other partnership exchanges through which people within each state could purchase health insurance.

According to the U.S. Census Bureau, in 2012, 48 million people aged 18 and older (15.4 percent of the population) had no health insurance. In mid-2016, the Census Bureau reported that only 9.1 percent of the population went without health insurance in 2015. While more people obtaining health insurance was good news, separate Census Bureau data showed that medical out-of-pocket expenses (higher insurance premiums, co-payments, and higher deductibles) caused an additional 11.2 million people to be classified at the poverty level—a figure determined by one's income as compared to the current cost of living index. (The poverty-level annual income for a family of three in 2014 was $19,055.) Thus, even though median income for U.S. wage earners increased to $56,516 in 2015 and even with government subsidies available to help pay the cost of health insurance, many individuals were still struggling to pay health care costs in 2016.

Job-based health insurance coverage remained strong in 2015, with 55.7 percent of the population receiving health insurance through work. Work-based health insurance in the United States began after World War II, when competition was strong for qualified workers. The government encouraged the practice by exempting employers from paying taxes on employer-provided health insurance programs. However, because the ACA contains a "Cadillac tax" provision, which is a 40 percent surcharge on the value of employer-based health premiums above certain specified thresholds, by 2016, many employers had converted to insurance plans with high deductibles.

With the election of Donald Trump as president of the United States in November 2016, the continued implementation of the provisions of the Affordable Care Act was dependent upon the act remaining in force. President Trump had campaigned on the promise to repeal the act but had also expressed the desire to keep some of the provisions of the ACA in force, such as the requirement for insurance companies to insure people with previous conditions and the ability of children to remain on their parents' health insurance policies until age 26. The status of the ACA and of the people who obtained insurance under its administration will depend entirely upon future acts of President Trump and the two houses of Congress.

COURT CASE Suit Brought over ACA Requirement to Buy Insurance

In a case argued on appeal in May 2015 and decided in August 2015, a resident of Pennsylvania sued the U.S. Department of Health and Human Services when he lost his health insurance. His policy was discontinued because it did not meet the requirements of the 2010 Patient Protection and Affordable Care Act. He objected to being "forced" to purchase health insurance or pay a fine.

The plaintiff was presented in court as "financially stable," with "an annual income that requires him to file federal tax returns." He maintained that he "could afford health insurance if he wanted to obtain such coverage." The plaintiff said he was "non-observant in his religion, and does not qualify for the Affordable Care Act's religious exemption" but "does not want to be forced to purchase health insurance."

The plaintiff originally filed suit in the U.S. District Court for the District of Columbia, challenging the ACA as unconstitutional, both "facially" and as applied to him. His complaint alleged that the religious exemption in the act violates the First Amendment's guarantee of religious freedom and constituted an unconstitutional establishment of religion. The plaintiff also claimed violation of his rights under the Equal Protection Clause in the Fourteenth Amendment because all states did not implement provisions of the act equally.

The appeals court concluded that the plaintiff had standing to litigate his Establishment Clause claim, but his argument failed "on the merits." Furthermore, the plaintiff lacked standing "to press his equal protection challenge."

Published as part of the court's decision was the argument that unless, as mandated in the ACA, people were provided incentives to purchase health insurance, they would wait until they got sick to buy insurance, which results in "adverse selection," an economic term describing a situation in which the insurance pool is skewed toward predominantly sick people using more insurance benefits than others in the pool.

The appeals court decision proclaimed that effectively, the plaintiff in this case was not exempt from the ACA provision requiring him to purchase health insurance or pay a fine.

Source: Cutler v. US Dept. of Health and Human Services, 797 F.3d 1173 (2015) – United States Court of Appeals, Dist. of Columbia Circuit.

Check Your Progress

5. The largest percentage of the nation's health care dollar comes from what source?
6. Ultimately, who is the primary funder of the nation's health care dollar?
7. Name six factors that have contributed to increases in health care costs.
8. The ACA prohibited insurance companies from excluding potential clients with preexisting conditions. What did the authors of the act foresee as a measure to balance out the insurance pool in order to pay for clients using more health care services?
9. What is the purpose of the "shared responsibility" established by the ACA?

13.3 Access and Quality

ACCESS

Access to health care means that people are able to use appropriate health care services when necessary in order to maintain and improve their health. For access to exist:

1. Adequate services, such as primary physicians and specialists, hospitals, medical clinics, urgent care, emergency services, and so on, must exist, and members of a population must physically be able to reach them. In certain areas, such as inner cities and rural areas, there are often too few health care practitioners and diagnostic facilities. In addition, there can be structural barriers to obtaining health care services, such as lack of transportation to health care providers, mobility limitations, an inability to obtain convenient appointment times, or lengthy waiting room times. All of these factors reduce the likelihood of a person successfully making and keeping health care appointments.
2. If adequate health care services and facilities exist and members of a population are able to reach them, they must also be able to *utilize* the health care system. Sometimes social or cultural barriers exist that can hinder utilization of health care services. For example, language barriers, such as poor English language skills, can make it difficult for people to understand basic information about health conditions or to determine when they should visit their doctor.

   Most often utilization depends upon affordability. Health insurance facilitates affordability and, therefore, utilization of the health care system. Uninsured people are less likely to have entry into the health care system to seek treatment when it is most helpful for treating or preventing major illnesses.

   Utilization of the health care system is also more likely if people can access health care providers who meet their needs. Seeing primary care providers—doctors, nurse practitioners, physician assistants—regularly helps increase the likelihood that people will receive appropriate care. Primary care providers who see patients over time learn about their diverse health care needs and can coordinate care to better meet those needs. Studies have shown that patients with regular primary care providers receive higher-quality care, have better health outcomes, and maintain better health than those without such primary providers.
3. Access to regular primary care providers also ensures that people receive ongoing health care. "Ongoing" means that patients can continue to see their chosen providers over time, ensuring that patients with conditions requiring more than one source of care will be able to see other providers as necessary. For example, women of childbearing age and older people tend to have more than one doctor. Specific facilities providing ongoing care include urgent care/walk-in clinics, doctors' offices, medical clinics, health center facilities, hospital outpatient clinics, health maintenance organizations/preferred provider organizations, military or other Veterans Affairs health care facilities, or other similar sources of care. (Hospital emergency rooms are excluded as sources of *ongoing* care.)

QUALITY

Historically, the quality of the health care services delivered to individuals has varied based on race, ethnicity, socioeconomic status, age, sex, disability status, sexual orientation, gender identity, and residential location. With the passage of the ACA in 2010, the Department of Health and Human Services was charged with identifying national disparities and developing and implementing a National Quality Strategy (NQS) to achieve better care, healthier people and communities, and affordable care.

The National Quality Strategy has set three broad aims for the improvement of health care in the United States:

- Better care: Improve the overall quality by making health care more patient-centered, reliable, accessible, and safe.
- Healthy people and healthy communities: Improve the health of the U.S. population by supporting proven interventions to address behavioral, social, and environmental determinants of health in addition to delivering higher-quality care.
- Affordable care: Reduce the cost of quality health care for individuals, families, employers, and government.

Source: National Quality Strategy.

To advance these aims, the NQS focuses on six priorities:

1. Making care safer by reducing harm caused in the delivery of care
2. Ensuring that each person and family is engaged as partners in their care
3. Promoting effective communication and coordination of care
4. Promoting the most effective prevention and treatment practices for the leading causes of mortality, starting with cardiovascular disease
5. Working with communities to promote the wide use of best practices to enable healthy living
6. Making quality care more affordable for individuals, families, employers, and governments by developing and spreading new health care delivery models

In addition to tracking the success of the NQS aims, the **Agency for Healthcare Research and Quality (AHRQ),** the lead federal agency responsible for assessing the health care system and recommending improvements for the quality, safety, efficiency, and effectiveness of health care for Americans, publishes the *National Healthcare Quality and Disparities Report*. Data for the report are obtained through:

Agency for Healthcare Research and Quality (AHRQ)
The lead federal agency responsible for tracking and improving the quality, safety, efficiency, and effectiveness of health care for Americans.

- Surveys of patients, patients' families, and providers
- Administrative data from health care facilities and home health agencies
- Abstracts of clinical charts
- Registry data
- Vital statistics

The most recent AHRQ report, titled *2015 National Healthcare Quality and Disparities Report and 5th Anniversary Update on the National Quality*

Strategy, lists the following findings under the six goals set by the National Quality Strategy:

1. **Patient safety** improved substantially, led by a 17 percent reduction in hospital-acquired conditions between 2010 and 2014. Patient safety disparities were uncommon.

   Source: AHRQ report, titled 2015 *National Healthcare Quality and Disparities Report and 5th Anniversary Update on the National Quality Strategy*

2. **Person- and family-centered care.** Successful person-centered care entails more than just the successful completion of clinical care; it also means that patients achieve their own desired outcomes. Studies show that patient-centered primary care delivered in the patient-centered medical home (PCMH) model led to sustained decreases in the number of annual emergency department visits and primary care visits, as well as increased screening for some types of cancer. However, person-centered care needs to be integrated outside of medical homes in the fee-for-service settings in which most patients receive care. Person-centered care improved quickly from 2010 to 2014, but disparities were common, especially for Hispanics and poor people. As is true for access, disparities by income are larger than disparities by race or ethnicity.

3. **Effective communication and coordination of care across the health care system.** Navigating today's health care system is complicated. Patients receiving care often interact with many physicians, nurses, medical assistants, and other trained professionals across multiple settings, a situation especially true for the sickest populations. For example, more than two-thirds of Medicare patients have at least two chronic conditions, and 14 percent have more than six chronic conditions. Nearly 50 percent of Medicare patients with more than six chronic conditions have more than 13 doctor visits per year and account for up to 70 percent of Medicare hospital readmissions.

   The data collected show that when health care providers coordinate with each other, medication errors decrease, and there is a decrease in unnecessary or repetitive diagnostic tests, unnecessary emergency department visits, and preventable hospital admissions and readmissions. These improvements lead to higher quality of care, improved health outcomes, and lower costs. Because delivery of coordinated care necessarily brings together disparate sectors of the health and health care system, improving care coordination offers a potential opportunity for drastically improving care quality that could save $240 billion a year. Improvement in care coordination lagged behind other priorities, and disparities were common.

4. **Promoting the most effective prevention and treatment practices for the leading causes of mortality, starting with cardiovascular disease.** The prevalence of cardiovascular disease risk factors and lack of public awareness compound the problem. According to the Centers for Disease Control and Prevention, in 2012, 29 percent of American adults had hypertension and another third had prehypertension—both early warning signs of cardiovascular disease—but only 52 percent of those people with hypertension had their condition under control. Successful prevention and treatment of cardiovascular disease could significantly improve the nation's clinical

and economic health. Awareness of risk factors and treatment strategies are improving, and there are fewer disparities in this area.

5. **Healthy living: Working with communities to promote wide use of best practices to enable healthy living.** Although the United States spends more per capita on health care than any developed country in the world, its citizens as a whole are the least healthy. Nearly 45 percent of Americans have at least one chronic condition; such conditions are responsible for 70 percent of the nation's deaths and 75 percent of health care spending. Many illnesses associated with chronic conditions are related to unhealthy lifestyle behaviors, environmental hazards, and poor social supports, and can be prevented by increasing access to effective clinical preventive services and promoting community interventions that advance public and population health. Increasing public health spending and improving access to immunizations and preventive care hold promise as cost-efficient ways to create healthier communities, reduce the personal and economic burden of chronic illnesses, and improve quality of life while reducing disparities throughout the United States. Studies show that promoting healthy lifestyles that prevent disease and disability is better for people and more efficient than treating conditions after organ damage has been done. Measures of healthy living are long term and difficult to evaluate. As a result, measures of healthy living used in the 2015 AHRQ report focus on receipt of indicated counseling and preventive services rather than actual achievement of a healthy lifestyle. Disparities continue to exist along racial and socioeconomic lines.
6. **Making quality care more affordable for individuals, families, employers, and governments by developing and spreading new health care delivery models.** From 2011 to the first half of 2015, the percentage of people under age 65 in families having problems paying medical bills decreased overall and for all poverty status and racial/ethnic groups. In all the years for which data was collected, people in poor and near-poor families were more likely to have problems paying medical bills than people in families that were not poor. However, the gaps between people in poor and not poor families and between near-poor and not poor families have continued to narrow over time. In all years, compared with whites, blacks and Hispanics were more likely to have problems paying medical bills, while Asians were less likely to have problems. None of these racial gaps were changing over time.

You can access the entire 2015 AHRQ report at: www.ahrq.gov/sites/default/files/wysiwyg/research/findings/nhqrdr/nhqdr15/2015nhqdr.pdf.

Population Changes Affecting Cost, Access, and Quality Other population changes affecting cost, access, and quality include the following:

- *Declines in national fertility and birth rates*: The **fertility rate** is defined by the National Center for Health Statistics as the total number of live births per 1,000 women aged 15 to 44 years. These rates are based on the most recent population estimates from the Census Bureau. **Birth rates** are different from fertility rates in that the

fertility rate
The total number of live births per 1,000 women aged 15–44 years.

birth rates
Total number of live births per 1,000 women in a specific age group.

denominator is not all women aged 15 to 44 but rather a specific age group. Statistics for fertility rates show a decline over time in the United States from high to low fertility. The fertility rate for all U.S. women is now the lowest it has been since the data have been recorded, standing at 63 births per 1,000 women in 2013.

In one major measure of a country's health system—infant mortality—the United States ranks near the bottom, with an infant mortality rate of 6.1 deaths for every 1,000 live births, which is well below the average for wealthy countries. In Iceland, 1.6 babies out of every 1,000 die; in Sweden, Japan, and Finland, the number is about 2 per 1,000. Cost and access are most often listed as the reasons for America's too-high infant mortality rate, as well as too few resources devoted to public health and primary care. (The high percentage of uninsured Americans has been listed as a cause, but infant mortality rates could decrease as more women of childbearing age gain health insurance coverage.)

- *A steady increase in life expectancy at birth and life span at older ages.* **Life expectancy** refers to the number of years one can expect to live at birth, and **life span** is the number of years one actually lives. Whereas most babies born in 1900 in the United States did not live past age 50, life expectancy at birth for Americans in 2015 was approximately 78.8 years. The rising life expectancy within the older population itself is increasing the number and proportion of people at very old ages. The "oldest old" (people aged 85 or older) constitute 8 percent of the world's 65-and-over population: 12 percent in more developed countries+ and 6 percent in less developed countries. In many countries, the oldest old are now the fastest growing part of the total population. On a global level, the 85-and-over population is projected to increase 351 percent between 2010 and 2050, compared to a 188 percent increase for the population aged 65 or older and a 22 percent increase for the population under age 65.

  The global number of centenarians is projected to increase 10-fold between 2010 and 2050. In the mid-1990s, some researchers estimated that, over the course of human history, the odds of living from birth to age 100 may have risen from 1 in 20,000,000 to 1 in 50 for females in low-mortality nations such as Japan and Sweden. This group's longevity may increase even faster than current projections assume; previous population projections often underestimated decreases in mortality rates among the oldest old.

life expectancy
The number of years an individual can expect to live, calculated from his or her birth.

life span
The number of years an individual actually lives.

- *A shift in the leading causes of death and illness from infectious and parasitic diseases to noncommunicable diseases and chronic conditions.* In early nonindustrial societies, the risk of death was high at every age, and only a small proportion of people reached old age. Public health projects of the twentieth century, which immunized millions of people against smallpox, polio, and major childhood killers such as measles, are responsible for extending life spans in most developed countries. Better living standards over time, especially more nutritious diets and cleaner drinking water, have also greatly reduced serious infections and prevented deaths in populations. Consequently, in modern societies, most people live past middle age, and deaths are highly concentrated at older ages.

Check Your Progress

10. Check the 10 amendments to the U.S. Constitution called the Bill of Rights at www.archives.gov/exhibits/charters/bill_of_rights_transcript.html. Is health care listed as a right for all Americans?
11. What are the three main goals of the National Quality Strategy for health care in the United States?
12. What were three areas of improvement in the nation's health care, as noted in the 2015 AHRQ report?
13. What is the difference between life expectancy and life span? Between fertility rate and birth rate?
14. In your opinion, why has life expectancy in the United States increased over time, while infant mortality rate has remained higher than in many other countries?

13.4 Health Care Trends

Trends that are swiftly advancing as health care moves into the twenty-first century include, but are not limited to, health/medical technologies and personalized medicine. The World Health Organization defines health/medical technologies as "the application of organized knowledge and skills in the form of devices, medicines, vaccines, procedures and systems developed to solve a health problem and improve quality of lives." Personalized medicine is a type of medical care in which treatment is customized for each individual patient.

HEALTH/MEDICAL TECHNOLOGIES

New health/medical technologies are a major driving force within the health care industry. The following health/medical technologies, many of which are already in use and/or production, will create value and impact our lives and the practice of medicine in the near future:

- Advances in imaging
- Biologics
- Clinical-grade wearables
- Gene-editing techniques
- Point-of-care testing
- Rational and pharmacogenomic drug design
- Three-dimensional bioprinting

Advances in Imaging Imaging equipment continues to improve in resolution and maneuverability, and, in some cases, equipment is becoming smaller as function improves.

Three-dimensional (3D) images are now possible via X-rays. The process, called 3D tomographic X-ray, has been in use over at least the past five years for breast imaging, and its use is expected to expand quickly into other specialty areas, such as orthopedics. In 2015, the technology was assigned a current procedural terminology code; these codes are used to report and bill for medical, surgical, and diagnostic procedures and services, indicating that the technology's use will continue to expand.

Magnetic resonance imaging (MRI) scanners are also undergoing a revolution in size and strength. To simplify a complex machine, an MRI scanner is a large, strong magnet. A patient lies in the machine containing the magnet, and a radio wave is used to send signals to bounce off the body, which are then converted into images by a computer attached to the scanner. MRIs come in different magnet field strengths measured in teslas (T). Scanners between 0.5T and 3.0T have been the norm, but as of 2016, MRI scanners at 7T were for sale. Clarity of images and less time required for patients to be in the scanner are advantages associated with the stronger machines.

Ultrasound machines have also been undergoing revolutionary change. By 2011, ultrasound devices had shrunk to the size of a laptop computer. As of 2016, the machine was further miniaturized to a handheld device, and development was headed toward a pocket-sized device predicted to one day replace the stethoscope. Newer designs are app-based and pair with a smartphone or tablet.

Biologics Biologics are medical products made from a variety of natural sources (human, animal, or microorganism). Like chemical drugs, some biologics are intended to treat diseases and other medical conditions, whereas other biologics are used to prevent or diagnose diseases. Examples of biological products include:

- Vaccines
- Blood and blood products for transfusion and/or manufacturing into other products.
- Allergenic extracts, which are used for both diagnosis and treatment (for example, allergy shots).
- Human cells and tissues used for transplantation (for example, tendons, ligaments, and bone).
- Gene therapies
- Cellular therapies
- Tests to screen potential blood donors for infectious agents such as HIV.

Biologics developed to suppress the human immune system have shown great progress in treating such diseases as inflammatory arthritis, psoriasis, some forms of cancer, and some neurological diseases.

Clinical-Grade Wearables Health monitoring trackers had a big year in 2015. Several devices designed for tracking what some critics called "trivial" metrics such as steps and sleep were available. However, more sophisticated sensors and advanced analytics were in development that will make health-monitoring wearables more meaningful in the health care spectrum. For example, clinical-grade wearable heart monitoring systems paired with advanced analytics software have already been launched, and more biotechnology companies are likely to follow suit in offering wearable monitoring devices for other disease states. Along those lines, a digital contact lens was to become available possibly in late 2016 that would measure blood glucose from tears. Predictions were that such a device, if widely available, could significantly change diabetes treatment and management for the 29.1 million diabetes-afflicted patients in the United States.

Gene-Editing Techniques Chapter 11 introduced the rapidly advancing concept of modifying an organism's genome by "cutting out" genes responsible for disease and other malfunctions and inserting functional sequences for mutations. Research in such types of genetic engineering took a huge step forward in 2016 with the development of CRISPR-Cas9, a unique technology that lets geneticists cut out, replace, or add parts to a cell's DNA sequence. In simplest terms, it works like this: The system consists of two key molecules with specific functions. An enzyme called Cas9 (the first molecule) cuts through the two targeted DNA strands at specific locations. Bits of DNA can then either be added or removed. A piece of RNA (the second molecule) makes sure that the enzyme cuts at the right point in the genome. Scientists can use the technique to target and mutate one or more genes in targeted cells. Other DNA-altering techniques have been developed, but as of 2016, CRISPR-Cas9 had rapidly become the fastest, simplest, cheapest, most versatile and precise method of genetic manipulation.

Point-of-Care Testing Point-of-care testing, or bedside testing, is defined as medical diagnostic testing that takes place at the time and place of patient care. The routine for check-up appointments has been: When scheduling a doctor's appointment, a patient must also schedule a laboratory visit during which the phlebotomist draws blood for the tests the doctor wants run. The patient leaves the facility and waits—often up to a week or more for a routine check-up—for test results to reach the doctor. A follow-up appointment with the doctor may be necessary for the patient's treatment to be adjusted. Point-of-care testing allows patient diagnoses in the physician's office, ambulance, home, field, or hospital. The results of point-of-care testing are timely and allow rapid treatment of the patient. Point-of-care testing has the potential to significantly impact health care delivery and to address the challenges of health disparities. The success of a potential shift from curative medicine to predictive, personalized, and preemptive medicine could rely on the development of portable diagnostic and monitoring devices for point-of-care testing.

In the cancer treatment field, researchers have already developed a microfluidic device that can separate circulating cancer tumor cells from whole blood, a technology that has broad applications for fast diagnoses of cancer and appropriate yet immediate treatment of the various types of cancer. The microfluidic technology also shows promise for point-of-care testing for infectious diseases, such as strep, influenza, and HIV. The miniaturization of some imaging devices, as discussed in this section, may also contribute to the point-of-care testing trend.

Rational and Pharmacogenomic Drug Design Rational drug design refers to the use of increasingly powerful computers to develop new drugs by looking at the molecular structure and chemical composition of target cells and creating substances that will bind to certain molecules, affecting their function inside the body. For example, drugs now in development for antiviral use will prevent viruses from using the body's protease enzymes to chop up amino acids that viruses use as building blocks for replicating. These new antiviral drugs may be used to combat such diseases as HIV, encephalitis, measles, and influenza.

Drugs are also in development that can bind with receptors for various neurotransmitters in the nervous system, helping to reduce symptoms in patients suffering from neurological and mental diseases. Similarly, drugs in development to combat cancer will target cancer cells for destruction but will not destroy normal cells in the body, thus eliminating many of the noxious side effects cancer patients often suffer during chemotherapy.

pharmacogenomics
The science that defines how individuals are genetically programmed to respond to drugs.

Drug design has also profited from research in **pharmacogenomics,** the science that defines how individuals are genetically programmed to respond to drugs. Many drugs that are currently available are "one size fits all," but they don't work the same way for everyone. It can be difficult to predict who will benefit from a medication, who will not respond at all, and who will experience negative side effects (called adverse drug reactions). Adverse drug reactions are a significant cause of hospitalizations and deaths in the United States. The field of pharmacogenomics is still in its infancy. Its use is currently quite limited, but new approaches are under study in clinical trials. In the future, pharmacogenomics will allow the development of tailored drugs to treat a wide range of health problems, including cardiovascular disease, Alzheimer disease, cancer, HIV/AIDS, and asthma.

Three-Dimensional Bioprinting Three-dimensional (3D) printing, also called additive manufacturing, is a process that allows a printer to re-create solid objects from a digital file. The technology has been around for a while, revolutionizing such industries as manufacturing, art, education, and medicine, and allowing individuals to print a multitude of useful household objects, as well as a multitude of not-so-useful doodads. The latest development in 3D printing is the bioprinter, which allows living tissue to be reproduced by a specially adapted machine—the bioprinter. Bioprinters were first offered for purchase in 2014. As of 2016, the machines were being used to produce a variety of tissues, such as bone, lung, liver, heart, skin, and brain, for use in research. They hold the potential to reproduce human organs and tissues from donor cells for transplantation, without the rejection side effects inherent in person-to-person organ and tissue donation. The tissue "printed" with the machines will also be invaluable in drug testing and in researching tissue and organ structure.

PERSONALIZED MEDICINE

personalized medicine
The products and services that leverage the science of genomics and proteomics.

genomics
The branch of molecular biology concerned with the structure, function, evolution, and mapping of genomes.

proteomics
The study of proteins that genes create or express to create tailored, individual approaches to disease prevention and health care.

You may have noticed that most, if not all, of the medical and biotechnological trends discussed thus far mark another overriding trend in health care: personalized medicine. **Personalized medicine** is defined as the products and services that leverage the science of **genomics** and **proteomics**—the study of the proteins that genes create or express—to create tailored, individual approaches to disease prevention and health care.

The hope with personalized medicine is that there will be better patient outcomes, not just in disease management but also in maintaining wellness and improving each patient's participation in his or her own care. Most experts believe that personalized medicine can only become reality with coordination of services and long-term business strategies consistent among all of the players.

Check Your Progress

15. Choose three of the medical technologies that are emerging as health care progresses, and give specific examples of how each might be applied in medical/health care situations.
16. Briefly describe two ways tests might be ordered during a patient's routine physical if personalized medicine were fully utilized.

HEALTH CARE AND QUALITY OF LIFE

We can measure who has access to health care in the United States, study the cost of health care, and evaluate the quality of health care administered to patients, but one result of receiving quality health care at an affordable cost, when and where we need it is difficult to measure. That result is **well-being,** defined as the perception that one's life is going well, a physical and mental state that vastly improves quality of life—the ultimate end goal of the administration of health care, both for individuals and for the population as a whole.

well-being
Perception that one's life is going well, a physical and mental state that vastly improves the quality of life.

Well-being definitely derives partly from enjoying good physical health, but other markers—employment, adequate housing, satisfying social contacts and personal relationships—contribute to the feeling.

Well-being is a state of mind that is more difficult to measure than other aspects affecting quality of life, such as the overall administration of health care, where statistics and data collection can reveal disparities, short-comings, and solutions. Because well-being is most often revealed through self-reporting, Healthy People 2020, an ongoing initiative of the federal Office of Disease Prevention and Health Promotion, approaches the measurement of health-related quality of life and well-being by collecting data for the Patient-Reported Outcomes Measurement Information System (PROMIS). Survey participants are asked more than 1,000 questions about fatigue, pain, emotional distress, and social activities. Most of the questions ask about a person's experience "in general" and assess self-reported symptoms within the previous seven days. The PROMIS survey has proved to be an efficient measure of participants' assessment of their own quality of life.

Data collected from studies such as the PROMIS survey and followed over time reveal that individual and population well-being is associated with such positive results as:

1. Fewer incidents of physical and mental illness
2. Healthier behaviors
3. Social connectedness
4. Increased productivity
5. Longevity

These positive outcomes align with the long-term goals of Healthy People 2020, which include:

- Attain high-quality, longer lives for the population, free of preventable disease, disability, injury, and premature death.
- Achieve health equity, eliminate disparities, and improve the health of all groups.

- Create social and physical environments that promote good health for all.
- Promote quality of life, healthy development, and healthy behaviors across all life stages.

Ensuring access to the American health care system, providing health care at affordable cost, and ensuring high-quality health care delivery are the keys to achieving a sense of well-being and a high quality of life for every individual.

Chapter Summary

Learning Outcome	Summary

LO 13.1 Identify the expectations of the major stakeholders in the U.S. health care system.	Who are health care *stakeholders?*
	• Anyone with a vested interest in the health care industry
	Who are the major stakeholders in the U.S. health care industry, and what are their concerns?
	• Consumers—the patient and family
	  • Readily available health care at an affordable price
	• Employers
	  • Low-cost health insurance and healthy employees
	• Health care facilities and practitioners
	  • Provide the best care possible to patients
	• Federal, state, and local governments
	  • Easily accessible health care at an affordable cost
	  • Private insurers
	    • Good reimbursement for providers and positive bottom line for an organization
	• Volunteer facilities and agencies
	  • Obtain immediate care for patients in need
	• Health care practitioner training institutions
	  • Attract competent and dedicated students
	• Professional associations and other health care industry organizations
	  • Attract members, maintain standards, and provide professional news
	• Biotechnology companies
	  • Offer products consumers buy and make a profit
	• Pharmaceutical companies
	  • Investigate and market medications and make a profit
	• Companies related to health care
	  • Sell health care services and products to the industry and the consumer for a profit

LO 13.2 Describe the major factors influencing the cost of health care.	What are major considerations in health care costs?
	• Cost: The amount individuals; employers; local, state, and federal governments; HMOs; and insurers spend on health care in the United States
	  • Approximately $3 trillion in 2014
	  • American taxpayers, through taxes and health insurance premiums, absorb the cost
	  • Fifty percent of the total U.S. population account for 97 percent of health care costs
	  • Factors adding to health care costs annually include:
	    • Fee-for-service reimbursement
	    • Fragmentation in payment and care delivery
	    • Administrative costs
	    • Aging population, rising rates of chronic disease, and lifestyle choices
	    • Advances in medical technology
	    • Tax treatment of health insurance
	    • Changing trends in health care market consolidation
	    • Higher physician, facility, and drug costs
	    • Legal and regulatory environment of health care

What are the costs for individuals?

- Patient Protection and Affordable Care Act of 2010
  - Established shared responsibility among federal and state governments, employers, and individuals for access to affordable health care
  - Intent was that younger, healthier people would anchor the system
  - Subsidies based on income
  - Penalty for taxpayers who do not enroll in any health insurance
  - As of mid-2016, only 9.1 percent of the population were without health insurance

LO 13.3 Examine the major components of both access and quality in health care.

What are the steps necessary for access to exist?

- Access: The availability of health care and the means to purchase health care services
- Three steps for attaining access:
  1. Adequate services must exist, and consumers must be able to reach them
  2. Consumers must be able to utilize them, that is, barriers such as language should not exist
  3. People receive ongoing health care

What is quality?

- Quality: The degree of excellence of health care services offered

What is the National Quality Strategy?

- Developed by the Department of Health and Human Services to:
  - Improve the quality of care
  - Improve the health of the U.S. population by addressing proven interventions in behavioral, social, and environmental determinants of health
  - Reduce the cost of health care

What is the Agency for Healthcare Research and Quality?

- The lead federal agency responsible for tracking and improving the quality, safety, efficiency, and effectiveness of health care for Americans
- Latest AHRQ report shows:
  - Patient safety improved substantially
  - Overall quality is improving; however, disparities are not changing
  - More effective communication and coordination of care are necessary
  - Attention is warranted to ensure continued improvements in effective prevention and treatment practices, starting with cardiovascular disease
  - Working with communities to promote wide use of best practices enabling healthy living is critical
  - Quality care must be more affordable

What other population changes affect cost, access, and quality?

- Declines in national fertility and birth rates
- A steady increase in life expectancy at birth and life span at older ages
- A shift in the leading causes of death and illness from infectious and parasitic diseases to noncommunicable diseases and chronic conditions

LO 13.4 Discuss those trends in medical research and treatment that may affect the delivery of health care in the future.

What are some significant health care trends in research and treatment?

- New medical technologies:
  - Advances in imaging
  - Biologics
  - Clinical-grade wearables
  - Gene-editing techniques
  - Point-of-care testing
  - Rational and pharmacogenomics drug design
  - Three-dimensional bioprinting
- Personalized medicine

What is a significant indication for quality of life?

- Well-being: One's perception that life is going well
- Well-being's positive results:
  - Fewer incidents of physical and mental illness
  - Healthier behaviors
  - Social connectedness
  - Increased productivity
  - Longevity

What is Healthy People 2020?

- An ongoing initiative of the federal Office of Disease Prevention and Health Promotion that attempts to measure quality of life

Chapter 13 Review

Applying Knowledge

LO 13.1

1. Those who have a vested interest in the American health care industry are called
   a. Employers
   b. The public
   c. Stakeholders
   d. Insurers
2. Which of the following is *not* true of a nonprofit organization?
   a. Nonprofits work for a positive income at the end of the year.
   b. It has shareholders.
   c. It has goals in service of its mission statement.
   d. It operates under different laws than for-profit companies.
3. Three key issues of concern to everyone within the American health care industry are
   a. Cost, access, quality
   b. Cost, availability, insurance
   c. Competition, education, quality
   d. Cost, access, hospitalization

LO 13.2

4. What is the largest contributor to the health care dollar?
   a. Taxes
   b. Private donations
   c. Health insurance
   d. Employers

5. What area of health care spends the largest amount of the health care dollar?
   a. Physician services
   b. Hospital care
   c. Prescriptions
   d. Nursing homes
6. Which of the following is *not* true under ACA?
   a. Everyone can get health care insurance for free.
   b. Preexisting conditions must be allowed.
   c. Consumers can get health insurance through their employer if offered.
   d. There are tax penalties if you do not have health insurance.

LO 13.3

7. List three steps vital for access to health care to exist.
8. Which of the following is *not* a reason for the relatively high rate of infant mortality in the United States?
   a. High cost
   b. Restricted access to health care
   c. Fewer births than other nations
   d. High rate of uninsured
9. What is the name of the lead federal agency responsible for tracking and improving the quality, safety, efficiency, and effectiveness of health care for Americans?
   a. AHRQ
   b. HIPAA
   c. PPACA
   d. NHQR
10. Which of the following, established via implementation of the 2010 ACA, set goals for improving health care quality?
   a. HIPAA
   b. National Quality Strategy
   c. Department of Health and Human Services
   d. Social Security
11. What is the term for the statistically probable number of years a newborn ought to live, based on environment, heredity, lifestyle and health practices, risk factors, and so on?
   a. Lifetime
   b. Life expectancy
   c. Life span
   d. Adulthood
12. What is the number of years an individual actually lives called?
   a. Life span
   b. Life expectancy
   c. Adulthood
   d. Childhood

13. Which of the following is listed as a major population change affecting the cost, access, and quality of health care in the United States?

a. People are healthier.

b. Affordable care has been achieved for all income levels of society.

c. People no longer die of heart disease.

d. Life expectancy and life span have increased across the U.S. population.

14. Which of the following best defines the term *fertility rate* within a population?

a. The total number of live births recorded in each state for one year.

b. The total number of live births per 1,000 women aged 15 to 44 years.

c. The total number of live births within a specific population group.

d. The total number of births in an entire country for one year.

LO 13.4

15. What is the process called that involves correcting defective genes responsible for disease?

a. Genetics

b. Genomics

c. Pharmacology

d. Gene editing

16. Which of the following does not involve a technique using a biologic?

a. A child is vaccinated against polio.

b. A person receives an allergy shot.

c. A patient receives a bone transplant.

d. A cancer patient receives radiation treatment.

17. Which of the following is a medical technology likely to increase its current trend toward miniaturization?

a. 3D printing

b. Gene therapy

c. Imaging

d. Pharmacogenomics

18. What is the process called that is currently revolutionizing gene manipulation?

a. The endeGene therapy

b. Pharmacogenomics

c. CRISPR-Cas

d. Genomics

LO 13.1 to LO 13.4

19. As an employee working in a job with health care benefits, who pays for your care?

20. Who pays for the health care of the remaining uninsured?

21. How will increasing numbers of older people affect health care services in the future?

22. In your opinion, what are the implications for future health care practitioners in the United States if health care costs continue to rise?

23. Ultimately, who pays for health care services in the United States?

24. How has implementation of the 2010 ACA affected the number of uninsured Americans to date?

Ethics Issues Health Care Trends and Forecasts

Use your critical thinking skills to answer the questions that follow each ethics issue.

Ethics ISSUE 1:

As the world progresses into the twenty-first century, one aspect of health care—disaster planning—requires urgent attention. Not only does each year bring killer tornadoes, hurricanes, blizzards, floods, and wildfires, the threat of spreading diseases and terrorist attacks continues to loom. Health care practitioners are on the front lines during any disaster, and the logistical and ethical concerns associated with caring for populations during these events fall heavily on their shoulders. If all assigned health care practitioners can't report for duty, who will take charge? Should triage (an assessment of which of the injured should receive treatment first) proceed as in normal times, and who will be responsible for deciding? Will nurses be expected to perform as surgeons, technicians as pharmacists, or aides as nurses?

Every health care facility should have a disaster plan and should practice implementation of the plan periodically.

Discussion Questions

25. In your opinion, would it be ethical, in case of a disaster, for triage personnel to recommend treating only those injured individuals who could recover?

26. If materials were sorely lacking and some health care team members were unable to report in during a disaster, in your opinion should ethics be suspended and volunteers used to perform patient care duties?

27. Which patient care duties could reasonably be suspended during an extreme emergency, if materials, personnel, and perhaps even the usual medical facility were not available?

Source: For a thorough accounting of health care practitioners under stress during a disaster (Katrina), read *Five Days at Memorial: Life and Death in a Storm-Ravaged Hospital,* by Sheri Fink, Crown Publishers, New York, 2013.

Case Studies

Use your critical thinking skills to answer the questions that follow each case study.

LO 13.3

Medical tourism is a recent trend in health care. Patients go to a different country for either urgent or elective medical procedures. The procedures are the same procedures being done in U.S. hospitals and outpatient surgery centers, often by American-trained physicians who have moved back home. Medical tourism is fast becoming a worldwide, multibillion-dollar industry. In fact, some insurance companies are paying for the cost of the procedures, as costs are far less than those charged in the United States. Sometimes the insurance company even pays for the plane fare and hotel costs. The reasons patients travel for treatment vary from the lower costs (for Americans) to shorter waiting times (for those in countries where there is national health insurance). There is no regulation by the U.S. government of medical tourism. Many patients come back enthusiastic about not only the success of their treatment and the integrity and skill of all the providers, but also the high-class hotel-like accommodations while in the foreign hospital. India is one of the major countries advertising these services.

28. If other countries are able to do similar procedures as those done in the United States for lower fees and with the same or better outcomes, why can't the United States offer the same?

29. If your insurance company wanted you to go to another country for a procedure because it was less expensive, would you do it? Explain your answer.

In 2014, American patients with recurring head and neck cancers were traveling to China to receive gene therapy via a drug designed to activate the p53 gene, which is supposed to turn off cells that multiply abnormally but often malfunctions, letting cancerous tumors grow. Because the drug was not FDA-approved in the United States, patients traveled to China to receive it at a cost of $20,000 for the 2-month treatment. No studies had yet been conducted to determine the efficacy of the treatment, but many patients believed their tumors were receding. A genetic research company in the United States was threatening to sue the Chinese company manufacturing the drug, alleging patent infringement.

30. In your opinion, should American patients be prohibited from traveling to foreign countries to receive unproven and possibly dangerous medical treatment? Explain your answer.

Moore's law, which said that the number of transistors that can be packed into a given space would roughly double every 18 months to 2 years, has largely come to pass, resulting in faster and more powerful, yet cheaper computers. Antonio Regalato, writing for *MIT Technology Review*, posited a few years ago that Moore's law can and should be applied to medical technology in order to facilitate access and bring down the cost of modern technological advances used in health care. The more medical technology becomes digital, Regalato proposed, the lower health care costs will go. Some ideas along this line are mentioned in Chapter 13, as in the discussion of ultrasound machines small enough to replace stethoscopes. Regalato's article mentions others: eyeglass prescriptions from a smartphone app that require no optometrist middle person; diagnoses obtained by sending photos taken with a smartphone to a medical practitioner; and online bidding sites for physician's fees.

Source: www.technologyreview.com/s/518871/we-need-a-moores-law-for-medicine/.

31. In your opinion, would the further digitalization of medical technology lower health care costs in the long run?
32. In your opinion, what ethical considerations would arise with the further digitalization of medical technology?
33. Can you think of other instances in which digitalizing medical technology has entered the health care industry or might apply in the future?

Internet Activities

LO 13.2 and LO 13.3

Complete the activities and answer the questions that follow.

34. Visit the following Web site: http://nhqrnet.ahrq.gov/inhqrdr/state/select.

    Select your state and explore the quality of your state's health care. Where does your state stand compared with those states with "highest quality" health care?

35. Visit the following Web site for Healthy People 2020: www.healthypeople.gov/.

    What are Leading Health Indicators? What is the current Leading Health Indicator Topic?

36. Visit the Web site for the National Center for Health Statistics: www.cdc.gov/nchs/fastats/health-insurance.htm.

    What are the latest statistics for the number of uninsured Americans? Is this an improvement over the previous year, are numbers roughly the same, or have the numbers gone down?

Resources

LO 13.2

Health care costs:

http://khn.org/news/health-care-costs/

www.allhealth.org/publications/Cost_of_health_care/Cost_Drivers_in_Health_Care_109.pdf

www.beckershospitalreview.com/finance/9-drivers-of-high-healthcare-costs-in-the-u-s.html

Local (counties and cities) health care spending: www.library.unt.edu/gpo/acir/Reports/information/m-192.pdf

Health care spending (changes over time): http://www.healthsystemtracker.org/chart-collection/u-s-spending-healthcare-changed-time/?_sft_post_tag=health-spending#item-start

www.pbs.org/newshour/rundown/new-peak-us-health-care-spending-10345-per-person/

www.cms.gov/research-statistics-data-and-systems/statistics-trends-and-reports/nationalhealthexpenddata/nhe-fact-sheet.html

Health spending: http://www.healthsystemtracker.org/chart-collection/u-s-spending-healthcare-changed-time/?_sft_post_tag=health-spending#item-start

U.S. health care spending: http://bipartisanpolicy.org/wp-content/uploads/sites/default/files/BPC%20Health%20Care%20Cost%20Drivers%20Brief%20Sept%202012.pdf

Lifetime distribution of health care costs: www.ncbi.nlm.nih.gov/pmc/articles/PMC1361028/

LO 13.3

2015 National Healthcare Quality and Disparities Report and 5th Anniversary Update on the National Quality Strategy. Agency for Healthcare Research and Quality, April 2016. AHRQ Pub. No. 16-0015. www.ahrq.gov/sites/default/files/wysiwyg/research/findings/nhqrdr/nhqdr15/2015nhqdr.pdf

Global health and aging: www.nia.nih.gov/research/publication/global-health-and-aging/preface

Point-of-care diagnostic testing: https://report.nih.gov/nihfactsheets/ViewFactSheet.aspx?csid=112

Life expectancy in 2015: www.cdc.gov/nchs/

National Quality Strategy: www.ahrq.gov/workingforquality/about/index.html

www.ahrq.gov/workingforquality/about/index.html

LO 13.4

Definition of health/medical technologies: www.who.int/topics/technology_medical/en/

Ten medical technologies: http://medicalfuturist.com/top-10-medical-technologies-of-2016/

Bioprinting: www.ncbi.nlm.nih.gov/pubmed/25093879

Genome editing: www.thermofisher.com/us/en/home/life-science/genome-editing/geneart-crispr/crispr-cas9-based-genome-editing.html

Pharmacogenomics: https://ghr.nlm.nih.gov/primer/genomicresearch/pharmacogenomics

Healthy People 2020: www.healthypeople.gov/2020/topics-objectives/topic/health-related-quality-of-life-well-being

Well-being: www.cdc.gov/hrqol/wellbeing.htm

Glossary

A

access The availability of health care and the means to purchase health care services.

accountable care organization (ACO) A health care payment and delivery model that could reward doctors and hospitals for controlling costs and improving patient outcomes by allowing them to keep a portion of what they save if standards of quality are met.

accreditation Official authorization or approval for conforming to a specified standard.

active euthanasia A conscious medical act that results in death.

addendum A significant change or addition to the electronic health record (EHR).

administer To instill a drug into the body of a patient.

administrative law Enabling statutes enacted to define powers and procedures when an agency is created.

advance directive A written statement of a person's wishes regarding medical treatment, often including a living will or power of attorney or both. These documents are done to make sure the patient's wishes are carried out should the person be unable to communicate them to a doctor.

affirmative action Programs that use goals and quotas to provide preferential treatment for minority persons determined to have been underutilized in the past.

affirmative defenses Defenses used by defendants in medical professional liability suits that allow the accused to present factual evidence that the patient's condition was caused by some factor other than the defendant's negligence.

Agency for Healthcare Research and Quality (AHRQ) The lead federal agency responsible for tracking and improving the quality, safety, efficiency, and effectiveness of health care for Americans.

alternative dispute resolution (ADR) Settlement of civil disputes between parties using neutral mediators or arbitrators without going to court.

Amendments to the Older Americans Act A 1987 federal act that defines elder abuse, neglect, and exploitation, but does not deal with enforcement.

American Medical Association Principles A code of ethics for members of the American Medical Association written in 1847.

American Recovery and Reinvestment Act (ARRA); also called the Recovery Act. A 2009 act that made substantive change to HIPAA's privacy and security regulations.

artificial insemination The mechanical injection of viable semen into the vagina.

assumption of risk A legal defense that holds the defendant is not guilty of a negligent act, since the plaintiff knew of and accepted beforehand any risks involved.

autonomy (or self-determination) The capacity to be one's own person and make one's own decisions without being manipulated by external forces.

autopsy A postmortem examination to determine the cause of death or to obtain physiological evidence, as in the case of a suspicious death.

B

background check The process of reviewing criminal and/or financial history to confirm information about an applicant for employment.

beneficence Refers to the acts health care practitioners perform to help people stay healthy or recover from an illness.

bioethicists Specialists who consult with physicians, researchers, and others to help them make difficult ethical decisions regarding patient care.

bioethics A discipline dealing with the ethical implications of biological research methods and results, especially in medicine.

birth rate Total number of live births per 1,000 women in a specific age group

brain death Final cessation of bodily activity, used to determine when death actually occurs; circulatory and respiratory functions have irreversibly ceased, and the entire brain (including the brain stem) has irreversibly ceased to function.

breach Any unauthorized acquisition, access, use, or disclosure of personal health information that compromises the security or privacy of such information.

breach of contract Failure of either party to comply with the terms of a legally valid contract.

business associates Individuals and/or organizations that provide certain functions, activities, or services on behalf of covered entities that involve access to, or the use of, disclosure of protected health information.

C

case law Law established through common law and legal precedent.

categorical imperative A rule that is considered universal law binding on everyone and requiring action..

certification A voluntary credentialing process whereby applicants who meet specific requirements may receive a certificate.

Chemical Hygiene Plan The Standard for Occupational Exposures to Hazardous Chemicals in Laboratories, which clarifies the handling of hazardous chemicals in medical laboratories.

Child Abuse Prevention and Treatment Act A federal law passed in 1974 requiring physicians to report cases of child abuse and to try to prevent future cases.

chromosomes Units within cell nuclei where genetic material is stored.

civil law Law that involves wrongful acts against persons.

claims-made insurance A type of liability insurance that covers the insured only for those claims made (not for any injury occurring) while the policy is in force.

Clinical Laboratory Improvement Act (CLIA) Also called Clinical Laboratory Improvement Amendments. Federal statutes passed in 1988 that established minimum quality standards for all laboratory testing.

clone An organism begun asexually, usually from a single cell of the parent.

cloning The process by which organisms are created asexually, usually from a single cell of the parent organism.

code of ethics A system of principles intended to govern behavior—here, the behavior of those entrusted with providing care to the sick.

coma A condition of deep stupor from which the patient cannot be roused by external stimuli.

common law The body of unwritten law developed in England, primarily from judicial decisions based on custom and tradition.

common sense Sound practical judgment.

comparative negligence An affirmative defense claimed by the defendant, alleging that the plaintiff contributed to the injury by a certain degree.

compassion The identification with and understanding of another's situation, feelings, and motives.

confidentiality The act of holding information in confidence, not to be released to unauthorized individuals.

Confidentiality of Alcohol and Drug Abuse Patient Records A federal statute that protects patients with histories of substance abuse regarding the release of information about treatment.

consent Permission from a patient, either expressed or implied, for something to be done by another. For example, consent is required for a physician to examine a patient, to perform tests that aid in diagnosis, and/or to treat for a medical condition.

consequence-oriented (or teleological) theories Consequence-oriented or teleological theories judge the rightness of a decision based on the outcome or predicted outcome of the decision.

constitutional law Law that derives from federal and state constitutions.

contract A voluntary agreement between two parties in which specific promises are made for a consideration.

contributory negligence An affirmative defense that alleges that the plaintiff, through a lack of care, caused or contributed to his or her own injury.

Controlled Substances Act The federal law giving authority to the Drug Enforcement Administration to regulate the sale and use of drugs.

coroner A public official who investigates and holds inquests over those who die from unknown or violent causes; he or she may or may not be a physician, depending on state law.

cost In this context, the amount individuals, employers, state and federal governments, HMOs, and insurers spend on health care in the United States.

courtesy The practice of good manners.

covered entity Health care providers who conduct administrative and financial transactions in electronic form. This includes all employees, volunteers, trainees, and all others who are under the control of the entity.

Criminal Health Care Fraud Statute A section of the United States Code that prohibits fraud against any health care benefit program.

criminal law Law that involves crimes against the state.

critical thinking The ability to think analytically, using fewer emotions and more rationality.

curative care Treatment directed toward curing a patient's disease.

D

damages Court-ordered monetary awards to patients, given as a result of legally recognized injuries to patients

defendant The person or party against whom criminal or civil charges are brought in a lawsuit.

de-identify To remove all information that identifies patients from health care transactions.

denial A defense that claims innocence of the charges or that one or more of the four Ds of negligence are lacking.

deontological (or duty-oriented) theory Decision-making theory that states that the rightness or wrongness of the act depends on its intrinsic nature and not the outcome of the act.

deposition Sworn testimony given and recorded outside the courtroom during the pretrial phase of a case.

discrimination Prejudiced or prejudicial outlook, action, or treatment.

dispense To deliver controlled substances in some type of bottle, box, or other container to a patient.

DNA (deoxyribonucleic acid) The combination of proteins, called nucleotides, that is arranged to make up an organism's chromosomes.

doctrine of informed consent The legal basis for informed consent, usually outlined in a state's medical practice acts.

doctrine of professional discretion A principle under which a physician can exercise judgment as to whether to show patients who are being treated for mental or emotional conditions their records. Disclosure depends on whether, in the physician's judgment, such patients would be harmed by viewing the records.

do-not-resuscitate (DNR) orders Orders written at the request of patients or their authorized representatives that cardiopulmonary resuscitation not be used to sustain life in a medical crisis.

Drug Enforcement Administration (DEA) A branch of the U.S. Department of Justice that regulates the sale and use of drugs.

durable power of attorney An advance directive that confers on a designee the authority to make a variety of legal decisions on behalf of the grantor, usually including health care decisions.

duty of care The obligation of health care professionals to patients and, in some cases, nonpatients.

duty-oriented (or deontological) theory See *deontological (or duty-oriented) theory.*

E

electronic health record (EHR) Contains the same information as any medical record, but in electronic form and is a collection of all the medical records for a single patient.

electronic medical record (EMR) Contains all patient medical records for one practice or one organization.

emancipated minors Individuals in their mid- to late teens who legally live outside their parents' or guardians' control.

emergency A type of affirmative defense in which the person who comes to the aid of a victim in an emergency is not held liable under certain circumstances.

employment-at-will A concept of employment whereby either the employer or the employee can end the employment at any time, for any reason.

ethics Standards of behavior, developed as a result of one's concept of right and wrong.

ethics committee Committee made up of individuals who are involved in a patient's care, including health care practitioners, family members, clergy, and others, with the purpose of reviewing ethical issues in difficult cases.

ethics guidelines Publications that detail a wide variety of ethical situations that professionals (in this case, health care practitioners) might face in their work and offer principles for dealing with the situations in an ethical manner.

etiquette Standards of behavior considered to be good manners among members of a profession as they function as individuals in society.

exclusive provider organization (EPO) A managed care plan that pays for health care services only within the plan's network of physicians, specialists, and hospitals (except in emergencies).

executive order A rule or regulation issued by the president of the United States that becomes law without the prior approval of Congress.

F

Federal Anti-Kickback Law Prohibits knowingly and willfully receiving or paying anything of value to influence the referral of federal health care program business.

Federal False Claims Act A law that allows for individuals to bring civil actions on behalf of the U.S. government for false claims made to the federal government, under a provision of the law called *qui tam* (from Latin meaning "to bring an action for the king and for oneself").

federalism The sharing of power among national, state, and local governments.

felony An offense punishable by death or by imprisonment in a state or federal prison for more than one year.

fertility rate The total number of births per 1,000 women aged 15 to 44 years.

fidelity Being faithful to the scope of practice for your profession, as in role fidelity.

Food and Drug Administration (FDA) A federal agency within the Department of Health and Human Services that oversees drug quality and standardization and must approve drugs before they are released for public use.

forensics A division of medicine that incorporates law and medicine and involves medical issues or medical proof at trials having to do with malpractice, crimes, and accidents.

fraud Dishonest or deceitful practices in depriving, or attempting to deprive, another of his or her rights.

G

gene A tiny segment of DNA found on a chromosome in a cell. Each gene holds the formula for making a specific enzyme or protein

gene therapy The insertion of a normally functioning gene into cells in which an abnormal or absent element of the gene has caused disease.

General Duty Clause A section of the Hazard Communication Standard that states that any equipment that may pose a health risk must be specified as a hazard.

genetic counselor An expert in human genetics who is qualified to counsel individuals who may have inherited genes for certain diseases or conditions.

genetic discrimination Differential treatment of individuals based on their actual or presumed genetic differences.

genetic engineering Manipulation of DNA within the cells of plants and animals, through synthesis, alteration, or repair, to ensure that certain harmful traits will be eliminated in offspring and that desirable traits will appear and be passed on.

genetics The science that accounts for natural differences and resemblances among organisms related by descent.

genome All the DNA in an organism, including its genes.

genomics The branch of molecular biology concerned with the structure, function, evolutions, and mapping of genomes.

Good Samaritan acts State laws protecting physicians and sometimes other health care practitioners and laypersons from charges of negligence or abandonment if they stop to help the victim of an accident or other emergency.

gross domestic product (GDP) America's total value for all goods and services produced.

H

Hazard Communication Standard (HCS) An OSHA standard intended to increase health care practitioners' awareness of risks, to improve work practices and appropriate use of personal protective equipment, and to reduce injuries and illnesses in the workplace.

Health Care Education and Reconciliation Act (HCERA) Enacted in 2010, a federal law that added to regulations imposed on the insurance industry by the Patient Protection and Affordable Care Act.

health care power of attorney A legal document that specifically identifies a person to take responsibility for a patient's health care decisions when a patient is not able to do so.

health care practitioners Those who are trained to administer medical or health care to patients.

health information technology (HIT) The application of information processing, involving both computer hardware and software, that deals with the storage, retrieval, sharing, and use of health care information, data, and knowledge for communication and decision making.

Health Information Technology for Economic and Clinical Health Act (HITECH) A section of the American Recovery and Reinvestment Act (ARRA) that strengthened certain HIPAA privacy and security provisions.

Health Insurance Portability and Accountability Act (HIPAA) of 1996 A federal law passed in 1996 to protect privacy and other health care rights for patients. The act helps workers keep continuous health insurance coverage for themselves and their dependents when they change jobs, and protects confidential medical information from unauthorized disclosure and/or use. It was also intended to help curb the rising cost of health care fraud and abuse.

health maintenance organization (HMO) A health plan that combines coverage of health care costs and delivery of health care for a prepaid premium.

health savings account (HSA) Offered to individuals covered by high-deductible health plans, these accounts let these individuals save money, tax free, to pay for medical expenses.

heredity The process by which organisms pass on genetic traits to their offspring.

heterologous artificial insemination The process in which donor sperm is mechanically injected into a woman's vagina to fertilize her eggs.

Hippocratic oath A pledge for physicians, developed by the Greek physician Hippocrates circa 400 B.C.E.

homologous artificial insemination The process in which a man's sperm is mechanically injected into a woman's vagina to fertilize her eggs.

hospice A facility or program (often carried out in a patient's home) in which teams of health care practitioners and volunteers provide a continuing environment that focuses on the emotional and psychological needs of the dying patient.

Human Genome Project A scientific project funded by the U.S. government, begun in 1990 and successfully completed in 2000, for the purpose of mapping all of a human's genes. This Web site is an excellent resource: www.ornl.gov/sci/techresources/Human_Genome/home.shtml.

I

independent practice association (IPA) A type of HMO that contracts with groups of physicians who practice in their own offices and receive a per-member payment (capitation) from participating HMOs to provide a full range of health services for HMO members.

infertility The failure to conceive for a period of 12 months or longer due to a deviation from or interruption of the normal structure or function of any reproductive part, organ, or system.

interrogatory A written set of questions requiring written answers from a plaintiff or defendant under oath.

in vitro fertilization (IVF) Fertilization that takes place outside a woman's body, literally, "in glass," as in a test tube.

involuntary euthanasia The act of ending a terminal patient's life by medical means without his or her permission.

J

jurisdiction The power and authority given to a court to hear a case and to make a judgment.

just cause An employer's legal reason for firing an employee.

justice What is due an individual.

L

law Rule of conduct or action prescribed or formally recognized as binding or enforced by a controlling authority.

law of agency The law that governs the relationship between a principal and his or her agent.

legal precedents Decisions made by judges in the various courts that become rule of law and apply to future cases, even though they were not enacted by legislation.

liability insurance Contract coverage for potential damages incurred as a result of a negligent act.

liable Legally responsible or obligated.

licensure A mandatory credentialing process established by law, usually at the state level, that grants the right to practice certain skills and endeavors.

life expectancy The number of years an individual can expect to live, calculated from his or her birth.

life span The number of years an individual actually lives.

limited data set Protected health information from which certain specified, direct identifiers of individuals have been removed.

litigious Prone to engage in lawsuits.

living will An advance directive that specifies an individual's end-of-life wishes.

M

malfeasance The performance of a totally wrongful and unlawful act.

managed care A system in which financing, administration, and delivery of health care are combined to provide medical services to subscribers for a prepaid fee.

managed care organization (MCO) A corporation that links health care financing, administration, and service delivery.

mature minors Individual in their mid- to late teens, who, for health care purposes, are considered mature enough to comprehend a physician's recommendations and give informed consent.

meaningful use A process by which health care providers use an electronic health record according to guidelines set by the federal government.

medical boards Bodies established by the authority of each state's medical practice acts for the purpose of protecting the health, safety, and welfare of health care consumers through proper licensing and regulation of physicians and other health care practitioners.

medical ethicists Specialists who consult with physicians, researchers, and others to help them make difficult ethical decisions regarding patient care.

medical examiner A physician who investigates suspicious or unexplained deaths.

medical practice acts State laws written for the express purpose of governing the practice of medicine.

medical record A collection of data recorded when a patient seeks medical treatment.

medical services organization (MSO) A physician group purchases a hospital, which then contracts with employers to provide full health care services.

Medical Waste Tracking Act The federal law that authorizes OSHA to inspect hazardous medical wastes and to cite offices for unsafe or unhealthy practices regarding these wastes.

minor Anyone under the age of majority: 18 years in most states, 21 years in some jurisdictions.

misdemeanor A crime punishable by fine or by imprisonment in a facility other than a prison for less than one year.

misfeasance The performance of a lawful act in an illegal or improper manner.

moral values One's personal concept of right and wrong, formed through the influence of the family, culture, and society.

multipotent stem cells Stem cells that can become a limited number of types of tissues and cells in the body.

mutation A permanent change in DNA.

N

National Childhood Vaccine Injury Act A federal law passed in 1986 that created a no-fault compensation program for citizens injured or killed by vaccines, as an alternative to suing vaccine manufacturers and providers.

National Organ Transplant Act Passed in 1984, a statute that provides grants to qualified organ procurement organizations and established an Organ Procurement and Transplantation Network (OPTN).

National Vaccine Injury Compensation Program (VICP) A no-fault federal system of compensation for individuals or families of individuals injured by childhood vaccinations.

needs-based motivation Human behavior is based on specific human needs that must often be met in a specific order. Abraham Maslow is the best-known psychologist for this theory.

negligence An unintentional tort alleged when one may have performed or failed to perform an act that a reasonable person would not or would have done in similar circumstances.

nonfeasance The failure to act when one should.

nonmaleficence As paraphrased from the Hippocratic oath, means the duty to "do no harm."

Notice of Privacy Practices (NPP) A list provided by all covered entities that demonstrates adherence to HIPAA's privacy practices rules.

O

Occupational Exposure to Bloodborne Pathogen Standard An OSHA regulation designed to protect health care workers from the risk of exposure to bloodborne pathogens.

Occupational Safety and Health Administration (OSHA) Established by the Occupational Safety and Health Act, the organization that is charged with writing and enforcing compulsory standards for health and safety in the workplace.

occurrence insurance A type of liability insurance that covers the insured for any claims arising from an incident that occurred, or is alleged to have occurred, during the time the policy is in force, regardless of when the claim is made.

P

palliative care Treatment of a terminally ill patient's symptoms to make dying more comfortable; also called comfort care.

parens patriae A legal doctrine that gives the state the authority to act in a child's best interest.

passive euthanasia The act of allowing a patient to die naturally, without medical interference.

patient portal A secure online Web site that gives patients 24-hour availability to health care providers.

Patient Protection and Affordable Care Act (PPACA) A federal law enacted in 2010, to expand health insurance coverage and otherwise regulate the health insurance industry. Many provisions of the law were scheduled to take effect in 2014 and 2015.

Patient Self-Determination Act A federal law passed in 1990 that requires hospitals and other health care providers to provide written information to patients regarding their rights under state law to make medical decisions and execute advance directives.

permissions Reasons under HIPAA for disclosing patient information.

persistent vegetative state (PVS) Severe mental impairment characterized by irreversible cessation of the higher functions of the brain, most often caused by damage to the cerebral cortex.

personalized medicine The products and services that leverage the science of genomics and proteomics to create tailored, individual approaches to disease prevention and health care.

pharmacogenomics The science that defines how individuals are genetically programmed to respond to drugs.

physician-hospital organization (PHO) A health care plan in which physicians join with hospitals to provide a medical care delivery system and then contract for insurance with a commercial carrier or an HMO.

plaintiff The person bringing charges in a lawsuit.

pluripotent stem cells Stem cells that can become almost all types of tissues and cells in the body.

precedent Decisions made by judges in the various courts that become rule of law and apply to future cases, even though they were not enacted by a legislature; also known as case law.

preferred provider organization/association (PPO/PPA) A network of independent physicians, hospitals, and other health care providers who contract with an insurance carrier to provide medical care at a discount rate to patients who are part of the insurer's plan. Also called preferred provider association (PPA).

prescribe To issue a medical prescription for a patient.

primary care physician (PCP) The physician responsible for directing all of a patient's medical care and determining whether the patient should be referred for specialty care.

principle of utility Requires that the rule used to make a decision bring about positive results when generalized to a wide variety of situations.

prior acts insurance coverage A supplement to a claims-made policy that can be purchased when health care practitioners change insurance carriers.

privacy Freedom from unauthorized intrusion.

privileged communication Information held confidential within a protected relationship.

procedural law Law that defines the rules used to enforce substantive law.

professional corporation A body formed and authorized by law to act as a single person.

prosecution The government as plaintiff in a criminal case.

protected health information (PHI) Information that contains one or more patient identifiers.

proteomics The study of the proteins that genes create or "express."

protocol A code prescribing correct behavior in a specific situation, such as a situation arising in a medical office.

public policy The common law concept of wrongful discharge when an employee has acted for the "common good."

Q

quality The degree of excellence of health care services offered.

quality assurance See *quality improvement (QI).*

quality improvement (QI) A program of measures taken by health care providers and practitioners to uphold the quality of patient care. Also called quality assurance.

quarantine Used in connection to infectious diseases and illnesses, states may separate and restrict the movement of people with infectious diseases if they are a threat to public health. A court order is required.

R

reasonable person standard That standard of behavior that judges a person's actions in a situation according to what a reasonable person would or would not do under similar circumstances.

reciprocity The process by which a professional license obtained in one state may be accepted as valid in other states by prior agreement without reexamination.

registration A credentialing procedure whereby one's name is listed on a register as having paid a fee and/or met certain criteria within a profession.

release of tortfeasor A technical defense to a lawsuit that prohibits a lawsuit against the person who caused an injury (the tortfeasor) if he or she was expressly released from further liability in the settlement of a suit.

res ipsa loquitur Literally, "the thing speaks for itself"; a situation that is so obviously negligent that no expert witnesses need be called. Also known as the doctrine of common knowledge.

res judicata Literally, "the thing has been decided"; legal principle that a claim cannot be retried between the same parties if it has already been legally resolved.

respondeat superior Literally, "let the master answer." A doctrine under which an employer is legally liable for the acts of his or her employees, if such acts were performed within the scope of the employees' duties.

right-to-know laws State laws that allow employees access to information about toxic or hazardous substances, employer duties, employee rights, and other workplace health and safety issues.

risk management The taking of steps to minimize danger, hazard, and liability.

S

safe haven laws State laws that allow mothers to abandon newborns to designated safe facilities without penalty.

scope of practice The determination of the duties/procedures that a person may or may not perform under the auspices of a specific health care professional's license.

self-insurance coverage An insurance coverage option whereby insured subscribers contribute to a trust fund to be used in paying potential damage awards.

Smallpox Emergency Personnel Protection Act (SEPPA) A no-fault program to provide benefits and/or compensation to certain individuals, including health care workers and emergency responders, who are injured as the result of the administration of smallpox countermeasures, including the smallpox vaccine.

social media Forms of electronic communication through which users create online communities to share information, ideas, personal messages, and other content.

stakeholders Those who have a vested interest in the health care industry in the United States, and in any efforts to reform the industry.

standard of care The level of performance expected of a health care worker in carrying out his or her professional duties.

Stark Law Prohibits physicians or their family members who own health care facilities from referring patients to those entities if the federal government, under Medicare or Medicaid, will pay for treatment.

state preemption If a state's privacy laws are stricter than HIPAA privacy standards, state laws take precedence.

statute of frauds State legislation governing written contracts.

statute of limitations That period of time established by state law during which a lawsuit may be filed.

statutory law Law passed by the U.S. Congress or state legislatures.

stem cells Cells that have the potential to become any type of body cell.

subpoena A legal document requiring the recipient to appear as a witness in court or to give a deposition.

subpoena *duces tecum* A legal document requiring the recipient to bring certain written records to court to be used as evidence in a lawsuit.

substantive law The statutory or written law that defines and regulates legal rights and obligations.

summary judgment A decision made by a court in a lawsuit in response to a motion that pleads there is no basis for a trial.

summons A written notification issued by the clerk of the court and delivered with a copy of the complaint to the defendant in a lawsuit, directing him or her to respond to the charges brought in a court of law.

surrogacy The process by which a woman becomes pregnant by artificial insemination or surgical implantation of a fertilized egg for the purpose of carrying a fetus to term for another woman.

surrogate mother A woman who becomes pregnant, usually by artificial insemination or surgical implantation of a fertilized egg, and bears a child for another woman.

T

tail coverage An insurance coverage option available for health care practitioners: When a claims-made policy is discontinued, it extends coverage for malpractice claims alleged to have occurred during those dates that claims-made coverage was in effect.

technical defenses Defenses used in a lawsuit that are based on legal technicalities.

telemedicine Remote consultation by patients with physicians or other health professionals via telephone, closed-circuit television, or the Internet.

teleological (or consequence-oriented) theories See *consequence-oriented (or teleological) theories.*

terminally ill Referring to patients who are expected to die within six months.

testimony Statements sworn to under oath by witnesses testifying in court and giving depositions.

tort A civil wrong committed against a person or property, excluding breach of contract.

tortfeasor The person guilty of committing a tort.

U

Unborn Victims of Violence Act Also called Laci and Conner's Act, a federal law passed in 2004 that provides for the prosecution of anyone who causes injury to or the death of a fetus in utero.

Uniform Anatomical Gift Act A national statute allowing individuals to donate their bodies or body parts, after death, for use in transplant surgery, tissue banks, or medical research or education.

Uniform Determination of Death Act A proposal that established uniform guidelines for determining when death has occurred.

Uniform Rights of the Terminally Ill Act A 1989 recommendation of the National Conference of Commissioners on Uniform State Laws that all states construct laws to address advance directives.

United Nations Globally Harmonized System of Classification and Labeling of Chemicals Led to a 2012 revision of the Hazard Communication Standard in order to transform "right to know" to "right to understand," in line with GHS.

utilitarianism A person makes value decisions based on results or a rule that will produce the greatest balance of good over evil, everyone considered.

V

veracity Truth telling.

virtue ethics Focuses on the traits, characteristics, and virtues that a moral person should have.

vital statistics Numbers collected for the population of live births, deaths, fetal deaths, marriages, divorces, induced terminations of pregnancy, and any change in civil status that occurs during an individual's lifetime.

void Without legal force or effect.

voluntary euthanasia The act of ending a patient's life by medical means with his or her permission.

W

well-being A physical and mental state that vastly improves quality of life.

workers' compensation A form of insurance established by federal and state statutes that provides reimbursement for workers who are injured on the job.

wrongful death statutes State statutes that allow a person's beneficiaries to collect for loss to the estate of the deceased for future earnings when a death is judged to have been due to negligence.

wrongful discharge A concept established by precedent that says an employer risks litigation if he or she does not have just cause for firing an employee.

X

xenotransplantation Transplantation of animal tissues and organs into humans.

Index

Note: Page numbers followed by f indicate figures; those followed by t indicate tables.